Change Processes in Child Psychotherapy

Change Processes
in Child Psychotherapy
Revitalizing Treatment and Research

STEPHEN R. SHIRK
ROBERT L. RUSSELL

THE GUILFORD PRESS
New York   London

©1996 The Guilford Press
A Division of Guilford Publications, Inc.
72 Spring Street, New York, NY 10012

Printed in the United States of America

This book is printed on acid-free paper.

Last digit is print number: 9 8 7 6 5 4 3 2 1

Library of Congress Cataloging-in-Publication Data

Shirk, Stephen R.
   Change processes in child psychotherapy : revitalizing treatment
and research / Stephen R. Shirk, Robert L. Russell.
      p.   cm.
   Includes bibliographical references and index.
   ISBN 1-57230-095-7
   1. Child psychotherapy.   2. Personality change.   3. Child
psychiatry—Differential therapeutics.   4. Adjustment
(Psychology) in children.   I. Russell, Robert L.   II. Title.
   [DNLM: 1. Psychotherapy—in infancy & childhood.   2. Mental
Disorders—in infancy & childhood.   3. Mental Disorders—therapy.
4. Child Psychiatry.   WS 350.2 S558c 1996]
RJ504.S535 1996
618.92'8914—dc20
DNLM/DLC   96-15603
                                                               CIP

To Donna, Emmy Kate, and Anna Gabrielle
–S.R.S.

To the memory of my parents
–R.L.R.

Acknowledgments

W E WOULD LIKE to acknowledge the contributions of numerous colleagues and clinical supervisors who have both supported and challenged our understanding of child psychotherapy. This work reflects many exchanges with researchers and clinicians whose insights and cumulative experience we have tried to express in these pages. We are grateful for the tireless word-processing and editorial assistance provided by Anne Warner. And finally, we thank Seymour Weingarten for his enduring support of this project.

Preface

CHILD PSYCHOTHERAPY is entering a critical period. The traditional child treatments, especially psychodynamic and play therapies, which have been widely practiced by child clinicians for decades, are being challenged from one side by the development of promising behavioral and family interventions, and from another by the press for empirically validated and cost-effective treatments. This critical period could determine whether traditional child psychotherapy continues to thrive or whether it is relegated to the archives of treatment history.

It is noteworthy, however, that the traditional child therapies are not only challenged by external sources, which could potentially serve as an impetus for conceptual and technical growth, but also are threatened from within the tradition itself. One of the most glaring weaknesses in this tradition is the absence of systematic dialogue between child practitioners and clinical researchers. To a great degree, this dialogic gap reflects the paucity of research on nonbehavioral child psychotherapy. But the problem runs much deeper. A vast literature on the development of basic psychological processes such as language, play, emotion regulation, and self-esteem, to name but a few, has not been integrated into this therapeutic tradition. In essence, the failure of child psychotherapy to absorb new insights emerging from both clinical and developmental research threatens its vitality. Interestingly, as our review of the literature will reveal, this lack of exchange did not always characterize traditional child psychotherapy. In fact, over 40 years ago, the practice of these therapies was accompanied by a lively research enterprise that examined, among other things, comparisons of children's language behavior in therapeutic and other caregiving contexts.

It is our contention that the growth, perhaps even the survival, of traditional child psychotherapy hinges on opening the flow of ideas between practicing child clinicians and researchers in clinical and developmental psychology. Viewed most broadly, the principal goal of this book is to reopen this dialogue.

In order to bring coherence to such a conversation, a number of tasks must be accomplished. These tasks represent the main aims of this book. First, and consistent with one of the basic notions of traditional therapy, in order to know where we want to go it is useful to assess where we have been. To this end, the first aim of the book is to reexamine the basic theory and research that have guided the practice of child psychotherapy. Our review of this literature reveals many false starts and repetitions of problems, as well as a number of conceptual and methodological advances along the way. One of the most important insights to emerge from this review is that child psychotherapists have been keenly interested in the complex linguistic, emotional, and interpersonal processes that constitute therapeutic interactions. To understand *how* or *why* therapy works requires specification of *what* actually transpires in the therapy session. Unfortunately, little effort has been expended in studying what actually occurs during child therapy. Instead, much of the research has focused on relating whole therapies, what we will refer to as "brand-name" treatments, to indices of outcome. Part of the problem, it seems, is that traditional child psychotherapy has not systematically elaborated its postulated change mechanisms. Thus, a second major aim of this book is to explicate the basic interpersonal, emotional, and cognitive change processes implicit in models of child psychotherapy.

Furthermore, despite the existence of a rich literature on interpersonal, emotional, and cognitive processes, insights from basic research have not been imported into the conceptualization or investigation of child treatment processes. Instead, much of the child psychotherapy literature has evolved in isolation from basic psychological research. It is our belief that the vitality of child psychotherapy hinges on the integration of research, especially developmental research, on interpersonal, emotional, and cognitive processes. Thus, a third major aim of this book is to link basic research on such processes with the complex interactions that constitute child psychotherapy.

Another core insight to emerge from our review of the child psychotherapy literature is that methods of intervention have developed in connection with theories of etiology and pathogenesis. In striking contrast to this perspective, the prevailing approach to child treatment research severs the conceptual link between models of pathogenesis and methods of intervention. Instead, research is largely organized around the evaluation of "brand-name" treatments, such as psychodynamic and cognitive-behavioral therapies, for specific diagnostic groups, such as conduct or dysthymic disorders. Although this approach represents an important advance over earlier studies that included poorly defined treatments and mixed groups of troubled children, this research paradigm is flawed in two respects.

First, the use of psychiatric diagnoses as the principal, and at times, the only classification and inclusion criterion tends to ignore substantial within (diagnostic) group variation in underlying pathogenic processes that contribute to child psychopathology. Second, treatments are complex phenomena and are typically composed of diverse interactions and multiple interventions. Too much of the literature has shown too little concern with the specific processes that constitute "brand-name" treatments, and very few studies have examined the relationship between specific treatment procedures or interactions, what we call *change processes,* and treatment outcomes. In brief, we propose that the current approach to child treatment research, with its emphasis on treatment brands and psychiatric disorders, is not focusing on those features of treatment that hold the greatest promise for advancing the practice of child psychotherapy. Thus, a fourth, and perhaps most important, aim of this book is to reorient treatment research to the specification of both the underlying pathogenic processes, such as the conflicts, deficits, or distortions that contribute to the child's presenting problems, and to the change processes that constitute psychosocial treatments. In other words, in keeping with the assumptions of traditional child psychotherapy, we aim to restore the fundamental link between formulations of pathogenesis and methods of intervention. In this respect, not only is research used to inform clinical practice, but also insights from clinical practice are utilized to redirect research. One of the basic tenets of this book is that formulations of pathogenic process, a critical component of clinical practice, provide a better framework for the selection or design of psychosocial treatments than symptom clusters or psychiatric diagnoses.

In order to provide an alternative framework for the conduct and investigation of child psychotherapy, a substantial portion of the book is devoted to an examination of postulated change processes and to the basic formulations that guide treatment selection. A fifth, and possibly most challenging, aim of this book is to develop a framework for the classification of cases that complements traditional psychiatric diagnosis. Although psychiatric diagnoses serve a variety of classificatory and prognostic functions, diagnoses based exclusively on the covariation of symptoms are simply inadequate for the selection or design of psychosocial treatments.

Instead, psychotherapeutic interventions are guided by an understanding of the pathogenic mechanisms that produce or maintain the child's overt presenting problems. Thus, formulations of pathogenic processes are essential to the design and delivery of interventions, and should be integrated into the taxonomy of childhood psychopathology.

Although the importance of case formulations for treatment planning is widely recognized, it is often argued that case formulations are too idiosyncratic to provide a reliable framework for the classification of cases, and for making judgments about the usefulness of treatment procedures across cases. Drawing on prototype theory, we propose that it is possible to identify basic-level case formulations that distinguish different *classes* of pathogenic processes, and that offer an alternative to symptom-based classification. In other words, we contend that there are meaningful clusters of pathogenic processes that can be reliably identified and used to guide treatment selection. Furthermore, we elaborate a set of principles for the development of case formulations.

The book is divided into three sections. The first section examines the theoretical and empirical foundation of child psychotherapy and provides a working definition of child *psychotherapy*. Based on these reviews, the section concludes with a reformulation of the essential ingredients of child psychotherapy. The second section is devoted to a close analysis of postulated change processes in child psychotherapy. Three related, but analytically distinguishable, types of change processes are examined in separate chapters—interpersonal, emotional, and cognitive. In each of these chapters, a developmental perspective is brought to bear on the process of change. Finally, the third section focuses on the importance of formulations of pathogenic process for treatment planning, and on the development of formulation prototypes that could be used to guide individual case conceptualizations. Case studies are presented to illustrate the integration of change processes with case formulations. The last chapter considers this model of child treatment in the broader contexts of development, family, and culture.

Some would argue that traditional child psychotherapy is not merely entering a critical period, but is already in "critical condition." It is our contention that the prognosis for child psychotherapy is bleak if clinical practice remains isolated from an evolving conceptual and empirical literature that could reshape its future development. However, by opening a dialogue between practitioners and researchers, it is our hope that child psychotherapy will thrive as a vital, and effective, form of psychosocial treatment for troubled children.

Foreword

How do we think about child psychotherapy research in a way that will advance the knowledge base in the field and improve treatment approaches? *Change Processes in Child Psychotherapy* provides a strong blueprint for how to accomplish both of these goals. It presents a sophisticated integration of research and clinical literature in child development, developmental psychopathology, and child psychotherapy. The book offers innovative suggestions about what the next steps should be in child psychotherapy treatment and research.

In this age of managed care, it is tempting to abandon what we know about the complexities of child development and underlying internal psychological processes, and opt for the easiest, most observable symptom reduction techniques. In some cases, of course, this is the appropriate course of action, but in many cases it is not. One of the key concepts in this book is that internal processes—cognitive, affective, and interpersonal—determine behavior and symptoms. Interventions should focus on the specific processes that are problematic for the child. This coherent framework is a true integration of developmental psychology and child psychotherapy.

The reviews of child psychotherapy outcome and process research presented here are comprehensive, as are the reviews of various theoretical approaches. In a sense, this book cuts across different theoretical treatment approaches because it focuses on specific internal processes and intervention strategies that can bring about change in them. Some theoretical approaches work better than others, depending on the goal of treatment and the context. Additionally, there are state-of-the-art reviews of the research literature in the areas of children's cognitive, emotional, and interpersonal development. A recent innovation is the linking of psychotherapeutic change to specific cognitive, emotional, and interpersonal problems. This is the direction for future research and treatment Shirk and Russell call for. It is an approach that goes against the grain of pressures from managed care systems and program evaluation approaches, but it is a logical extension of the general consensus in the field of psychotherapy that we need to become focused, look at specific processes, and stop carrying out global outcome studies. Shirk and Russell's model also adheres to the idea that therapeutic change in children must be studied and understood from a developmental perspective.

As in any science, the field of child psychotherapy must first develop theoretical frameworks, that is, identify crucial variables and the logical research questions necessary for real advancement. Then, it should find creative solutions to real-world obstacles that interfere with progress in the field. This is a time in which there are many real-world obstacles, but the synthesis that this book provides could be very helpful in pointing us in the right direction.

I think that this text will be valuable to the practicing clinician in that the case formulation approach presented here is practically useful in making treatment decisions. The researcher will find a host of ideas and up-to-date literature reviews. Most important to the field is the message of the book: Use what we know about developmental processes to guide treatment and treatment research with children. It is a challenge to the field to act on this message and to use the framework provided here.

SANDRA W. RUSS
Case Western Reserve University

Contents

Change Processes in Child Psychotherapy

I

___

THEORETICAL AND EMPIRICAL FOUNDATIONS OF CHILD PSYCHOTHERAPY

PART I CONTAINS four chapters. The purpose of these chapters is (1) to circumscribe a distinctive set of child treatment theories and practices that constitute "child psychotherapy" (Chapter 1), (2) to provide a detailed review of the empirical research assessing the outcomes and processes of child psychotherapy (Chapters 2 and 3), and (3) to provide a rationale, based on the theoretical and empirical history of child psychotherapy, for an alternative research and treatment model that links case formulations of pathogenic processes to specific intervention strategies (Chapter 4). The reader will not only be introduced to our rationale for offering an alternative model to revitalize child psychotherapy theory, research, and practice, but will also be guided through a half century of research.

Chapter 1 explicates the diversity of etiological and treatment models that comprise the field of child psychotherapy. For each of three major systems of child psychotherapy (psychodynamic, client-centered, and cognitive), we show how models of pathogenesis are linked with models of intervention. Furthermore, we show how each of the three systems of psychotherapy has spawned several different, and sometimes competing, models of pathogenesis and processes of intervention. Such diversity within "brand-name" treatments effectively causes such labels to become, at best, obsolete or, at worst, mystifying and misleading. Consequently, a shift in focus, from brand names to concrete descriptions of intervention strategies and differentiated case-based models of pathogenesis is recommended. Chapter 1 concludes with the explication of several dimensions along which intervention strategies can be concretely described and compared.

Chapter 2 reviews a half century of research on key child psychotherapy *outcome* questions: "Are treated children better off at outcome than untreated children?," "Are some brand-name treatments better than others?," and "Can treatments be optimized by matching intervention strategy to type of diagnosis, or better to the case-based pathogenic process?" By reviewing the major narrative and meta-analytic reviews of child treatment as they appeared chronologically in print, a colorful history of the assessment of child treatment emerges. Three conclusions were dominant in the field: (1) child psychotherapy does not work any better than spontaneous remission, (2) child psychotherapy works better than spontaneous remission, although all brand names work about equally well, and (3) some types of behavioral therapies work better for some disorders than nonbehavioral child therapies. As many of the reviews indicate, even in circumstances in which treatments prove to work better than controls, we have very little idea as to why they worked or how or for whom (even successful treatments, as measured by average posttreatment scores, have some children who do not improve and some who actually get worse). One of the main problems is the dearth of studies that link specific treatment processes with treatment outcomes. Such problems with the outcome literature suggest that outcomes cannot and should not be considered in isolation from treatment processes.

Chapter 3 reviews the much smaller set of studies that have addressed key *process* questions: "Of what is this or that brand-name therapy comprised?," "Which of the many therapeutic ingredients, including client activities, is responsible for client progress and ultimate change at outcome?," and "Given this hypothesized pathogenic process, which intervention strategy given in what dose is most potent for achieving positive change?" Review of the 50-year history of such process research not only reveals serious shortcomings in the number and quality of studies in the literature, but also reveals some repeated and possibly enduring findings. Chapter 3 concludes with suggestions on how to build on this body of research to improve our scientific base and our clinical practices.

Chapter 4 develops and summarizes themes in the first three chapters to present an extended rationale for (1) abandoning the "diagnosis by brand name" method of conducting child psychotherapy research and treatment, and (2) adopting a case-based model of "pathogenesis by specific intervention strategy" in its place. The complexity of diverse treatment processes within "brand-name" therapies is compounded by multiple pathways to specific diagnoses. Thus, rather than matching treatment brands to diagnoses, we recommend the specification of underlying pathogenic processes, such as cognitive, emotional, or interpersonal deficits or deviations, that contribute to the child's presenting problems, and then develop interventions that address such processes. It is proposed that matching formulations of pathogenetic processes to specific strategies of intervention refocuses researchers and clinicians at a unified level of analysis, and will lead to swifter identification of effective treatments. Perhaps more importantly for the attainment of this latter goal, the new model invites both researcher and clinician to revitalize their interest in systematic areas of psychology that present models of emotional, cognitive, and interpersonal functioning that can and should inform theories of pathogenesis and strategies of intervention.

1

The Domain
of Child Psychotherapy

T HE ORIGINS of modern child therapy are frequently traced to two early treatment cases. The first is Freud's treatment of "Little Hans" (Freud, 1909). In this case, Freud treated a phobic 5-year-old boy through psychoanalytic consultations with the child's father. Although the case has been described as a prototype for childhood neurosis (Anthony, 1986), for many child clinicians it represents one of the first demonstrations of the therapeutic utility of children's play. The second case is the treatment of "Little Peter" by Mary Cover Jones (Jones, 1924). In this case, a 3-year-old boy who apparently was well adjusted in most circumstances evinced marked fears of furry objects. Jones treated the boy by "direct unconditioning," that is, through gradual exposure to the feared objects. For John Watson, the father of behaviorism, and many who followed, this case demonstrated that emotional problems could be understood and successfully addressed without recourse to the murky and unverifiable constructs of the introspectionists and psychoanalysts.

Although both of these "classic" cases involve the treatment of childhood phobias, the formulations and interventions presented in the two approaches differ dramatically. For Freud, Hans's phobic reactions were the expression of internal conflict. By contrast, Peter's fear of rabbits, fur coats, and cotton was viewed as the result of simple contiguity learning, and treated through the systematic manipulation of the conditions that evoked his fear. In these two cases we find the origins of two enduring, alternative approaches to child therapy. In one, the child's inner life is viewed as the source of emotional distress and the focus of treatment. In the other, the origins of and solutions to the child's emotional problems are found in the environment. In the former we find the beginnings of child *psychotherapy;* in the latter, the roots of child *behavior therapy.*

Much has changed in the field of child therapy since these early cases. Like most evolving conceptual systems, psychoanalytic and behavioral approaches have been marked by increasing differentiation during the intervening decades. Within both camps there is now considerable diversity in practice. Moreover, it is no longer possible to equate behavioral treatments with environmental interventions, and psychodynamic approaches with intrapsychic interventions. The burgeoning interest in cognitive mediators among "cognitive-behaviorists" and the growing concern with the "facilitating environment" among analytic theorists have obscured this simple distinction. In addition, the rise of other therapeutic orientations such as client-centered, cognitive, and rational–emotive therapies has contributed to a proliferation of child treatments. Therefore, it is not possible to define child psychotherapy in terms of the assumptions and practices of a single theoretical orientation.

A view through the one-way mirror at a typical child psychiatry clinic reveals some of the heterogeneity in the current practice of child psychotherapy. Looking into the first therapy room we find a 7-year-old boy strategically placing commandoes for a devastating raid on what appears to be a middle-class, suburban home. The doll figures, caught up in their mundane household chores, appear to be oblivious to the imminent attack. His therapist sits back and remains quiet as the boy prepares for the frontal assault. Throughout the siege the therapist makes few statements, occasionally commenting on the ferocity of the attack. As we move down the corridor to the second room, we find a therapist and 10-year-old girl in what appears to be a tense conversation. The therapist is gently, but persistently, asking the child to reflect on some apparent misconduct. She asks, "And what were you feeling when you walked out of class?" The child looks out the window, folds her arms, and murmurs, "Nothing." The therapist pauses, "Nothing at all, you mean you were just blank?" The child walks to the window, then turns and looks at the door. For a moment it appears that she might bolt from the therapy room. The therapist sits back and offers another comment, "I get the sense this is really hard to talk about. Like you feel pressured by me." She hesitates, then adds, "I almost get the idea you want to walk out of here, too. I wonder if this is how it felt when you walked out of class?" The child makes no comment. Instead, she sits down and reaches for a checkerboard on the shelf. "Let's play checkers," she offers with a slight smile. We arrive at the next room just as the child and therapist are leaving. Both have their coats on; the child has a large ball under one arm. The therapist grins, "So what's the record this season?

I think you're undefeated in our kickball tournament so far!" We follow them outside. For the entire session the child and therapist engage in one-on-one kickball, with the child the clear winner in all but one game. On the way back to the therapy room, they stop at a soda machine, and the therapist buys the child a Coke. We decide to visit one last room. Here we find the therapist reminding his child patient that after they practice their "thinking games," then they'll continue to work on the model car. The child appears to concede, "Okay, but just one more time." "All right, what else could you do when the guys in your class tease you?" The child thinks hard, "I guess I could walk away." Then after a moment's reflection he adds with a grin, "But I'd rather slug them!" The therapist nods and asks, "And then what would happen?"

Our brief tour through these observation rooms points to the simple fact that a diverse range of practices are subsumed under the label child psychotherapy. In some sessions it appeared that expressive play was the principal therapeutic medium; in others, conversation and language seemed to play a far greater role. Some therapists appeared to structure the activities of the therapy sessions; others followed the child's direction. Some appeared to focus on "problems"; others principally concerned themselves with the quality of the ongoing relationship.

Was this apparent diversity in practice simply a function of the idiosyncrasies of this particular treatment setting? It seems unlikely. Surveys of child practitioners reveal a plurality of theoretical orientations and a broad range of therapeutic techniques (Koocher & Pedulla, 1977; Snow & Paternite, 1986). Similarly, Kazdin (1988) has identified over 230 "published" forms of child therapy. Thus, demarcating the boundaries of child psychotherapy and mapping its terrain can prove to be a daunting task.

DEFINING CHILD PSYCHOTHERAPY

Previous efforts to define child psychotherapy have relied on one of two strategies. The first involves extracting common elements from diverse approaches in order to arrive at a working definition. For example, Reisman (1973) advances seven "generic" principles common to the practice of child psychotherapy. These include the following: The therapist listens to the child and encourages the expression of feelings and beliefs; the therapist communicates understanding and respect; and the therapist clarifies unusual aspects of the child's behavior, feelings, or beliefs. Although these principles may be common to most forms of child psychotherapy, generic definitions tend to obscure important differences in practice.

The second alternative has been to identify child psychotherapy with a single theoretical orientation. For example, Nuffield (1988) distinguishes psychotherapy, "which is based on psychodynamic principles," from behavior therapy, which is grounded in learning theory. Such reductionism seems unwarranted in the face of multiple, competing theories of child psychotherapy. No doubt the many practitioners of nondirective forms of child therapy, such as experiential and relationship therapies, would find their exclusion from the domain of child psychotherapy to be unjustified.

The question, then, is how to meaningfully delimit the field of child psychotherapy without obscuring important differences in theory and practice. One solution is to move below the surface, where important differences in practice are evident, to a deeper level of analysis. Despite considerable diversity in practice, we propose that child psychotherapies are unified by a set of core assumptions. For the child psychotherapist, children do not respond directly to their social environments. Instead, it is assumed that *internal psychological processes* mediate between the social world and the child's emotional experience and overt behavior. In essence, children orient their actions and emotions to psychologically constructed situations. This "mediational assumption" appears to be shared by all forms of child psychotherapy. However, the mediational or constructive processes that are deemed critical for understanding child psychopathology and intervention vary across therapeutic systems. These include, to name a few, defense mechanisms, coping strategies, interpersonal representations, and narrative schemas. In turn, child maladjustment is understood in terms of distortions, deficiencies, or compromises in these internal, mediational processes. Although environmental influences are not ignored by child psychotherapists—in fact, pathogenic deficits, distortions, and compromises are often viewed as the residual effects of interpersonal transactions—therapeutic interventions aim at restructuring or remediating internal, psychological processes. Approaches that focus on overt behavior and emphasize environmental interventions represent the major alternative to child psychotherapy and are properly labeled child behavior therapy. For the child psychotherapist, the modification of behavior is predicated on changes in the child's internal psychological processes.

One implication of this conceptualization of child psychotherapy is that it does not exclude treatment approaches on the basis of theoretical origins. Treatments that have developed from a variety of theoretical sources can conceptually cohabit within the domain of child psychotherapy, provided they share the basic assumption that internal psychological processes mediate behavior and emotions, and are the principal focus of therapeutic interventions. Given this conceptualization, many cognitive-behavioral interventions that focus on internal constructs can be viewed as a form of psychotherapy.

The major risk of an inclusive definition of child psychotherapy is the potential for "leveling" important differences in theory and practice. Such leveling represents the worst form of eclecticism. By no means does our conceptualization imply that divergent therapeutic models are essentially "talking about the same thing, but in different languages." For example, coping strategies are not necessarily equivalent to defense mechanisms, nor are interpersonal schemas the same as interpersonal negotiation strategies. Nor is it assumed that treatments are interchangeable or equally effective with all problems. For example, learning new interpersonal negotiation strategies may be more effective than eliciting unexpressed emotion for remediating peer-relationship problems. Finally, it is not assumed that differences in technique are unimportant because "nonspecific" factors such as warmth and respect account for therapeutic change. Instead, we propose that child psychotherapy is *not* a unitary process.

At a molar level of analysis, child psychotherapies share the assumption that internal psychological processes mediate between the social environment and the child's emotional experience and behavior; and these mediating constructs are the principal targets of intervention. This core assumption defines the outer boundary of child psychotherapy. But when the domain of child psychotherapy is viewed more closely, there is far less agreement about the nature of the critical mediating constructs and the therapeutic processes that facilitate their change. Thus, in order to adequately map the terrain of child psychotherapy, it is important to consider the major theoretical sources that have contributed to its diversity.

SOURCES OF THEORETICAL INFLUENCE

Methods of intervention in childhood psychopathology tend to be derived from models of etiology. As Cowan (1988) notes, theories of psychopathology and intervention come in "matched sets" such that etiological theories typically identify core pathogenic processes that become the target for intervention. Models of intervention, then, are typically linked to conceptions of pathogenic process. For example, a history of child abuse is often regarded as a critical etiological factor in various forms of child maladjustment. The link between etiology, in this case, past maltreatment, and current maladjustment is through an ongoing and underlying pathogenic process such as social skill deficits or emotion regulation problems. In turn, the type of treatment, for example, social skills training or emotion expression, depends on the identified pathogenic process.

We propose that much of the diversity in the practice of child psychotherapy has its origins in rival etiological theories and their corresponding models of pathogenesis. Variations in prescribed therapeutic interventions follow from differences in models of pathogenic process, although at times, this connection has become obscure in clinical practice. In this section, we will examine the relationship between pathogenesis and intervention in three major child therapeutic frameworks—psychodynamic, client-centered, and cognitive.

Psychodynamic Approaches

Although Freud often is credited with drawing attention to the childhood origins of adult psychopathology, most of his clinical work was not conducted with children. In fact, in his best-known child case, the treatment of "Little Hans," Freud worked indirectly with the child through the boy's father. It was left to the followers of Freud to elaborate a theory of child psychopathology and intervention. Clearly, the most influential contributor to this effort is Anna Freud.

Because Anna Freud's work developed over an extended period of time, one encounters not one but a number of models of child psychopathology. Tolpin (1978) observes that Anna Freud distinguished two pathogenic models. The first might be termed the internal conflict model, in which psychological conflicts give rise to maladaptive symptoms. The second could be called the deficiency model. Here parental deficits act as the primary pathogenic agent and produce deficiencies in the child's personality. For Anna Freud (1968), the differential diagnosis of these two sources of disturbance carries significant implications for therapeutic intervention.

The Internal Conflict Model

A basic premise of the conflict model is that emotional disturbance cannot be understood by reference to observable symptoms alone. Instead, emotional and behavioral symptoms are manifestations of underlying emotional conflicts. In contrast to current empirical classification systems of child psychopathology, which define syndromes on the basis of symptom constellations, disorders are discriminated on the basis of shared underlying processes. As Anna Freud (1971) points out, two children may present with identical symptoms but differ widely in terms of their underlying emotional conflicts. Thus, the process of diagnosis is closely linked to uncovering precipitating conflicts.

What types of conflict give rise to symptoms of childhood psychopathology? Although psychoanalytic theory contains a number of conceptualizations of conflict, Anna Freud (1971) adopts the structural model. In analytic theory, three internal structures are posited—the id, ego, and superego. In the id one finds everything that is inherited, including the instincts. The id is viewed as an aggregate of sexual and aggressive impulses, each seeking immediate gratification and obeying one rule, the pleasure principle. By and large, the id is not coordinated with external reality. In infancy, impulses seeking discharge give rise to hallucinatory satisfaction. Because these self-generated satisfactions are incompatible with survival, the id's demands must be brought into conformity with the requirements of reality. According to Freud (1949), a portion of the id, modified by contact with the external world, develops to mediate between the id's demands and the requirements of reality. As the representative of survival, the ego attempts to substitute the reality principle for the pleasure principle. Behavior is regulated not just on the basis of maximizing pleasure, but also on minimizing pain as well. In order to meet the demands of reality and serve the reality principle, a variety of ego functions develop. For example, cognitive development is in the service of impulse regulation. Similarly, memory develops to provide a record of pleasurable and painful situations. In brief, higher order cognitive and perceptual processes principally function to coordinate the expression of drives with the demands of reality.

The differentiation of the ego from the id establishes a new arena for conflict. At its core is conflict between the pleasure principle and the reality principle. The id presses for unencumbered discharge of sexual and aggressive urges, while the ego struggles to maintain control. Because the ego develops from the id, early in its genesis the ego is at the mercy of the id's powerful impulses. In order to subdue these threats, the ego resorts to primitive defensive maneuvers. Childhood, then, is a period during which the ego attempts to gain mastery over the expression of powerful impulses. From this perspective, one of the primary tasks of early development is impulse control.

Internal conflict is further complicated by the development of the superego. The superego is formed through the process of identification with a special part of reality, namely the demands of society as represented by parental authority. Freud (1946) maintains that young children's first objects of sexual interest are their parents. These sexual wishes bring the child into conflict with the same-sex parent, who is viewed as a sexual rival. Resolution of this conflict requires abandoning the original love object and identifying with the same-sex parent. The superego is born from this process of identification; that is, the parental regulatory functions of monitoring and punishing impulse expression are internalized as part of superego formation. Consequently, conflicts between impulse expression and the demands of external reality are represented internally as conflicts between personality structures. The ego is caught in the middle of opposing internal demands, menaced on one side by the id's impulses, and threatened on the other by sanctions of the superego.

Conflict is conceptualized in terms of impulses and constraints, between drives and defenses. Prototypically, conflict involves a clash between urges or wishes and a set of prohibitions. In early development, conflict is between impulse expression and parental sanctions. For example, a young child might experience aggressive wishes toward a newborn sibling who represents a rival for parental affection. These wishes come in conflict with parental imperatives to be "nice" to the baby. This conflict could potentiate the development of symptoms that reflect the young child's tendency to regress in the face of conflict.

With increasing development, parental sanctions are internalized, and conflict occurs between internal structures. Ironically, not all development is an unmitigated blessing. For example, hostile feelings toward a parent can produce conflict, even in the absence of parental response, because the prohibitions against hostility are part of the child's personality. Defensive processes are mobilized in order to contain the hostile feelings and the anxiety aroused by their potential expression. Symptoms result as a compromise solution to the conflict between impulse and defense. Consider, for example, the school-age child who feels anger toward his parents. Internal sanctions against the expression of anger engender conflict. In order to manage these feelings, the anger is transformed by defensive processes. In this case, the child experiences fear that something dreadful will happen to his parents and feels that it is imperative to monitor their safety. The child presents to the clinician as anxious and unable to separate from home in order to attend school. In turn, the child's school avoidance is extremely upsetting to the parents, who feel manipulated by their child. The direct expression of anger has been transformed; however, the indirect effect of the defensive process accomplishes its aim. Moreover, as this example illustrates, internal conflicts interfere with the child's capacity to master normative developmental tasks. The progressive movement of development is blocked, and according to Anna Freud (1965), the aim of treatment is to return the child to the path of normal development.

From a psychodynamic perspective, beneath the overt expression of symptoms and outside the child's awareness lie disruptive internal conflicts. These conflicts drain the ego of its strength; defensive processes aimed at warding off anxiety and containing drives restrict the ego's flexibility; and anxiety undermines the efficient operation of ego functions (A. Freud, 1968). In summary, the ego is weakened and besieged by internal conflict. The goal of treatment is to rescue the ego.

By what method is the ego strengthened and its influence restored? In *An Outline of Psychoanalysis,* Freud (1949) addresses this question directly. He says, "The method by which we strengthen the weakened ego has as a starting point an extending of self-knowledge. The loss of such knowledge signifies for the ego a surrender of power and influence" (p. 34). Implicit in this formulation is the assumption that unconscious contents, in the form of impulses, infantile wishes, or distorted beliefs, press for control over behavior. Limitations on the ego's capacity for control correspond to the degree to which these influences are outside of awareness. The ego is strengthened by expanding the sphere of self-awareness. As Anna Freud (1965) notes, "The aim of [child] analysis remains the widening of consciousness without which ego control cannot be increased" (p. 31). Psychoanalytic child treatment rests on the assumption that a causal relation exists between self-understanding and the capacity for self-regulation.

At the core of the analytic treatment process is the effort to increase insight into the unconscious determinants of experience and behavior. According to Kennedy (1971), "By drawing the child's attention to previously unconscious feelings and ideas and by establishing links between his present concerns and these feelings and ideas that may have been conscious but isolated, we give the child insight, that is, enlarge his self-awareness" (p. 400). Treatment aims at helping the child understand the feelings, motives, and beliefs that shape his or her experiences or dilemmas. Returning to the example of the school-avoidant child, an attempt would be made to uncover the origins of the child's fears about parental safety. As Sandler, Kennedy, and Tyson (1980) point out, "Insight refers to a kind of turning to observe oneself, as if to say, behind this that I see there must be something else going on." In this case, an attempt would be made to move beyond the presenting problem of fear. Uncovering the underlying anger would figure prominently in the process of treatment. However, the release of unexpressed emotion is not regarded as sufficient for therapeutic change in analytic therapy (Sandler et al., 1980). Although the expression of emotional or thematic material through symbolic play, activities, or talk is a critical aspect of analytic treatment, increased understanding of the expressed material is the eventual goal.

Insight involves expanding self-awareness by making connections between underlying conflicts and current dilemmas. However, extending self-understanding is not simply an intellectual process. Efforts to uncover conflicts and troubling feelings are met with resistance; that is, as the underlying conflict is approached in therapy, it arouses anxiety and leads the child to avoid emotionally evocative material. Common to all resistances is the child's holding back or unconsciously wanting to shut something out of awareness. Thus, the process of treatment involves overcoming resistance. As Freud (1940) suggests, the formation of a strong alliance between therapist and patient permits resistances to be surmounted, or, in his words, "the ego, emboldened by the certainty of our help," takes the offensive against defensive obstacles.

Insight in child therapy is facilitated on the child's side by the processes of verbalization and self-observation, and on the therapist's side by the process of interpretation.

Of course, children vary in their capacity for verbalization and self-observation, and limits in these functions constitute a formidable therapeutic constraint. Some therapists in the analytic tradition are undaunted by children's disinclination to verbalize in therapy. For example, Melanie Klein (1975) maintains that play serves the same function as language in child treatment, such that "the child expresses its fantasies, its wishes, and its actual experiences through play and games" (p. 7). According to Klein, the symbolic character of children's play can be understood as the therapeutic equivalent of adults' dreams. Similarly, Erikson (1963) contends that therapists can count on the child to reveal through play "whatever aspect of his ego has been ruffled most." He proposes that children's play is an early form of the human ability to master experiences by creating model situations. Anna Freud (1946) appears more skeptical about this issue. Commenting on the work of Klein, she argues that there is no justification for equating children's play with verbalization, particularly, free association. As she notes, "Instead of being invested with symbolic meaning it (play) may at times admit of a harmless explanation. The car collision may be reproducing some accident in the street" (p. 29). Although there is some disagreement in the analytic camp about the communicative value of play, there is considerable consensus that treatment involves going beyond the expression of thematic play to reflections on its meaning. Erikson (1964) expresses this perspective, saying: "Those children who transfer not the solution but the unsolvability of their problems into the play situation and onto the person of the observer need to be induced by systematic interpretation to reconsider, on a more verbal level, the constellations that have overwhelmed them in the past" (p. 265). As one would expect, Anna Freud (1965) maintains that the ego is strengthened when feelings and impulses are grasped and put into thoughts or words.

In the treatment of internal conflict, interpretation is an essential therapeutic tool. In the psychoanalytic tradition, this process parallels interpretation in literature or science; that is, it involves the application of a conceptual framework to perceive, organize, or describe data or text. According to Kennedy (1979), interpretations extend the child's self-awareness by organizing and articulating what the child is experiencing. Again, turning to the case of the school-avoidant child, a series of interpretations might be offered. First, in order to facilitate the expression of unacknowledged anger, an interpretation directed toward the child's resistance might be offered. The therapist may indicate that it is not uncommon for children to feel anger toward their parents. As the anger is more freely expressed and acknowledged by the child, interpretations aimed at connecting the anger and the child's fear would follow. As Kennedy points out, interpretations provide the child with a framework for understanding his or her experiences, and provide the basis for emotional and behavioral change.

The Ego Deficit Model

In her later work, Anna Freud (1968) begins to acknowledge the limitations of insight and interpretation as therapeutic processes. Some children simply did not appear to benefit from the interpretive process. In fact, many of these children did not appear to be suffering from the debilitating effects of internal conflict. Although they evidenced patterns of impaired ego functioning, reflected in poor impulse control, low tolerance of frustration, limited affect regulation, and turbulent social relations, the source of ego weakening could not be traced to internal conflicts. According to Anna Freud (1968), the "damage is not self-inflicted as the result of internal strife" (p. 40). The ego is in a weakened state, not because of internal conflicts, but because of *developmental deficits.*

For Anna Freud, developmental deficits must be traced to a new source. Drawing on the work of Hartmann (1939), she turns to the child's family environment. Under normal family conditions, the young child's developmental needs are met by an "expectable environment." However, when parents fail as agents of the expectable environment, developmental needs are frustrated and structural deficits in the ego emerge.

This formulation of child psychopathology introduces an important role for the environment in the genesis of child maladjustment. In the infantile neurosis, the prototype of internal conflict, distorted perceptions of the parents, arising from the child's wishes, anxieties, and defenses, contribute to symptom formation. Here the environment is essentially psychological. This perspective on the environment is explicit in the work of Melanie Klein (1975). For Klein, the infant is faced with raging conflict between the instincts, quite apart from environmental influences (Guntrip, 1971). This inner drama is projected onto the outer world as the child comes to recognize other persons. In this respect, other persons are not subjects, but "objects" of the child's own making. Actual parental behavior is veiled by the child's projections. The environment is essentially psychological, a projection of the child's instinctual life. In contrast to this view, the developmental influence of the social environment is restored in the deficit model. Psychopathology results from *actual* failures of environmental agents to meet the child's developmental needs.

This type of formulation—a needs fulfillment model—establishes continuity between normal and psychopathological development. All children have developmental needs. What distinguishes disturbed from nondisturbed children is the environmental response to those needs. Thus, the deficit model necessitates, on the one hand, an explication of normative developmental needs, and on the other, a conceptualization of the facilitating environment. The model is based on a culinary metaphor—the recipe for normal development calls for certain "essential ingredients."

What are the "essential ingredients" for normal emotional development? In her later work, Anna Freud (1968) begins to address this issue. For example, the child's self-esteem is seen as depending on the mother's undisturbed attachment to her infant. Stability in later interpersonal relations is based on the reliability and responsiveness of the child's initial caregivers. Impulse control requires consistent and nonpunitive parental guidance. The capacity for emotion regulation emerges from the mother serving as an auxiliary ego in early development. Tolpin (1978) summarizes this perspective by pointing out that in early childhood, parents are "needed to fulfill developmental requirements and to act in place of self-sustaining and self-regulating psychic structure which has not yet formed" (p. 174). For example, infants and young children lack the capacity to calm themselves when distressed. During early development, parents serve this function. Over time, the child's capacity for emotion regulation is built from the parental response to the child's emotions. However, parents vary in their sensitivity and responsiveness to their child's emotional signals. Individual variation in emotion regulation follows from variation in parental attunement and responsiveness. In essence, parental responses are "imported" as internal structure. We come to care for ourselves as we have been cared for by others. If developmental needs are unfulfilled or distorted, developmental vulnerabilities are created.

Perhaps the most extensive elaboration of this perspective can be found in the work of D. W. Winnicott. For Winnicott, individual development is inextricably tied to the social environment. Although the individual represents a biological potential, the development of a person depends on a facilitating environment in which to grow (Winnicott, 1965). This view is concisely captured in a comment by Winnicott (1964): "I once risked the remark, 'There is no such thing as a baby'—meaning that once you set out to describe a baby, you will find you are describing a *baby and someone*. A baby cannot exist alone, but is essentially part of a relationship" (p. 66). At the core of all development is the fact of dependence. Innate potentials do not develop, as Guntrip (1971) puts it, "in sublime indifference" to the outer world (p. 104). Instead, they depend on an environment that understands, supports, and nurtures individual growth.

For Winnicott, development involves far more than the growth of ego functions that regulate, modulate, and control impulse and emotion. Instead, maturation is essentially about the development of a self, that is, the emergence of a person who *experiences* impulse, emotion, and interpersonal relations. The self, in essence, is not equivalent to the ego. Whereas the ego can be viewed as a regulatory system, the self represents the individual's unique subjectivity. According to Winnicott, the achievement of a coherent sense of self can only take place in the context of "good enough mothering." Apart from this interpersonal relationship, a self cannot develop; in fact, as Spitz has made evident, the interpersonally neglected infant may die despite adequate biological provisions (Guntrip, 1971).

What constitutes "good enough mothering"? Winnicott addresses this question with the deceptively simple concept of "holding." The function of "holding" in psychological terms is to provide ego support during that phase of development when the infant lacks the capacity to organize and modulate experience, and consequently is threatened by the experience of emotional disintegration. Good enough mothering involves empathic attunement to the infant's internal states. Overwhelming impulses or bodily needs disorganize the infant's sense of continuity and create anxiety. The mother's close identification with her baby, referred to by Winnicott (1965) as the "primary maternal preoccupation," facilitates her capacity to be sensitive and responsive to these disruptive "impingements." The mother who is not attuned to her baby, perhaps because of other preoccupations, fails to provide essential ego support. Moreover, the mother can act as an external impingement herself, by disrupting the baby's experience of continuity. For example, the baby may be forced to react to the mother's intrusive affective states or to an unpredictable pattern of caregiving. At such times the baby's emotional equilibrium is disrupted and anxiety is created. As Winnicott (1965) points out, too much doing and not enough responding on the part of the primary caregiver can result in impingements that threaten the baby's sense of coherence. The accumulation of impingements constitutes trauma, and for Winnicott, represents the principal psychosocial source of psychopathology. In contrast, maternal attunement to the child's emotions and needs leads to the experience of security. This experience of connection becomes part of the developing infant's sense of self and provides the basis for both increased autonomy and the capacity for relationship.

The significance of early infant–caregiver relationships for later emotional functioning is underscored by Bowlby and his followers. On two fronts, Bowlby (1958, 1973) challenges the traditional psychoanalytic position on the development of early relationships. First, in explaining the infant's emotional tie with mother, Bowlby rejects the *secondary drive* formulation implicit in both psychoanalytic and learning theories. For Bowlby, emotional attachment is not derived from the satisfaction of other more basic needs (e.g., nourishment or touch), but is the product of a behavioral system that has proximity to the mother as the set goal. This behavioral system has been selected over the course of evolution for its adaptive function. As Bowlby (1973) notes, emotionally significant bonds have basic survival value and therefore deserve a primary status.

On the second front, Bowlby (1973) challenges the view, most notably held by Melanie Klein, that real-life relationships are of limited importance compared to the world of internal object relations. Instead, Bowlby's attachment model is based on the simple assumption that actual relationships have an important impact on development, and that it is possible to assess the quality of early relationships. Bowlby (1973) argues, "The varied expectations of the accessibility and responsiveness of attachment figures that individuals develop during the years of immaturity are tolerably accurate reflections of the experiences those individuals have actually had" (p. 235). Thus, although the attachment system with its goal of proximity-seeking is built into the infant, the infant's experience of relationship is shaped by the caregiver's actual responses.

Research by Ainsworth and others (Ainsworth, Blehar, Waters, & Wall, 1978) suggests that variations in the mother's sensitivity and responsiveness to the infant's distress and needs result in different attachment patterns. Bowlby proposes that expectations about the availability of attachment figures are built up over the years of immaturity through repetitions of caregiving–care-receiving interactions. Experiences concerning the caregiver's accessibility and responsiveness are organized into an "internal working model," which has an existence outside of awareness and a propensity for stability (Bowlby, 1980). In essence, the child develops a set of interpersonal beliefs about the self in relation to significant others. According to Bowlby (1973), these beliefs exert a powerful influence on future emotional functioning. He says, "When an individual is confident that an attachment figure will be available to him whenever he desires it, that person will be much less prone to either intense anxiety or chronic fear than will an individual who for any reason has no such confidence" (p. 235). Internal working models derived from early social interactions play an active role in the guidance of behavior and the organization of emotion. According to Bowlby (1988) the pathway followed by the developing child and the degree to which he or she is vulnerable to stressful life events is determined to a very significant degree by the pattern of early attachment and its internal representation.

In contrast to the internal conflict model of psychopathology, Anna Freud's ego deficit model, Winnicott's concept of "good enough mothering," and Bowlby's attachment theory redirect attention to early social relationships as the source of adaptation and maladjustment. The psychosocial roots of psychopathology are to be found in the child's history of interpersonal relationships. Specifically, the inability of caregivers to meet the developing child's emotional needs creates vulnerability to psychopathology. From this perspective, children's functioning is undermined, not by distortions emanating from internal conflict, but from deficits incurred in early social interaction.

Given this reformulation of child psychopathology, what are the implications for child psychotherapy? Anna Freud (1968) cautions against the utility of genetic interpretations, that is, against interpretations aimed at linking the child's problematic past with current difficulties. Uncovering the child's experience of environmental failure and connecting it with current difficulties is not likely to be sufficient for therapeutic change. According to Anna Freud, the therapeutic value of this type of interpretive activity is limited, because the child suffering from developmental deficits does not have sufficient ego strength to make use of such interpretations (Sandler et al., 1980). Although the ego is in a weakened state, as in the case of neurotic conflict, insight and the expansion of self-awareness are not sufficient remedies for structural deficits. Winnicott takes this view a step further. Viewed from his perspective, the therapist's interpretive activity represents "too much doing and not enough responding." As a result, efforts at uncovering and interpreting harmful events could actually constitute an "impingement" that is countertherapeutic. In essence, the interpretations themselves constitute emotional stressors rather than sources of relief. This position has been elaborated in the adult psychotherapy literature by Kohout and his followers, who maintain that interpretations can interfere with the therapeutic process and can "recapitulate the rejection and rebuffs" experienced in early childhood (Tolpin, 1978, p. 178).

When faced with a child who is struggling with ego deficits, Anna Freud (1968) suggests that the therapist consider two alternatives, "neither of which are truly analytic" (p. 43). The first alternative is to "turn the treatment situation itself into an improved version of the child's initial environment and within this framework aim at the belated fulfillment of the neglected developmental needs" (p. 43). Here the essential therapeutic processes are not interpretation and insight, but instead, a "corrective emotional (interpersonal) experience." Developmental needs that were neglected or thwarted in the child's family of origin are attended to by the supportive therapist. As Anna Freud observes, the deprived and traumatized child needs "help, support, encouragement, and sympathy" rather than a series of interpretations about the unconscious roots of behavior (Sandler et al., 1980, p. 255).

The second alternative suggested by Anna Freud is to work directly with the social environment that has undermined the child's development. This approach may be limited by the degree to which parental attitudes and personalities are open to change and the extent to which the harmful environment has been internalized by the child (A. Freud, 1968). Given significant internalization, as is often the case with older children, environmental change may not be sufficient for therapeutic progress. In such cases, the therapist is faced with both ongoing family relations and an *internal* family derived from past interactions. In other cases, environmental obstacles to development may be enduring, for example, the child who continues to be victimized by a parent. Here the effectiveness of individual treatment with the child is limited by ongoing, disruptive influences in the social environment. In this case, environmental change is a prerequisite for therapeutic progress.

In summary, two major etiological models of child psychopathology are prominent in the psychodynamic child treatment tradition. Corresponding to each etiological model is a set of therapeutic interventions. Interpretative interventions, with the aim of insight and expanded self-awareness, have their origins in the internal conflict model. Corrective interpersonal interventions, with the goal of remediating deficits in internal psychological structure, follow from a reconceptualization of the role of the social environment in the genesis of psychopathology. Here therapy aims at compensating for inadequate or inappropriate environmental provisions. Thus, even within the psychodynamic tradition, child psychotherapy is far from a unitary process.

Client-Centered Approaches

In contrast to psychodynamic treatment, client-centered therapy was not developed principally for adults and then later extended to children. Instead, client-centered therapy was discovered with children (Wright, Everett, & Roisman, 1986). Carl Rogers's original therapeutic formulations grew out of his early clinical experiences in child guidance (cf. Rogers, 1939, 1942). Although client-centered therapy has evolved as it has been applied to adults, the basic framework for client-centered *child* psychotherapy can be found in Rogers's early work (Wright et al., 1986).

Client-centered therapy represents a challenge to the claim that models of intervention are "paired" with theories of etiology and pathogenesis. Unlike other models of intervention, client-centered child therapy appears to be based on a number of basic principles of therapy process rather than on an explicit model of psychopathology. However, a close reading of the client-centered child therapy literature reveals implicit formulations of child psychopathology. The outlines of one formulation can be found in the early work of Virginia Axline (1947).

The Self-Esteem Model

At the heart of Axline's model is the assumption that positive adjustment is predicated on the unobstructed expression of one's inner sense of self. Child maladjustment reflects an incongruence or split between the child's inner self and the self presented in everyday interaction. As Axline (1947) notes, "When the behavior and concept of self are consistent, and when the self-concept that is built up within the individual finds adequate outward expression, then the individual is said to be well adjusted. There is no longer a split focus. There is no longer inner conflict" (p. 14). Psychopathology reflects a distortion of the true self. She goes on to say, "The further apart the behavior and the concept, the greater the degree of maladjustment" (p. 14).

For Axline, the source of incongruence between inner experience and outer expression is to be found in the child's caregiving relationships. Children who have encountered caregivers who fail to value them become unable to value themselves. For Axline, self-esteem and self-acceptance are essentially social phenomena, the consequences of parental acceptance or rejection. This perspective has been elaborated by contemporary client-centered child clinicians, who maintain that "the correlation is quite high between the degree of psychopathology and the degree of self-depreciation, rejection of self, and lack of self-esteem" (Wright et al., 1986, p. 53). Wright and his colleagues go on to say, "As a rule all (child) psychotherapy clients either consciously or unconsciously feel unwanted or unworthy" (p. 53). Thus, from a client-centered perspective, one expects to find vulnerabilities in self-worth behind the myriad forms of child maladjustment.

The significance of self-esteem and self-acceptance for child psychopathology is underscored by Clark Moustakas (1959). According to Moustakas, the development of self-esteem is severely impaired in emotionally disturbed children. Because the child has been "severely rejected by others, he comes to reject himself" (p. 3). As a result, the child develops deep feelings of personal unworthiness and inadequacy. Usually these feelings are not directly expressed but surface as undifferentiated feelings of anxiety or hostility. As Moustakas (1959) notes, "Wherever hostility is expressed in the child's overt behavior, anxiety is potentially a strong internal attitude and significantly affects the child's behavior. Wherever anxiety is the primary outer expression, hostility usually lies beneath it" (pp. 24–25). Although anxiety and hostility have their roots in the experience of inadequacy and the devaluation of the self by significant others, the connection between these feelings and the situations that aroused them is often lost for disturbed children. Instead, the child simply is overwhelmed by fear or anger which in turn restricts the range and flexibility of behavior. For Moustakas, beneath the child's emotional distress and behavioral turmoil lies the loss of self-esteem.

This conceptualization of the relationship between self-worth and psychopathology is a cornerstone of client-centered child psychotherapy; however, the foundation for this therapeutic approach is a set of assumptions about the nature of "normal" development. Drawing on both ontogenetic evidence and evolutionary theory, Rogers (1951) hypothesizes:

Man like every other living organism, plant or animal, has an inherent tendency to develop all his capacities in ways that serve to maintain or enhance the organism. This is a reliable tendency, which when free to operate, moves the individual toward what is termed growth, maturity, and life enrichment. (p. 488)

For Rogers, development involves self-propelled change processes arising from within the individual. Moreover, development is inherently self-directed. The "directional trend," as Rogers refers to it, is toward greater differentiation of function, greater self-regulation, and increased complexity. Developmental processes do not merely maintain the organism, but expand its capacities and increase its autonomy. In essence, development is propelled by an internally originating growth process that moves the individual toward actualization of potential capacities.

This view of development is embraced by Axline (1947), who states, "There seems to be a powerful force within each individual which strives continuously for complete self-realization. This force may be characterized as a drive toward maturity, independence, and self-direction" (p. 10). According to Axline, if the child is provided with "good growing ground," much like a plant requires rich soil, self-regulating growth processes will enable the child to attain maturity and realize his or her potential.

This conceptualization of development provides the basis for the practice of client-centered child psychotherapy. According to Rogers (1942), therapy is not a matter of doing something to children or even attempting to induce children to do something about themselves. Instead, therapy involves freeing the child for normal growth and development. Rather than directly attending to specific problems or issues, the therapist attempts to provide the conditions for growth. According to Axline (1947), therapy is an *opportunity* offered to the child to experience growth under the most favorable conditions. Given the appropriate, facilitating conditions, the inherent tendency toward growth and self-actualization produces therapeutic change. The basic assumption of this therapeutic orientation is that internally originating processes of growth are also, under appropriate circumstances, self-correcting processes. Gendlin captures this perspective with a medical analogy. He says, "We cleanse wounds or sew stitches, and that helps, but the healing comes from inside" (Wright, Everett, & Reisman, 1986, p. iv).

Given the emphasis on self-correcting, developmental processes, it is not surprising that one of the fundamental aims of treatment is to avoid obstructing the child's tendency toward growth. As Dorfman (1951) points out, the therapist provides warmth, understanding, and company, but not leadership. Similarly, Moustakas (1959) reminds us that the origin of the word therapy comes from the Greek noun meaning servant, the verb for which is "to wait." As Moustakas notes, the therapist waits for the child to express his or her difficulties and to find new ways of relating. Waiting is viewed as a positive force, as a commitment to the assumption that children have within themselves the capacity to solve their own problems and the tendency to move toward greater maturity. In this assumption, we find the roots of nondirective child psychotherapy. As Axline (1947) states in her principles of child treatment, "The therapist does not attempt to direct the child's actions or conversation in any manner. The child leads the way; the therapist follows" (p. 75). Not surprisingly then, the emphasis in client-centered child therapy is not on specific therapeutic interventions but on the interpersonal conditions that facilitate growth. Thus, the process of change is closely tied to the quality of the therapeutic relationship. And for client-centered child therapists, the essential ingredient of the therapeutic relationship is permissiveness.

According to Rogers (1942), all therapeutic techniques aim at developing a "free and permissive" relationship. Similarly, Axline (1947) advises child therapists to establish "a feeling of permissiveness in the relationship so that the child feels free to express his feelings completely" (p. 75). As this principle implies, the permissive relationship is not an end in itself, but a means to emotion expression. The therapist-offered conditions of warmth, nonjudgmental acceptance, and genuineness provide the basis for the therapeutic process. For Rogers, these conditions are not established through technique alone, but are a reflection of attitudes embedded in the therapist's personality. This is not to say that the therapeutic value of treatment is determined solely by the therapist's attitudes; however, no set of techniques or methods can compensate for the absence of warmth, acceptance, and genuineness. Without these therapist-offered conditions, the process of therapy is blocked.

How does the permissive therapeutic relationship promote growth and change? Two models of therapy process can be found in early client-centered theory. By no means are they incompatible; instead they appear to differ in emphasis. For Axline (1947), the process of change is closely linked with the child's experience of an accepting and validating relationship. Children are maladjusted because they have encountered obstacles to the full expression of the real self. The discrepancy between real self and presented self is accompanied by emotional conflict. The therapist-offered conditions of warmth, respect, and most importantly, acceptance, allow the child to reveal his or her real self to the therapist. The child discovers that feelings, thoughts, and wishes that have been denied expression can, in fact, be accepted. Through the process of acceptance by a nonjudgmental therapist the child reestablishes connection with denied or rejected aspects of the self. The experience of revealing the self in an accepting relationship increases the child's confidence to act on the basis of his or her concept of self. With this increase in self-acceptance, mediated by the therapist's validating response, the discrepancy between real and presented selves diminishes and symptoms of maladjustment abate.

The Emotional Obstruction Model

A second therapy process model can be found in Rogers's (1942) early work. In this formulation, emotion expression is viewed as a pivotal mechanism of therapeutic change. Conversely, child psychopathology is conceptualized in terms of obstructed emotion. According to Rogers, "Maladjustments are not failures in *knowing*" (p. 29). Instead, obstructed or unexpressed emotions have the potential to undermine adaptive functioning. Of early client-centered therapy Rogers (1942) says, "This newer therapy endeavors to work as directly as possible in the realm of feeling and emotion rather than attempting to achieve emotional reorganization through an intellectual approach" (p. 29). The warm, receptive attitude of the therapist serves to establish the appropriate conditions for emotion expression. The essential function of the permissive relationship is to reduce the child's defensiveness in order to facilitate the expression of feelings. The fundamental role of the therapist is to create an atmosphere in which the child can recognize positive, negative, and ambivalent feelings and accept them as part of the self rather than hiding them behind defensive processes.

In his early work, Rogers (1942) provides an outline of a sequential model of therapy process. Therapy is structured by a set of therapist-offered conditions. The therapist offers a warm, nonjudgmental relationship to the child and supports the free expression of feelings. Although the therapist is neutral in relation to the valence of the expressed emotion, therapy provides a unique opportunity for the expression of negative feelings. When such feelings are expressed, the therapist accepts, recognizes, and clarifies them. However, the origins and meaning of the feelings are not interpreted by the therapist. According to Rogers, "When the individual's negative feelings have been quite fully expressed, they are followed by the faint and tentative expressions of the positive impulses which make for growth" (p. 39).

Consequently, interpretation is not required to bring about emotional change. Emotional discharge inherently leads to a change in emotional valence. Rogers cites the case of young boy who spent numerous sessions expressing rage through aggressive play. Following a sequence of sessions in which the boy tortured, beat, and killed father images, he began to express feelings of admiration for a father figure pictured in the newspaper. Rogers notes that this shift of emotion in therapy paralleled changes in the child's behavior at home. Thus, it appears that therapeutic change depends on the release of negative emotion by the child and the full acceptance of these feelings by the therapist. According to Rogers, "The more violent and deep the negative expressions (provided they are accepted and recognized), the more certain are the positive expressions of love, of social impulses, of fundamental self-respect, of desire to be mature" (p. 39). Given this view of emotion processes, it appears that catharsis constitutes the principle mechanism of therapeutic change. However, Rogers is quick to point out that the expression of emotion involves more than an experience of release. It leads to a reorganization of the child's experience, to new ways of perceiving self, others, and relationships. Insight is "inextricably linked to the experience of catharsis" (p. 174).

For Rogers, insight implies "the perception of new meaning in the individual's own experience" (p. 174). It involves the reorganization of the experiential field. However, insight is not based on the therapist's interpretive activity. Significant changes in experience follow from the client's expression of emotion, not from the therapist's insightful interpretations of the client's problems. As Rogers points out, the primary technique that leads to insight on the part of the client demands self-restraint on the part of the therapist. The therapist encourages and clarifies feelings until, as Rogers puts it, "Insightful understanding appears spontaneously" (p. 195).

Reorganizations in the experiential field create new opportunities for action. Consistent with the assumption that individuals have the means to solve their own problems under the appropriate conditions, the transformation of insight into action is client directed. The therapist's role is not to prescribe new behaviors but to clarify behavioral choices. Given the hypothesized developmental trend toward greater maturity and self-actualization, catharsis and insight represent the necessary and sufficient conditions for positive behavioral change.

Three basic tenets appear to capture the character of early client-centered child therapy. First, therapy is nondirective. Given the assumption that individuals, including children, have the capacity to solve their own problems, respect for this assumption demands that therapy be client directed. The locus of responsibility for sessions is the client and not the therapist. For the therapist to direct the session also involves the risk of not accepting the child completely, which could replicate the conditions responsible for maladjustment. In addition, the goal of client-centered therapy is to move the child toward greater reliance on his or her own experience for values and standards (Rogers, 1957). For the therapist to lead the way and assume responsibility for the child would undermine the very aim of treatment.

The second tenet is that the principal vehicle of change is the therapeutic relationship rather than specific therapeutic techniques. Therapy is viewed as an opportunity for growth rather than a sequence of well-timed interventions. The therapist's main aim is to provide the facilitating conditions for self-directed development. This does not mean that the therapist need not be skillful. Instead, the fundamental therapeutic skill involves the effective *communication* of the basic conditions for growth—warmth, acceptance, and genuineness.

The third tenet is that therapeutic change is predicated on emotional rather than cognitive processes. Client-centered therapists assume that when a child feels differently, he or she will act differently. In this connection, insight is viewed as a consequence rather than an antecedent of emotional reorganization. Similarly, the process of validation and acceptance of the child's real self cannot be communicated intellectually, but must be experienced in the context of an emotionally genuine relationship.

Much contemporary nondirective child psychotherapy is guided by these basic tenets. For example, Gumaer (1984) maintains that there is only one therapeutic procedure in child-centered therapy, "the establishment of a facilitative relationship which provides an atmosphere that encourages personal growth in the client" (pp. 37–38). However, client-centered therapy has undergone a significant evolution during the decades since its emergence in the 1940s and 1950s. According to Wright and his colleagues (1986), the process of client-centered therapy was transformed when Rogers attempted to apply the basic principles of nondirective therapy to severely disturbed adults. The therapist-offered conditions of acceptance, warmth, and genuineness did not appear to facilitate a self-directed therapeutic process. Instead, therapists were often confronted with silence, low levels of involvement in the process of self-exploration, minimal self-disclosure, and outright rejection. As Wright et al. note, some of these same frustrations are encountered by child therapists.

In working with severely disturbed adults, nondirective therapists began to experience marked disparity or incongruence between their expressed warmth and acceptance and their inner feelings of frustration, helplessness, and anger. From a client-centered perspective, this type of incongruity is countertherapeutic. In the first place, incongruity is presumed to be one of the conditions associated with maladjustment. Recapitulation in the context of therapy could hardly constitute an effective remedy. In the second place, incongruence is antithetical to genuineness, one of the necessary therapist-offered conditions for client growth. Caught between the conflicting demands of nondirective acceptance and genuineness, therapists began to take a more active role by disclosing their own feelings and experience (Wright et al., 1986). The increased emphasis on therapist congruence represents a significant turning point in the evolution of client-centered therapy.

The Emergence of Experiential Child Therapy

Two important changes appear to distinguish early forms of nondirective child therapy from contemporary practices. In experiential child psychotherapy, as Wright and his colleagues refer to it, a number of client-centered principles are realigned. The first involves a new balance between therapist congruence and locus of responsibility. Nondirective therapy proscribes the introduction of meaning and feelings by the therapist. This responsibility resides with the child alone. The therapist is cast as a sensitive responder to the child's emotional and behavioral initiatives. Experiential child therapy, with its emphasis on genuineness and therapist congruence, endorses the use of the therapist's experience, including the therapist's feelings in session, as an important therapeutic tool. Although the focus of therapy remains the client's experience, the principle of congruence requires the therapist to acknowledge feelings as they are experienced in therapy and to communicate persistent feelings that exist in the relationship. Therapy is no longer exclusively client directed; instead client and therapist share the responsibility for the treatment process.

The increased emphasis on therapist congruence entails a second, although no less significant, realignment of basic principles. In early client-centered therapy, the therapist's principal communicative function is reflective. Interpretive comments represent a basic threat to empathy and acceptance. According to Rogers (1951),

> It is the counselor's function to assume, in so far as he is able, the internal frame of reference of the client, to perceive the world as the client sees it, to perceive the client himself as he is seen by himself, to set aside all perceptions from the external frame of reference while doing so, and to communicate something of this empathic understanding to the client. (p. 29)

In contrast, congruence involves responding from the therapist's experiential process. It does not mean interpreting the child's experience from an external frame of reference, but it does imply responding to the child from the therapist's frame. Wright et al. maintain that congruence is a means by which the therapist can provide interactional feedback to the child concerning his or her impact on others.

What does this realignment of principles mean for the practice of experiential child psychotherapy? Like early nondirective child therapy, experiential therapy remains process oriented. The aim of treatment is not to solve specific problems but to facilitate the process of growth. For the experiential therapist this means using a full repertoire of techniques to maximize the child's experiential process (Wright et al., 1986). Unfortunately, an explicit model of what constitutes the experiential process for children has not been articulated. In the adult psychotherapy literature, Gendlin (1974) describes "experiencing" as the process of attending to and focusing on the implicitly felt meaning of experience and attempting to articulate it. Thus, the experiential process involves symbolizing that which is implicitly felt. As a process in therapy, experiencing is characterized by an emotionally involved, inward focus on feelings, attitudes, and meanings related to behavior and experience (Greenberg & Safran, 1987). The client's attention is directed toward internal rather than external referents, and the experience is a blend of cognitive and affective components. For example, if said in an emotionally involved manner, the statement, "I can't let myself get angry, I end up feeling so guilty and that makes me mad" reflects a high level of experiencing. Others suggest that "experiencing" entails an immediate experience of feeling, as well as reflective awareness of such feelings (Luborsky, Chandler, Auerbach, Cohen, & Bachrach, 1971).

Given these perspectives on experiencing, the process of therapy can no longer be conceptualized as catharsis or simple emotion expression. The emphasis on symbolization suggests that the discharge of feelings through behavior, what Axline referred to as the child's natural medium, is not a sufficient therapeutic process. Instead, it appears that experiential child therapy involves a greater emphasis on the *representation* of experience. Similarly, the importance of reflective awareness suggests that the process of self-observation is critical. Feelings are not simply expressed in therapy, they are also acknowledged and understood. However, a developmental model of these processes in experiential child psychotherapy still awaits elaboration.

In summary, the client-centered tradition directs the child therapist's attention to the child's felt experience. The essential "substance" of therapy is the child's immediate feelings and experience rather than beliefs, attitudes, and impulses lurking outside awareness. Emotional processes in the form of catharsis, validation, or experiencing constitute the principle vehicles of change. Although the role of the client-centered child therapist has undergone transformation over time—from reflector of the child's emotions to active facilitator of the child's experiencing—both early and contemporary forms of client-centered therapy underscore the importance of the therapist-offered conditions of warmth, nonjudgmental acceptance, genuineness, and empathy as the catalysts of therapeutic progress.

Cognitive Approaches

Although cognitive constructs such as insight, interpretation, and self-observation have been a part of the child psychotherapy literature for some time, cognitive therapies for children represent a relatively recent development. The offspring of the cognitive reformulation of social learning theory (Bandura, 1977; Mischel, 1973) and adult cognitive therapy, cognitive approaches to child psychotherapy share the assumption that *internal, mediational processes* are the principal target of therapeutic intervention. Although there have been a number of prominent contributors to the cognitive movement in psychotherapy, Beck's (1976; Beck, Rush, Shaw, & Emery, 1979) cognitive reconceptualization of emotional disorders captures many of the core assumptions of the cognitive approach.

The Cognitive Distortion Model

The basic tenet of Beck's theory is that the relationship between an event and an emotional reaction is mediated by the interpretive activity of the individual. As Beck (1976) notes, "The thesis that the special meaning of an event determines the emotional response forms the core of the cognitive model of emotions and emotional disorders" (p. 52). And for Beck, meaning is to be found in cognition, the product of the individual's interpretive activity. For example, a youngster who receives the highest grade in class may interpret this event as confirming his or her self-worth, or as a potential threat to fitting in with the peer group. Given the first interpretation, happiness or even euphoria is the likely reaction; given the second, anxiety is probable. According to Beck, these types of interpretation occur rapidly and quite spontaneously. From the perspective of the experiencing subject, such spontaneous thoughts do not appear to be the result of intentional activity; and of equal importance, they seem plausible. As a result, Beck refers to these rapid, mediating cognitions as "automatic thoughts."

The automatic thoughts that accompany interpersonal situations do not occur by accident. Instead, they originate in a set of assumptions about the self and social reality. These assumptions operate like rules that form the basis for specific interpretations, expectancies, and self-instructions (Beck, 1976). More abstract than specific automatic thoughts, assumptions consist of "equations, formulas, and premises that enable the person to order, classify, and synthesize his (her) observations of reality so that he (she) can come to meaningful conclusions" (p. 43).

Beck gives the example of a student who is corrected by her instructor for talking in class. Her emotional response is shame and sadness. Her interpretation of the situation is, "He has caught me doing something wrong and will dislike me from now on." Her underlying assumption is, "Correction by authority equals disapproval and the exposure of weakness." Beck notes that the operation of these assumptions is comparable to the function of a major premise in a syllogism. Given the major premise in the form of an underlying assumption, and a minor premise in the form of an interpersonal event, the interpretation or automatic thought "logically" follows. Unlike automatic thoughts that can be monitored, major premises, that is, assumptions about social reality, are typically less accessible to awareness. As Beck points out, these premises are part of the individual's cognitive organization and function like the rules of grammar during everyday speech.

Given this cognitive model of emotion, what processes account for emotional disorders? For Beck, emotional maladjustment results from distortions in the individual's interpretive activity. Inappropriate or excessive emotional reactions follow from "a web of incorrect meanings" attached to particular situations. As Beck (1976) states, "The deviant meanings constitute the cognitive distortions that form the core of emotional disorders" (p. 49). Normal emotional responses are based on reasonably accurate appraisals of reality. In contrast, emotional responses in psychological disorders are "determined to a far greater degree by internal (that is, psychological) factors that confound reality" (p. 75). The ideational content of emotional disorders contains a distortion of reality. Viewed from this perspective, emotional disorders are largely the result of poor reality testing.

The critical etiological question concerns the source of maladaptive assumptions. Interestingly, Beck provides relatively little insight into the origins of cognitive distortions. Comparing the development of maladaptive assumptions (rules) to the development of grammar, Beck notes that relatively little grammar is taught explicitly. Instead, general rules, in both the interpersonal and grammatical domains, are derived from concrete situations. According to Beck, "Insomuch as rules are part of the social heritage, they are probably absorbed to a large extent through observations of other people as well as from personal experiences" (p. 45). Although these comments suggest an etiological model of cognitive distortions, Beck's theory is not directed primarily toward issues of origins. Instead, as a model of intervention, the theory is principally concerned with the *maintenance* of emotional disorders. Consistent with this view, therapy does not focus on interpersonal history, but on uncovering and restructuring extant maladaptive assumptions and automatic thoughts.

Elaborating on Beck's references to the childhood origins of cognitive distortions, Guidano and Liotti (1983, 1985) provide a unitary etiological model of cognitive dysfunction. Two concepts form the foundation of this developmental model—self-knowledge and attachment.

According to Guidano and Liotti (1985), self-knowledge is constructed through interaction with significant others (p. 107). During infancy a "nucleus" of self-knowledge is formed long before the child is able to remember or reflect on it (Guidano & Liotti, 1983). This "tacit" knowledge structure contains "the rules with which the child comes to perceive and recognize the invariant aspects of self and other" (1985, p. 104). In other words, schemas or models of self and the environment are formed during early childhood. And like most cognitive schemas, these "tacit" rules or models provide a frame for the construction of subsequent knowledge. As Guidano and Liotti (1983) emphasize, the decoding of experience is biased by "a tendency first to recognize and then to shape incoming information into available, preexisting knowledge structures" (p. 105). Assimilation is the dominant principle in the organization of experience.

The most basic structures of self-knowledge are constructed out of patterns of caregiving interactions in early childhood. As the child comes to recognize the caregiving qualities of significant others, knowledge is gained about the self. As Guidano and Liotti (1985) put it, "Any information about the outside world always and inevitably corresponds to information about the self" (p. 108). Consequently, patterns of caregiving correspond to patterns of self-conception. In their words, "The qualitative aspects of attachment patterns between the child and his or her caregivers will reflect themselves in different structural aspects of the child's developing self- knowledge" (p. 109). Out of the quality of parental care, the young child derives a self-conception regarding fundamental aspects of identity, such as personal worth and lovableness. These deep, tacit knowledge structures provide the scaffolding for more explicit beliefs and expectations about the self and social reality. Moreover, early knowledge structures direct and coordinate the individual's emotional and imaginative life, and limit the range of assimilable experiences (Guidano & Liotti, 1985). Thus, the origins of cognitive dysfunction are to be found in distorted self-knowledge constructed in early childhood. The cognitive distortions described by Beck (1976) follow from these knowledge structures. As Guidano and Liotti (1983) contend,

> With respect to cognitive growth, these distorted self-conceptions, functioning as a set of tacit rules, will coordinate thinking and deductive reasoning on the basis of the mythical and dogmatic "logic" to which they are still bound. In this way, they can set into motion typical patterns of reasoning filled with all those inferential errors and disorders of thinking. (p. 106)

This perspective has been elaborated by Leahy (1985, 1988), who maintains that distorted self-conceptions will be characterized by the "logic" of the developmental period during which they were formed. Thus, distorted self-conceptions entail both maladaptive content—for example, "I am totally unlovable"—and problematic reasoning—for example, global, polarized thinking.

On the basis of this general model, Guidano and Liotti (1983) outline a set of relationships between abnormal patterns of attachment and specific emotional disorders. For example, in depression, the course of attachment is characterized by a relative lack of affective contact in the child's environment. Although a wide variety of family situations can lead to limited affective contact, the common experience for the child is "precocious and unwilling separation" from caregivers (Guidano & Liotti, 1983, p. 109). This attachment pattern gives rise to conflicting self-knowledge. The lack of affective contact engenders a sense of unworthiness, whereas the experience of isolation results in the belief that one can reliably count only on the self. This nucleus of self-knowledge forms a "biased" scaffolding for the progressive elaboration of attitudes toward the self and beliefs about the social world. Thus, for example, given their underlying sense of unworthiness, these individuals anticipate abandonment and are highly sensitive to rejection. At the same time, given their belief in the unreliability of others, they tend to rely on their own resources when faced with difficulties and often actively exclude the support of others (Guidano & Liotti, 1983). From a nucleus of self-knowledge, the early schemas, a destiny of loneliness and self-blame unfolds.

Implicit in this model is a hierarchical conceptualization of mediating cognitions. At the deepest level are the early schemas of self-knowledge. Formed prior to self-reflection, these early schemas represent tacit knowledge structures that provide the framework for beliefs about the self and others, or what has been termed "maladaptive assumptions." These assumptions, rooted in the biased structure of early self-knowledge, engender automatic thoughts that are elicited by interpersonal events. Consequently, for the cognitive therapist, interventions can be aimed at different levels of depth. Traditional cognitive therapy with adults has been directed largely toward restructuring maladaptive assumptions and automatic thoughts. Intervention principally involves identifying, monitoring, and challenging cognitive distortions (Beck, 1976). However, intervention is not entirely "intellectual." As Beck (1976) points out, the cognitive therapist employs both "experiential" and "behavioral" methods. In the former, the patient is exposed to experiences that may be powerful enough to change cognitive distortions. In the latter, new behaviors are taught, such as assertiveness, with the goal of changing self-perceptions. As these methods imply, the cognitive therapist is both active and directive in his or her interactions with patients. More recently, a number of cognitive theorists (Guidano & Liotti, 1985; Leahy, 1985; Mahoney, 1985) have proposed that intervention can be directed toward the early schemas that engender cognitive distortions. According to Guidano and Liotti (1983) many cognitive-behavioral interventions such as "thought stopping" and "rational restructuring" address important, but peripheral, maladaptive cognitions. Although these techniques are often sufficient to produce therapeutic effects, in more complex cases they fail to yield meaningful or sustainable change. This is not to say that these interventions are unnecessary for a cognitive treatment strategy. Instead, because these interventions often reveal deeper cognitive rules and beliefs, they represent the first step in the treatment process. As Guidano and Liotti (1983) contend, the initial cognitive-behavioral interventions frequently "bring to light deeper theories that usually need to be confronted with therapeutic techniques of a different logical level" (p. 151). This level of intervention is referred to by Guidano and Liotti as *developmental analysis.* Here the aim of treatment is to find the developmental origins of the patient's maladaptive assumptions. For Guidano and Liotti (1983), the process of psychotherapy "must fully acknowledge the life experiences on which the patient built his or her irrational beliefs and found a confirmation of their truth" (p. 152). Of particular importance is the evidence used by patients to support their beliefs about personal identity and social relations. As Leahy (1988) notes, the problem is not that something happened in the past, but that the patient still believes the conclusions drawn from it.

For example, an adopted adolescent expressed the belief, "I don't measure up to my friends," and was constantly driven by perfectionism and plagued by self-criticism. An exploration of the origins of this belief about his relative inadequacy revealed that this teen viewed his adoption as evidence to support his assumption of inadequacy. He expressed this view through the associated belief, "If only I had been perfect, my real parents wouldn't have given me up." This underlying assumption was expressed in a tacit interpersonal rule: "In order to maintain relationships (be accepted), one must be flawless." Lapses in flawless performances, for example, getting a B rather than an A on a school exam, resulted in harsh self-condemnation.

Unlike traditional insight-oriented therapy, recovery or reconstruction of the developmental origins of maladaptive beliefs or schemas is *not* regarded by cognitive therapists as sufficient for therapeutic change. Instead, the therapist collaborates with the patient to reevaluate the evidence upon which the maladaptive beliefs are based. A plausible, rival account of the evidence might be offered. For example, in the case of the troubled adolescent, the patient was encouraged to develop other possible accounts of his early adoption and ultimately was supported in his efforts to uncover the "true" story. Leahy (1985) recommends a reintroduction of traditional cognitive methods at this point to enable the patient to dispute deeper beliefs.

In addition to isolated or networked propositions and concepts, narrative schemas also have been identified as a fundamental unit of cognitive organization (Anderson, 1980). Such narrative schemas have been shown to be at work in memory processes early in toddlerhood and to develop and change throughout the school-age years. Russell and van den Broek (1988) have proposed a structural model of narrative schemas and have explicated three dimensions as targets for clinical intervention. For example, a child may experience difficulties because of inaccurate causal or temporal organization in their narrative schema of a series of events. On the other hand, a child's difficulties might be the result of an inaccurate or deficient representation of the subjectivities of the persons or characters in their schematic representation—their narrative schema might be devoid of the theories of mind that animate humans with intentions, hopes, desires, empathy, and will.

In the model of therapy presented by Russell and van den Broek (1988), exposing the child to alternative narrative representations of problematic episodes can help to correct or augment the child's cognitive–emotional organization of episodic information. Armed with an altered narrative representation of events, the child can entertain new behavioral options and experience new forms of interpersonal engagement. Although the authors have not developed a theory of the etiology of schematic malformation, it is clear that such schemas often represent, accurately and inaccurately, events that have been encountered repeatedly or that have been traumatic. Unlike many forms of cognitive intervention, this theory stresses holistic and not piecemeal changes in cognitive organization as necessary for deep restructuring of a child's everyday experience.

The application of the cognitive distortion model to the psychotherapy of children is a relatively recent phenomenon. DiGiuseppe (1981) proposes that many of the techniques of adult cognitive therapy can be adapted for the treatment of children. Consistent with the assumptions of the cognitive distortion model, DiGiuseppe (1981) emphasizes the role of distorted judgments about social reality and unrealistic self-appraisals in children's maladjustment. However, recognizing that children are often "unwilling consumers of mental health services," DiGiuseppe (1981, p. 53) suggests that child cognitive therapy requires a preliminary phase during which the child's motivation for change must be established. According to DiGiuseppe, in order to ensure collaboration, the initial task of therapy is to establish or support two basic cognitive beliefs: first, that change is possible, and second, that change is desirable. As DiGiuseppe notes, "The inability to perceive an alternative behavioral or emotional response to the troublesome situation keeps the child from recognizing even the possibility of behavior change" (p. 58). Similarly, the inability to recognize the desirability of change may reflect deficits in consequential thinking; that is, the child fails to acknowledge some of the painful consequences of his or her behavior or attitudes. However, as DiGiuseppe (1981) cautions, failure to acknowledge the desirability of change might not be due to cognitive deficits but rather to patterns of reinforcement or modeling in the child's environment.

With the establishment of therapeutic collaboration, the cognitive therapist "moves along to the crucial step in cognitive therapies, challenging or disputing the child's troublesome beliefs" (DiGiuseppe, 1981, p. 61). Here the child's developing cognitive capacities represent an obstacle to the direct application of cognitive techniques. For example, in his discussion of the treatment of childhood depression, Leahy (1988) draws attention to several potential constraints. First, limitations in abstract reasoning will constrain younger children's ability to think about and to evaluate rational versus irrational thoughts. Similarly, lacking well-developed concepts of internal psychological processes, the link between cognition and emotion may be difficult for young children to grasp. Finally, the child's ability to monitor and challenge maladaptive thoughts entails self-reflective capacities that may exceed the cognitive abilities of young children. Given these potential obstacles, Leahy proposes that cognitive therapy must be adapted to the cognitive developmental level of the child. For example, the therapist is likely to emphasize teaching rational self-verbalizations through modeling rather than dialogue. Similarly, the therapeutic task of challenging maladaptive assumptions may need to be preceded by perspective-taking training to enable children to observe their own psychological processes.

Although children's developing cognitive capacities make the application of cognitive techniques challenging, there is increasing evidence that cognitive distortions play an important role in some forms of child psychopathology. For example, depressed children show a negative bias in their perceptions of self, world, and the future, typically found among depressed adults (Kazdin, French, Unis, & Esveldt-Dawson, 1983). The work of Kaslow, Rehm, and Siegel (1984) reveals that depressed children evidence more stringent standards for failure, exhibit lower expectations for performance, and evaluate the self more negatively than nondepressed children. Similarly, Seligman and his colleagues (1984) find that children with depressive symptoms overattribute negative events to internal, stable, and global causes. Finally, Leitenberg, Yost, and Carroll-Wilson (1986) provide evidence that depressed children overgeneralize negative outcomes, catastrophize the consequences of negative events, and selectively attend to negative features of events. Other types of biases and distortions are found among aggressive children. For example, Dodge and Frame (1982) show that these children overattribute hostile intentions to peers, even in situations in which a hostile attribution is unwarranted. These types of findings suggest that cognitive distortions represent an important target for therapeutic intervention with disordered children.

The Cognitive Deficit Model

Although cognitive distortions undoubtedly contribute to the maladjustment of many children, a different type of cognitive problem is often associated with child psychopathology. As Kendall (1981, p. 54) points out, the disordered child frequently "fails to engage in the cognitive, informa-tion-processing activities of an active problem solver, does not initiate the reflective thinking that can govern behavior, or essentially lacks the cogni-tive skills needed to perform certain high-level mental activity." In such cases, *cognitive deficits* rather than *cognitive distortions* are the primary contributors to child maladjustment.

Three types of internal, mediational deficits constitute the principal targets of cognitive interventions: (1) verbal mediation processes, (2) social problem-solving strategies, and (3) social perspective-taking abilities. Un-like behavioral skills training, which targets discrete, observable behaviors, the focus of cognitive interventions is the development of general, covert cognitive processes (Urbain & Kendall, 1980).

Perhaps one of the best examples of intervention into verbal mediation processes is Meichenbaum's (1977) approach to self-control training. Draw-ing on the work of Luria (1961) and Vygotsky (1962), who studied the role of language and symbolization in the regulation of behavior, Meichen-baum (1979) hypothesizes that habitual maladaptive behavior, for example, impulsiveness in the classroom, must be "deautomatized" by the introduc-tion of deliberate, mediating cognitions. According to Meichenbaum (1979, p. 9), "Forced mediation increases the likelihood of interrupting a chain of events that would otherwise lead to the maladaptive response." Thus, instead of the child immediately responding to some form of provocation, overt behavior is preceded by an "internal dialogue" that includes appraisals, attributions, and expectations. For Meichenbaum (1979) this internal dialogue plays a central role in the development of self-control. Two critical steps are involved: first, increasing the child's capacity to monitor situations that evoke maladaptive behavior (e.g., interpersonal contexts, affective cues, or verbal labels), and second, teach-ing the child sets of self-instructions that increase the likelihood of self-con-trol (e.g., assessing the consequences of behavior). Unlike the operant behavioral approach that emphasizes restructuring the environment to establish behavioral control, the cognitive approach helps children alter their internal processes to attain self-control.

A related approach that has emerged from the psychodynamic tradi-tion focuses on the development of cognitive controls. According to Santostephano (1985), adaptive functioning requires the individual to balance the demands of environmental circumstances with the internal world of fantasies, wishes, and representations of past experience. How-ever, unlike early psychoanalytic theory, which viewed these demands as quantities of energy, Santostephano reconceptualizes them as sources of information. Mediating between the two sources are cognitive controls that regulate the acquisition and utilization of information. Controls are viewed as the basic tools by which the individual structures experience. For example, one type of cognitive control, focal attention, concerns the way the child surveys a field of information. Child maladjustment can be understood in terms of deficits in specific cognitive controls. One prominent form of "pathological cognitive orientation" involves inefficient registering of information from both internal and external sources. These children frequently show deficits in delaying motor activity, being aware of social standards, monitoring their own reactions, and connecting thoughts, beliefs, or fantasies with action. For Santostephano, the aim of therapy is the rehabilitation of cognitive structures through a set of cognitive–affective exercises. For example, interventions directed at focal attention provide the child with experiences in tracking increasingly complex stimuli.

A second major target for cognitive intervention is children's social problem-solving strategies. Although a number of alternative approaches have emerged during the last 20 years (Alexander & Parsons, 1973; Kendall, 1984; Lochman & Curry, 1986), one of the most extensive programs is the Interpersonal Cognitive Problem-Solving approach (ICPS), developed by Spivack, Shure, and their associates (Shure & Spivak, 1978; Spivack, Platt, & Shure, 1976; Spivack & Shure, 1974). Three sets of interpersonal cognitions bear a consistent relationship with indices of behavioral adjustment: (1) alternative thinking, (2) consequential thinking, and (3) means–end thinking (Urbain & Kendall, 1980). The first refers to the child's ability to generate multiple potential solutions to an interpersonal problem; the second concerns the child's ability to see both immediate and long-term consequences for problem solutions; and the third involves the child's ability to plan a set of actions (means) to attain a specific goal. The aim of therapy is to facilitate the development of these cognitive processes through a structured set of activities and discussions (Spivack & Shure, 1974). For example, the child might be asked to link problem solutions with specific consequences in both hypothetical and real-life interpersonal situations. Although these types of approaches have been shown to be effective in improving children's problem-solving skills, their impact on interpersonal behavior is less clear (Urbain & Kendall, 1980).

A third major target for cognitive intervention is children's social perspective-taking ability. Drawing on the work of Mead (1934) and Piaget (1965/1932), social developmentalists have viewed perspective-taking processes as the cornerstone of social intelligence and as a critical contributor to adaptive social behavior (Chandler, 1973; Selman, 1980). Research indicates that maladjusted children show significant deficits in perspective-taking ability relative to nondisturbed peers (Chandler, Greenspan, & Barenboim, 1974; Selman, 1980). The inability to take another's point of view and/or to reflect on the self from another's perspective is thought to contribute to children's problems with self-regulation, aggression, and social relatedness.

One of the most frequently referenced approaches to perspective-taking intervention has been conducted by Chandler and his colleagues (Chandler, 1973; Chandler et al., 1974). In their work, perspective-taking training involves writing and videotaping skits of events involving agemates. Children play different roles during successive productions of the skit, thereby providing them with the opportunity to occupy different roles in relation to the same event. Videotapes are reviewed and discussed by members of the "cast." Approaches such as these have been effective in promoting children's social perspective-taking ability and in improving behavioral adjustment (Urbain & Kendall, 1980).

As a group, self-instructional, social problem solving, and perspective-taking training share the assumption that cognitive deficits figure prominently in various forms of child maladjustment. Children encounter interpersonal problems because they lack the information-processing capacities or social-cognitive skills needed for adaptive functioning. Intervention, then, aims at facilitating the development of missing cognitive processes. The *sufficiency* of this formulation has been questioned by Selman and Schultz (1988). According to their view, not all interpersonal cognitive problems can be understood as cognitive deficits. Instead, their research with disturbed children and adolescents points to another type of cognitive problem, namely the *translation* of cognitive strategies into effective action. This type of problem has been termed a "production deficiency" (Flavell, 1977).

For example, Selman and his colleagues (Selman & Demorest, 1984; Selman, Schorin, Stone, & Phelps, 1983) have examined children's interpersonal negotiation strategies in the controlled confines of a clinical interview and in the context of actual peer interaction. Interpersonal negotiation strategies represent qualitatively distinct, developmentally ordered approaches to the resolution of interpersonal conflicts. At the lowest level of negotiation strategies, impulsive solutions, such as physical aggression or withdrawal, involve the lack of coordination in social perspectives. At the highest level, strategies reflect an awareness of the need for an integration of social perspectives; thus conflict is viewed from a third-person perspective. Here action strategies involve compromise, dialogue, and efforts at mutual understanding.

Based on their observations of children in interviews and interpersonal situations, Selman and Schultz (1988) describe two types of social cognitive "pathology." The first refers to those children who evidence low-level performance in both contexts. Unable to generate high-level strategies in either the interview or social behavior, the "low–low" child represents the cognitive deficit prototype. Even in the supportive context of a clinical interview, these children are limited to a narrow repertoire of low-level interpersonal strategies. In contrast, the "high–low" child performs quite well in interview, suggesting the presence of adaptive strategies in his or her cognitive repertoire, but in the "heat" of interpersonal interaction, fails to employ such strategies. In essence, a gap separates the interpersonal thought and action of these children. Their problem does not reside in a cognitive deficit, but in the transformation of cognition into action.

The gap between effective interpersonal thought and maladaptive interpersonal action requires a different type of explanation. For Selman and Schultz (1988), the troubled child's inability to apply what he or she "knows" reflects the powerful influence of affective processes in social interaction. As they note, when cognitive processes are the focus of study or intervention, emotion often remains a background issue. However, when social interaction becomes the focus, affective processes occupy center stage. Although the presence of effective cognitive strategies is a necessary condition for adaptive interaction, it is by no means sufficient. Instead, Selman and Schultz suggest that the gap between thought and action, so frequently found among troubled children, must be considered in light of the child's interpersonal history. When the child has difficulty translating cognitive strategies into action, it may be more fruitful to focus on the unique meaning of the interpersonal event for the child. In this respect, the work of Selman and Schultz integrates aspects of both cognitive distortion and cognitive deficit models. Of equal importance, their work underscores the fact that interpersonal cognitive problems are not merely intellectual problems.

CONCLUSION

The domain of child psychotherapy is bounded by a set of shared assumptions. First, it is assumed that children's emotional experience and overt behavior are mediated by internal psychological processes. Second, child maladjustment is conceptualized in terms of distortions, deficiencies, or compromises in these internal, mediational processes. These disrupted processes are regarded as pathogenic, that is, as the source of the child's maladjustment. And third, interventions aim at the modification, remediation, or reorganization of these disrupted, internal processes. These assumptions represent the distinguishing features of the broad class of interventions properly labeled child psychotherapy.

Our brief survey of some of the major approaches to child psychotherapy has revealed a varied terrain within this vast domain. Competing approaches appear to have their origins in rival theories of etiology and pathogenesis. Not surprisingly then, one encounters not one, but multiple models of therapeutic change—even within "brand-name" therapeutic approaches. In fact, it appears that for each formulation of child psycho-pathology, there is a corresponding model of psychotherapy process. Furthermore, such diversity does not line up with variations in well-known treatment "brands." Instead, within each of the major systems of child psychotherapy one finds more than one model of pathogenesis and intervention. Thus, insofar as child psychotherapy does not appear to be a unitary process, even within the major approaches, it seems fruitless to attempt to homogenize the existing variability in practice to arrive at a generic model of child treatment. Our survey of several of the major approaches suggests a number of salient dimensions of variation.

First, treatments differ in *therapeutic focus*. At one end of this continuum are *process-focused* treatments and at the other are *problem-focused* treatments. For example, anchoring the problem-focused end are treatments aimed at remediating specific cognitive deficits. Here the focus of treatment is on facilitating the development of cognitive strategies. Interventions are aimed at a specific therapeutic target. In contrast, at the other end of the continuum are the client-centered approaches. Here treatment may proceed without explicit reference to the problems that led to the child's referral. Instead, the focus of treatment is on providing general conditions that are conducive to therapeutic change. A similar pattern is found in some psychodynamic treatments. As Anna Freud observes,

> The analyst reaches his aim only if he concentrates on the process. It is very much like driving somewhere. Your aim is to arrive, and if instead of looking at the road, you think how nice it will be when you arrive, you will probably have an accident. Concentrating on the driving process implies steering the car. (cited in Sandler et al., 1980, p. 251)

A second dimension of variation involves the degree of *therapeutic structure*. In practice, child psychotherapists vary in the degree to which they direct interactions in therapy sessions. At one end of the *directive–nondirective* dimension are the followers of Axline's play therapy. Here the imposition of any constraints on the child's spontaneous play is viewed by some as a practice that "undermines the very foundation of the therapeutic relationship" (Ginott, 1964, p. 148). The fundamental prescription is to follow the lead of the child. In essence, the structure of the therapy session is created, almost unilaterally, by the child. Psychodynamic child psychotherapy, with its emphasis on fixations and developmental arrests, appears less optimistic about the child's inherent ability to find solutions to emotional problems, given the appropriate therapeutic conditions. Consequently, the psychodynamic therapist may direct the child's attention to recurrent patterns of behavior or themes, introduce questions whose aim is to connect feelings with behavior, or offer interpretations of the meaning of feelings and behavior. In this respect, psychodynamic therapy is more directive than the client-centered approach. At the directive end of this continuum are treatments that emphasize specific therapeutic *tasks*. For example, Santostephano (1985) argues that many children are unable to make use of nondirective treatments because they lack the cognitive capacities to represent and symbolize emotionally significant events. The child who sticks to playing board games may need to learn in therapy how to represent events without becoming overwhelmed. In order to accomplish this goal, a therapist-directed treatment with highly structured cognitive tasks is prescribed. Similarly, social problem-solving interventions typically entail a series of structured tasks directed toward remediation of social-cognitive deficits. In turn, variations in therapeutic structure appear to imply important differences in the level of therapist activity. At one extreme, the therapist provides the supportive conditions that allow the child to direct the therapy session; at the other, the therapist actively organizes a set of tasks that directs the process of therapy.

A third dimension of variation in the practice of child therapy involves the *therapeutic medium*. As many child clinicians have discovered, literal conversation is not the preferred medium of communication for many children in therapy. Instead, a variety of nonliteral or "verbal substitutes" are employed in child treatment, including drawing, games, storytelling, and most importantly, thematic play. Treatments clearly vary in their emphasis on verbal communication. At one end of the continuum, the emphasis is on verbal interaction, analogous to adult psychotherapy; at the other, communication depends less on verbalization than other forms of representation, such as symbolic play. For example, client-centered approaches deemphasize the importance of verbal interaction. Play is seen as an adequate, and developmentally appropriate, medium for the expression of feelings and concerns. In contrast, approaches that emphasize the importance of language in self-regulation, such as some cognitive-behavioral and psychodynamic treatments, place a corresponding value on verbalization in the context of child treatment. Here play is not viewed as a sufficient medium for therapeutic change. Language use is both an essential part of the therapeutic process and as critical consequence of treatment.

The Problem of Treatment Selection

As the foregoing dimensions of variation imply, a generic model of child psychotherapy seems implausible. Although this broad class of therapies shares a set of critical assumptions, meaningful differences in the process of treatment cannot be ignored. This apparent diversity raises an important practical question. Given the fact that alternative approaches to child psychotherapy are not simply "talking about the same thing, but in different ways," how is the practitioner to choose which therapeutic approach to apply to the treatment of troubled children?

From a historical perspective, questions regarding differential treatment selection are relatively new. Typically, practitioners were trained within a single theoretical framework and their approach to child treatment reflected allegiance to a particular theoretical orientation. Treatments derived from a single theoretical orientation were applied to a broad range of childhood emotional disorders. For example, in the early child treatment literature we find psychodynamic methods being applied to childhood disorders as far ranging as simple phobias and reading problems to delinquency and autism (Barrett, Hampe, & Miller, 1978). A similar pattern is found in the client-centered literature, although early research rarely utilized diagnostic methods that could adequately distinguish the types of children receiving treatment (Shirk & Russell, 1992). In fairness, the broad application of a specific treatment approach, particularly in the early phase of its development, can be justified as part of the process of defining the limits of efficacy. However, the absence of systematic research on the differential effectiveness of child therapies maintained the early optimism that treatment approaches could be applied in a rather undifferentiated manner. Child therapy training, in turn, was often, and in many quarters still is, based on allegiance to a specific theoretical orientation.

The belief that therapies are equally effective across diverse disorders was dubbed "the uniformity myth" of psychotherapy as early as 1966 (Kiesler, 1966). In criticizing this view, Kiesler maintains that the effectiveness of a particular treatment method depends on a matrix of factors, including the type of problem treated, the context of treatment, and the characteristics of the therapist. This perspective has been extended to child treatment. Here the contention is that it is a myth to describe or apply treatments for an undifferentiated class of clients known collectively as "children." "Children" represents a diverse group of individuals with varied cognitive, emotional, and behavioral capacities, and to treat them as a homogeneous group is to succumb to the "developmental uniformity myth" (Kendall, Lerner, & Craighead, 1984). A similar warning was sounded by Kazdin (1988), who emphasizes that it is unreasonable to expect single conceptual models to "explain" child psychopathology, or, we might add, to provide the basis for interventions in all childhood disorders.

These perspectives mark a new era in the treatment of child psychopathology. Instead of fitting the child to the treatment, the treatment must be tailored to the developmental and psychopathological characteristics of the child. A basic principle of this new approach is that child treatment must be guided by the *selective application* of the most effective treatment for the type of problem presented by a child of a particular developmental level. This principle is central to the current search for *prescriptive treatments* for childhood disorders. The basic assumption of this perspective is that certain therapeutic approaches are better suited for some disorders than others. In other words, treatments are not equally effective across disorders and developmental levels. The clinical task for the child therapist, then, is to selectively apply treatments as a function of developmental, psycho-pathological, and contextual factors. Allegiance to a particular theoretical orientation is incompatible with the principle of selective application. As Achenbach (1990, p. 81) notes, "Multiple interventions are . . . needed in many cases, and the trainee must be prepared to use a greater variety of techniques than when treating only adults."

The question to be answered, then, is whether there is an empirical foundation for the differential effectiveness of child treatments across problem types and levels of development. In essence, does the existing literature provide support for prescriptive treatments for childhood disorders? Such evidence would provide the child practitioner with a clear basis for choosing the appropriate form of intervention from the varied domain of child therapies. To answer this question we must take a close look at the child psychotherapy outcome literature.

2

—

The Effects
of Child Psychotherapy:
Outcome Research

Controversy about the effectiveness of psychotherapy, including child psychotherapy, has a long history. In fact, unlike the question raised at the end of the last chapter, initial questions did not concern the relative efficacy of different treatments for different disorders, but reflected far greater skepticism about the usefulness of psychotherapy in general. The question was simple and direct: "Is psychotherapy effective at all?"

When the general effectiveness of psychodynamic psychotherapy was "empirically" challenged and rhetorically undermined by Eysenck (1952, 1961), the initial thrust to marshal forceful, empirical counterevidence for psychotherapy's superiority over no treatment was seriously stalled. The absence of a hard-boiled quantitative procedure that would allow researchers to combine and summarize all of the research evidence within a single formula meant that narrative polemics were pitted against each other, and there was no clear scientific way to adjudicate the validity of the arguments, pro or con, for psychotherapy's effectiveness. Thus, the responses to Eysenck were largely narrative critiques of his method of sampling and summarizing studies of psychotherapeutic effectiveness.

In addition, however, steps were taken in the empirical direction that Eysenck had first showcased: A rash of new narrative box-score reviews were undertaken where the number of therapeutic successes over the no-treatment control conditions were simply summed and compared to the number of null and negative findings. Like batting averages, these box scores seemed to change significantly, depending on which studies were included, who tallied the score, and just what was meant by a success or a failure. Such reviews did suggest, perhaps somewhat unconvincingly and perhaps in a way that seemed somewhat self-serving, that therapy was superior to no treatment more often than not, at least in the context of scientific studies.

Two of the four major reviews of the effectiveness of psychotherapy undertaken after Eysenck (1961, 1966) had box scores that were definitely in support of the efficacy of therapeutic treatments. Moreover, there was only one review, that by Rachman (1971), whose box scores suggested that most studies did not prove the efficacy of psychotherapy. These findings and their interpretation did not quell serious questioning of psychotherapy's effectiveness, nor did they allay doubts that perhaps the social cost and ideology of therapeutically induced health were floating above any cumulative and trustworthy basis in evidence. The field, in other words, was still in a struggle to prove its legitimacy, even to those who swore by its efficacy in their anecdotal accounts of therapeutic successes, but who also respected and ascribed to higher scientific standards.

It was not until the advent of meta-analysis in the late 1970s that largely narrative and box-score reviews of the literature could be replaced and much of their subjective and equivocal character purged from the review process. Meta-analysis, unlike the box-score method, was a technique that allowed reviewers to express the difference between treatment and control conditions in terms of a common metric, the effect size, and to average such effect sizes across the entire domain of studies of psychotherapy. The success or failure of psychotherapy could be boiled down and expressed in a single number, giving psychotherapy something like an average temperature on a scale ranging from effects that were highly positive to highly negative. Finally, here was a technique that gave legitimacy to such locutions as "On average, psychotherapy . . . ," or "The general effectiveness of psychotherapy over no treatment is estimated to be . . . ," or, better still, "The average treated patient is estimated to be better off than the average untreated patient by. . . ." Here, the whole enterprise of therapy could be appraised and its social and economic legitimacy tied to a number seemingly as immune to ideological and idiosyncratic distortion as temperature expressed in degrees Celsius.

Surely, a breath of relief and a sense of exhilaration, if not outright exoneration, could be gleaned in the field of research and practice when Smith and Glass (1977) published their pioneering meta-analysis: On all sorts of outcome measures, across all sorts of patients who had been treated with all sorts of modalities from within all sorts of orientations, the average psychotherapy patient improved significantly over the patient receiving no treatment. One number, the effect size, embodied the whole story. The average patient was about three-fourths of a standard deviation better off across all sorts of outcome measures at the end of treatment than those receiving no treatment.

At last, one would have thought, the question of psychotherapy's effectiveness had been proven; in fact, it could be expressed in hard-boiled quantitative terms, and all those practicing it and touting its heretofore controversial claims of efficacy could be vindicated. Not quite! Even though the meta-analytic finding was based on the scrutiny of 375 published and unpublished studies, the sheer newness of the technique and the seeming strength of the findings invited a healthy spate of scientific skepticism and fine-grained criticism, if not outright debunking (meta-analysis, from one critical vantage point, was redubbed mega-silliness (Eysenck, 1978). Some critics bristled at the thought of mixing all kinds of studies, differing on so many dimensions, into the same analyses (Shadish & Sweeney, 1991; Strube, Gardner, & Hartmann, 1985). Imagine estimating the average benefit of medical treatments, for diseases ranging from AIDS to the common cold. What could one such number possibly reveal that was scientifically worth knowing? Estimates concerning the average effectiveness of psychotherapy derived from such admixtures were likely to be as surreal as estimates of the average hardness of diamonds and cow chips combined! With the loss of the specificity of the individual study, so too inexorably followed the loss of believability and scientific warrant, at least in some critical quarters (Eysenck, 1995).

To answer such criticisms, there followed re-meta-analyses, new meta-analyses, and meta-meta-analyses employing increasingly sophisticated quantitative procedures. The aim now was to improve the psychometric and statistical properties associated with the technique of meta-analyses, to try to replicate the earlier findings of therapies' success on more stringently defined samples of therapies, and to specify in greater detail what characteristics of patients, therapists, orientations, and of the studies' designs that might mediate or moderate the overall average effect size (Shadish & Sweeney, 1991).

The finding that psychotherapy was superior to no treatment did and did not survive this critical onslaught. The finding has survived, in that meta-analysis after meta-analysis has reported that treatments do in fact produce larger positive effects over and above no treatments, to a degree that cannot be attributed to chance. The finding has not survived, in that critics are still questioning the validity of the technique and even producing "more sophisticated" meta-analyses with less positive findings for variables long associated with the key ingredients of therapy, such as techniques (Shapiro, 1985). Today, consequently, few researchers, clinicians, or aspiring initiates should be carelessly sanguine about the efficacy of psychotherapy per se: The question still deserves close attention.

Consider what happens when the initial question of the general effectiveness of psychotherapy for the average client is sharpened and readdressed at a less abstract level, one that distinguishes types and modalities of treatment along with types and age-levels of clients. Here, the results of meta-analyses can also be considered quite favorable, if somewhat puzzling, to the psychotherapeutic enterprise. The good news is as follows: Most meta-analyses that compared the effectiveness of different types of treatment, averaged across samples of clients at all age levels and with all types of psychopathology, revealed that they were all superior to the no-treatment control conditions. However, results also revealed that the many different brand-name treatments were all about equivalent to each other in remediating most types of presenting problems (Stiles, Shapiro, & Elliot, 1986). The puzzling or paradoxical kernel in this good news consists in the fact that decades of theory and research on psychotherapy had argued and empirically shown that the different therapies prescribed technical interventions that were strikingly dissimilar. Simplifying, Freudians tended to *interpret* what their clients had said, Rogerians tended to *reflect or acknowledge* what their clients had said, and Cognitivists tended to *contest* what their clients had said. How could such different therapeutic techniques lead to such overall equivalent results? Were the differing technical interventions superfluous relative to something that all of the therapies had in common, that is, warm, parent–child-like relationships that were naturally conducive to positive growth? Or was the sophistication of the field's research on process and outcome and their relationship so gross that the wheat could not yet be separated from the chaff?

Similarly perplexing is the nagging fact that several reanalyses of major outcome studies have shown that who the therapist is accounts for more outcome variance than what the therapist does (cf. Lambert, 1989). Can it really be believed that what we have taken to be techniques of intervention are simply inert, and what counts is the therapist's charisma, charm, and good old heartfelt care? Imagine what skepticism might be spawned by such a conclusion. How could we legitimately continue to warrant the development of differing theories of psychotherapy or the years and great sums of money spent by students in graduate schools and internships and postdoctoral programs, all of which are geared to imparting specific, often orientation-specific, technologies of treatment?

Leading researchers on the relationship of in-therapy patient and therapist behavior to outcome have produced quite controversial findings. In the most famous reviews of the adult process–outcome literature, Orlinsky and Howard (1986) reported several noteworthy positive relationships between techniques and positive outcomes. The more a therapist offered interpretations and clarifications, the more the patients seemed to benefit at outcome. On the other hand, in reviewing Orlinsky and

Howard's work, Shapiro et al. noted that the authors used an outdated box score technique and did not take into account study characteristics such as design quality. Using the same corpus of adult process–outcome studies, Shapiro et al. (1994) applied the more powerful meta-analytic techniques, calculating effect sizes and controlling for study characteristics. Their results are in striking contrast to Orlinsky and Howard's results. They found very little evidence supporting the notion that techniques are related to outcome, that is, that what the therapist did was related to how much improvement the patient made at the end of treatment. These and other such studies have led adult researchers to question whether we really know what helps in therapy and whether we have the right research techniques to find out (Stiles, 1988). After hundreds and hundreds of studies, there is movement afoot to go back to the drawing board!

When the corpus of psychotherapy research is parsed by the age level of the clients, the good and the bad news is reiterated for child and adolescent psychotherapy. The child or adolescent in psychotherapy reaps significantly greater benefits than the child or adolescent in control conditions, so the current meta-analyses seem to attest. This finding has been duplicated in two recent meta-analyses. Both Casey and Berman (1985) and Weisz, Weiss, Alicke, and Klotz (1987) have reported that the average child in treatment improves about 0.71 and 0.79 standard deviations over the average child in control conditions, respectively. Such good news has led child advocates and policy makers to proclaim:

> The available research appears to indicate that we have the appropriate facilities, methods of treatment, human resources, and systems of care (both mental health and nonmental health)—albeit in deficient quantities—to treat children in need. Outcome research indicates that the various therapies work, that the various facilities along the continuum of intensiveness and restrictiveness work, and that prevention services work, and even preliminary amounts of research indicate that mental health care delivered in other systems works. (Tuma, 1989, p. 198)

A rash conclusion from such an evaluation might be that all we need to do is proliferate all that has been shown to work! For taken at the most abstract and perhaps scientifically naive level, it could thus be confidently concluded that the average child or adolescent benefits from the average mental health or other system-delivered therapeutic treatment. The success of psychotherapy across age levels of clients (the life-span effectiveness of therapy!) adds clout to its claim to validity and efficacy!

Lest we become too intoxicated with the apparent success of therapeutic treatments for children, we should pause and ponder several questions. Does the equivalence paradox and charismatic therapist factor also re-emerge at the child and adolescent level? Do the "hip," "cool," "awesome," charismatic child therapists account for good outcomes, their techniques or lack thereof thrown to the wind? Are the hundreds of name brands of child therapies all equivalent, and if so, why? Perhaps there are other pitfalls and caveats that specifically arise and must be addressed when attention is turned to child and adolescent forms of psychotherapy, such as the problem of maturation (e.g., simply growing out of problematic behaviors or expressing the same disorder in a different form as one moves across developmental stages). Surely we will want to know what processes of treatment lead to success and what processes lead to no gains or even to negative effects. As in adult therapy research, we will want to find specific answers to our specific questions.

To hunt down the answers to these questions, or the lack of answers, it is necessary to take a closer look at the history and anatomy of child and adolescent psychotherapy research as it emerges from its reviews, both narrative and meta-analytic, over a span of about 40 years. To anticipate a little here, the results of such a review might well appear sobering, perhaps even a little shocking, especially to those familiar with the quite extensive and programmatic adult psychotherapy process and outcome literatures. The results might also puzzle all of those who believe in the wisdom of applying and learning about the results of early treatment interventions as a way to prevent, or at least to minimize, later sometimes chronic adult psychopathology. Perhaps it is not too hyperbolic to conclude that what we know about the efficacy of child and adolescent psychotherapy and its relationship to therapist–child in-session behavior is based on no more of a research bedrock than a few dozen studies of questionable quality. Perhaps going back to the drawing board is also indicated, not just for researchers of adult treatments, but for child therapy research as well. Here the trek back may not be so long or arduous.

THE EFFICACY OF CHILD PSYCHOTHERAPY

Historically, reviewers of psychotherapy outcome have not known what to do with data from child treatment studies. One review that included both adult and child studies was "purified" to contain only adult data (Rachman, 1971). As Smith, Glass, and Miller (1980) explain, "For the sake of comparability within the table, the results of studies on children and psychotics are excluded, as are studies of the effectiveness of behavior therapy" (p. 222). This "innocent" decision perhaps illustrates a bias operative in the psychotherapy research tradition: Adult studies of therapy effectiveness and their reviews are accorded more status than child studies, whose inclusion within the "larger" review literature may be seen as problematic.

As we will show to the contrary, there is a long tradition of reviews of studies of child and adolescent therapy, and we will show that they should be considered seriously. Later, in the same book, Smith et al. (1980) illustrate another common bias, the obverse of the one noted previously: They include both child and adult studies in the same analyses. In fact, the mean age of their hundreds of clients is only 22.9, with a standard deviation of over 9 years of age! A very large proportion of the studies of psychothera-peutic effectiveness must have indeed been conducted on child and adolescent clients. Although Smith, Glass, and Miller report near zero correlations of age with outcome effect sizes across all the modalities of treatment, we can expect with near certainty that, even if the outcome effect sizes are consistent across age levels, the processes of treatment must be different.

Clinical and developmental wisdom also suggests that lumping chil-dren with adults is like mixing oranges and apples; that is, whereas we can be sure that there are some continuities across age levels, across children, adolescents, and adults, we can also be sure that there are discontinuities. Not only do types of problems differ, as even the DSMs recognize, but the expression of the same underlying problem (e.g., depression) may take shape in radically different ways at different age/developmental levels. Moreover, the rapid developmental changes that we can expect across the childhood years must interact differently with pathological processes than the slower consolidations of development in the young adult years—even when the same disorder afflicts both groups. Clearly, we had better expect therapists to interact differently with clients of differing developmental and age levels! Nothing is more striking and perhaps more common in a supervisory session than to hear the supervisor identify inappropriately complex communications in the therapists-in-training's verbal interaction with a cognitively/linguistically immature child; or conversely, the identi-fication of inappropriately flat intonation when interacting with a younger child who looks and is bored to death.

For all of the foregoing reasons, then, it is not only convenient, but warranted, both developmentally and clinically, to focus exclusively on psychotherapeutic processes and outcomes in the treatment of children and adolescents. In fact, over a 40-year period, from 1953 to 1993, there have been numerous reviews of the effectiveness of child therapy. By way of preview it is worth noting that there are both broadly inclusive reviews and reviews that focus on a specific type (e.g., play therapy) or on a specific modality (e.g., group) of psychotherapy. There are no reviews in the 40-year history of assessing child and adolescent therapy that are exclusively devoted to process research or to the investigation of process–outcome relationships. When we review the reviews in chronological sequence, a sense of the development of research problems and substantive findings will become apparent. To be sure, we will also obtain a sense of enduring shortcomings in the field's research and its applicability to improving the delivery of therapeutic care to children and adolescents!

Early Reviews of Child Therapy Outcome

The first review was conducted by Lebo (1953). It seemed to be motivated by frustration with the disparity between claims of the effectiveness of nondirective play therapy with children and the lack of any sound research base. Research in nondirective therapy with adults is sound and extensive. Research in nondirective play therapy with children is still meager, unsound, and frequently of a cheerful, persuasive nature. As Lebo noted, it seemed that such articles could be more correctly classified as propaganda than as research (p. 177). He summarized the reported effectiveness of play therapy in studies of diverse populations: mentally deficient, allergic, those with personality problems, those with reading difficulties, and physically handicapped children. Although the individual studies purport to show the effectiveness of play therapy, or at least promise, in treatments that were prematurely terminated, Lebo concluded that the evidence for effectiveness was extremely shaky. The results were compromised because of the lack of appropriate control groups with which to compare treatment outcomes, and because the technical procedures of play therapy had not been differentiated in operational detail from heightened attention from an adult.

In the second review, by Levitt (1957), substantial improvement occured in the review itself and in the attempt to assess the question as to whether child psychotherapy is effective or not. Both of these improvements can be attributed to the influence of Eysenck's (1952) landmark study of the effectiveness of dynamically oriented adult therapy. In fact, Levitt basically applied the methods Eysenck used in his review of adult treatment efficacy to studies of child treatment, with a few technical modifications. Like Eysenck, Levitt wanted to compare rates of improvement of untreated groups with rates of improvement of treated groups. For this purpose, he found two studies that had follow-up data on children who were accepted for treatment at child guidance centers but never received treatment. In one study (Witmer & Keller, 1942), a group of such children were assessed at between 8 and 13 years after clinic contact and 78% were judged to be improved. In the second study (Lehrman, Sirluck, Black, & Glick, 1949), similar children were assessed at 1 year after clinic contact, and 70% were judged to be improved. The overall improvement percentage was 72.5% for the 160 cases evaluated across the two studies. For psychotherapy to be deemed effective, then, the improvement percentage of treated children would have to significantly exceed this 72.5%.

Levitt (1957) compiled the results of treatment garnered from 18 studies, which included data on 3,399 cases of child and adolescent treatment. The combined percent of cases that were judged to be much improved or partially improved at the end of treatment across all of the studies was 67.05%, less than the 72.5% of the baseline studies of untreated cases. However, 78.22% were reported to be much improved or partially improved at follow-up, slightly higher than the baseline figure. This figure is almost identical to the one baseline study in which follow-ups were spread across 8 to 13 years after clinic contact, as are some of the treated cases. This consideration led Levitt to conclude that "the present evaluation of child psychotherapy, like its adult counterpart, fails to support the hypothesis that treatment is effective" (p. 194). Wisely, Levitt added that this type of result "does not force the acceptance of the contrary hypothesis" and that this should be especially kept in mind, given "differences among the concerned studies and their generally poor caliber of methodology and analysis" (p. 194). In 1957, Levitt could advise that "until additional evidence from well-planned investigations becomes available, a cautious, tongue-in-cheek attitude toward child psychotherapy is recommended" (p. 157). In other words, the first two reviews of child treatment studies could only challenge future researchers and clinicians to provide evidence that therapy worked with children.

Just as Eysenck's (1952) provocative work stirred critical reaction from adult psychotherapy researchers, so too did the work of Levitt (1957). Two reviews appeared shortly after Levitt's, and each of them took his method and conclusions to task, one focusing on an empirical reanalysis and one focusing on a detailed critique of the quality of the data that formed the basis of comparison between treated and untreated groups. Not surprisingly, their conclusions seemed either to lend support to the notion that child psychotherapy was preferable to no treatment or that the finding of no significant difference between treated and untreated groups was itself spurious, based on bad methodology.

For example, Heinicke and Goldman (1960) employed basically the same analytic scheme as did Eysenck and Levitt, but introduced several modifications in the sample of treatment studies included in the review and in the studies used for baseline improvement rates. In their review, 17 studies were included that focus on eclectic treatments and that reported at least three criteria of outcome status. They reported that approximately 80% of the 4,010 cases were evaluated to be successfully adjusted or partially improved at outcome. Similarly, on a purified sample of 10 studies, formed by excluding 7 studies that had some major methodological flaw (e.g., treatments could not be called psychotherapy or a patient population was extremely restricted, as with juvenile delinquents), the authors reported a similar overall improvement rate.

Heinicke and Goldman (1960) noted that this rate of improvement might be obtained even with children with no treatment. They then picked three controlled studies to assess this question: Lehrman, Sirluck, Black, and Glick (1949) for both treatment and control percentages, Witmer and Keller (1942) for control percentages, and Witmer and students (1933) for treatment percentages. They justify this mix with the two Witmer studies because they learned that cases that closed as partially improved were not included in the follow-up analysis in the 1942 study. By combining the results of the three studies, Heinicke and Goldman could report that at treatment's close the overall percentage of successful and partially improved cases did not differ between treatment and control conditions, 73% for treatment and 74% for control groups. However, they noted two important refinements to this finding. First, they reported that the percent of successful cases of the treated group was larger than that of the untreated group at follow-up, 52% to 37%. They also reported that the percent of successfully adjusted cases increased from 34% at the close of treatment to the 52% at follow-up.

Obviously, such a finding only gives slim support to the idea that treatments were more successful than no treatments. Heinicke and Goldman (1960), however, bolstered this slim support by noting significant problems with the control groups. In actuality, the control groups received help from clinic staff, sometimes being seen for up to 6 weeks; the control groups were less severely impaired; and the parents of control-group children received higher ratings of adequacy. Some children in the control group were considered to be too well adjusted for treatment! Given these differences, the authors rightfully doubt the previous findings in the earlier reviews and use extreme caution in making anything out of their own findings. Interestingly, these authors in 1960 were not very impressed with the gross level of knowledge such reviews, even if methodologically clean, can provide in terms of obtaining an understanding of psychotherapy. Instead, they made a bold recommendation: "It is our impression that the carefully designed study of the process of therapy is at this point in our knowledge likely to be a more fruitful model to pursue" (p. 491). We will have occasion to come back to this recommendation, unfortunately noting how it basically has gone unheeded even to this day.

The second review in 1960 leveled a methodological broadside at the Levitt (1957) study. Hood-Williams (1960) isolated several methodological issues: (1) the problematic baseline studies, (2) the problem of history in selecting cases, (3) the problem of the length and intensity (indexed by noting the training of the therapist) of the treatment, and (4) the problem of including unsuitable cases. For example, the authors noted that many minor, transient child and adolescent problems clear up during the waiting period before treatment commences and that serious cases are often referred for treatment immediately. Could this not lead to the establishment of poor comparison groups, with the untreated children evidencing less serious pathology than the treated children? After noting this, the authors discovered a disturbing fact about the articles used in the previous review: After purifying the sample of obviously incomparable studies, it turned out that all of the studies reporting high success dated from before 1939, and six out of the seven studies reporting low success cases came after 1940. Surely, this cries out for extreme caution in interpreting the data. Even more surprisingly, Hood-Williams reported that length of treatment varies from 1 session to well over 40 across the studies, and there was a mix of providers from psychiatrists to social workers to unspecified providers simply instructing teachers how to better interact with the children in the classes! Finally, as many as 10% of the cases had diseases psychotherapy could hardly be expected to improve significantly (e.g., mongoloidism or endocrine dysfunction). Given these numerous serious methodological problems, the author concluded that "there is no satisfactory answer to the question of how effective psychotherapy is with children" (p. 87).

Naturally, Levitt (1963) defended his earlier conclusions. In the 1963 study, Levitt again conducted an evaluation of the effectiveness of psychotherapy with children by aggregating results from many (22) separate studies, with a total of 1,741 cases. He conceded that there are deep problems with the selection of appropriate control groups, for example, that individual authors vary in their definition of defectors (no treatment), from individuals having fewer than five sessions to individuals having fewer than 16 sessions. In addition, Levitt noted that previous critiques questioned the procedure of lumping every disorder into the same category. Here, Levitt begins to make some progress by reporting improvement rates by five different categories of disorders: Neurosis, Acting Out, Psychosis, Special (i.e., enuresis, tics, school phobia), and Mixed (i.e., cases unclassifiable). The improvement rates varied from a high of 77% for Special symptoms to a low of 55% for Acting Out. The combined overall rate of all categories combined was a mere 65.2%, significantly less than the 72.5% improvement base rate used in Levitt's (1957) initial study. He concluded that although there is significant variation in improvement across diagnostic categories, none of the improvement scores is significantly better than that expected, even of the no-treatment, baseline group. He concluded, "The inescapable conclusion is that available evaluation studies do not furnish a reasonable basis for the hypothesis that psychotherapy facilitates recovery from emotional illness in children" (p. 49).

Levitt gets another chance to refute his critics and raise the question of the effectiveness of psychotherapy with children again, but this time to a larger audience of psychotherapy researchers. In the first volume of the

Handbook of Psychotherapy and Behavior Change (Bergin & Garfield, 1971), Levitt summarized the findings of 47 outcome studies spanning 35 years of research on a total sample of 5,140 child cases at the end of treatment and 4,219 child cases at follow-up. The improvement rate for the 5,140 cases was 66.4%; for the 4,219, the improvement rate was 78.2%, after a median interval of 4.8 years after close. These rates did not represent a significant advantage over those expected by spontaneous recovery alone—with no treatment! Furthermore, Levitt pointed out two knotty problems, namely, that (1) variability in improvement rates is extensive, ranging from 43% to 86%, depending on both the treatment site and the "skill" of the individual therapist; and (2) evaluations of effectiveness may have been inflated, since many of the reports did not include a category for Worse, that is, for deterioration effects. The one study he cites reported that 16% of the treated children deteriorated, in comparison to only 9% of the control subjects. He noted that "the deterioration effect is now readily accepted by most psychotherapy researchers as the most probable expla- nation for the apparent failure of psychotherapy" (p. 476). The hypothesis to follow here is that some treatment processes work, some do not, and some even make the client worse. How does one set a new research agenda to begin to investigate this hypothesis in detail? Levitt, in accord with even his most vocal critics, suggested that

> the concepts of the psychonoxious therapist [note how similar this is to, but just the obverse of, the charismatic therapist] and the deterioration effect have turned the attention of psychotherapy researchers from unadorned outcome studies to investigations that seek to discover "what specific therapeutic interventions produce specific changes in specific patients under specific conditions." (Strupp & Garfield, 1969, pp. 476–477)

This is obviously a call for more detailed process and process–outcome research. Unfortunately, as of 1971, little interest in such research was evident; in over the 15- or 16-year history that the Annual Review of Psychology had been published, only six of the reviews of psychotherapy had subsections devoted to children, and the pages in these subsections amounted to only about 2% of the pages in the six chapters.

Based on 15 additional years of research, Heinicke and Strassmann (1975) offered a second round of responses to the findings of Levitt (1957) and Eysenck (1952). They begin by reviewing evidence that might serve to answer what they believe to be a woefully inadequate question: Is psycho- therapy more effective for the treatment of child and adolescent dysfunc- tion than no treatment? Again, they conclude that not only is this less than a scientifically interesting questioning, but also that the quality of the studies to date do not allow it to be answered with any degree of confidence. Instead, they suggest a question of more import: "Under what conditions is psychotherapy most effective in facilitating development?" (p. 565).

Unfortunately, even when addressing this new question, Heinicke and Strassman (1975) are struck by the veritable paucity of methodologically sound research: "This state of affairs is even more surprising when one realizes that as far back as ten to fifteen years ago, there were discussions as to what kind of research was needed for a meaningful comparison of the efficacy of treatment with children, and too little has been done in the interim" (pp. 565–566). They pinpoint a handful of studies that seem to meet minimal standards of methodological rigor and conclude that these studies do show treatments to be beneficial over and above the contrasting no-treatment control conditions. However, even in these studies they note that there is a question about what the clients actually received as treatment. For example, in studies showing differential impacts of treatments across diagnostic groups, they note that some therapies consisted of only four sessions of 30 to 45 minutes in length, and some were delivered by pediatricians.

Little focus on the in-therapy processes of treatment is noted to have taken place from the period spanning 1960–1975. Listen to the authors' level of frustration:

> Considering the fact that we have found few well-designed outcome studies, we should not be surprised that relatively little has been done with respect to assessing the nature of factors related to, or influencing, the results of the treatment process. . . . Here one quickly appreciates the very basic level of the kind of questions which need to be answered. Thus, one would think few would argue with the statement that how well a patient will do in treatment may have something to do with the qualities and skills of the therapist, what the patient is like, what is "wrong" with the patient, what is the nature of the environmental impact, and what is the interaction between these various elements. . . . Regrettably, however, the level on which much psychotherapy research has been done is somewhat analogous to giving a pharmacist some training in surgical techniques, having him do exploratory brain surgery, and then generalizing the results of his operation to what an experienced neurosurgeon might have accomplished with a specific disorder. (Heinicke & Strassman, 1975, pp. 568–569)

The authors make a strong plea for researchers to be especially sensitive to developmental level, frequency of session and duration of treatment, and to the use of meaningful outcome indices such as the Behavior Problem Checklist (Quay & Peterson, 1967), and the Developmental Profile (A. Freud, 1965). Their strongest stance, however, besides indicating that conclusions about the effectiveness of child and adolescent treatments are still premature, pertains to their assessment of the role of process evaluations in future research. They believe:

> It is indeed not possible to evaluate the meaning of outcome results without knowledge of the essential facets of treatment. Since, to our knowledge, reliable methods of observing this process have not yet been developed, and in any case are likely to be very complicated and time-consuming, it may well be most efficient in the next research strategies to rely on the daily reports of the therapist to capture the process and to expend more energies on the development of relevant and reliable measures of outcome. (Heinicke & Strassmann, 1975, p. 584)

Interestingly, in the 1970s, adult process researchers did come to rely on therapist and patient reports of the experiences in the therapy session (Orlinsky & Russell, 1994), but little of this exciting work spilled over into the child literature.

The case for psychotherapy's effectiveness with children and adolescents is not strengthened when special modalities are reviewed. In Abramowitz's (1976) review of group psychotherapy for children and adolescents, the results of 42 studies are reported. In brief, about one third of the studies reported generally positive results for group psychotherapy, one-third reported mixed results, and about one-third reported null findings. These percentages were upheld across studies of differing methodological quality and across problem areas (e.g., disruptive behavior, social isolation, poor self-concept, and academic underachievement). Interestingly, most of the null findings were reported in unpublished dissertations—which led Abramowitz to suspect that even the equivocal findings pertaining to group psychotherapy's effectiveness obtained in her review were positively biased, as many more dissertations and theses with null findings probably never were published. (This is a problem that has come to be known as the "file drawer problem," since these studies with null findings are likely to be locked away in some researcher or student's file, rather than in some journal, however obscure.) Unfortunately, most of the children included in the studies were identified on the basis of teacher nomination alone, and sometimes whole classrooms were targeted for intervention, even though individuals in them might have been very well adjusted! Moreover, although four types of group therapies were identified (verbal, play, activity, and behavioral), "not a single investigator has offered an empirical verification of the purported differences in treatment modalities (i.e., independent variables) studied" (p. 325). Are the outcome results due to poor treatment implementation rather than to the outright inert character of the delivered interventions? Clearly, this question could not begin to be addressed. Consequently, Abramowitz concluded that "definitive conclusions concerning the robustness of group psychotherapy in alleviating emotional and behavioral problems in children must await the refinements of further research. However, the present data base does not promise a favorable prognosis" (p. 325).

In 1978, the second edition of the *Handbook of Psychotherapy and Behavior Change* (Garfield & Bergin, 1978) was published. In it, Barrett, Hampe, and Miller (1978) published an extensive historical and empirical review of research on child psychotherapy. After a brief review of the child guidance movement, the authors quickly moved to reevaluate the basis for Levitt's (1957, 1963, 1971) earlier challenges to the field of child psychotherapy. Their first line of questioning naturally focused on the aptness of Levitt's baseline control groups, a common target of other review authors as well. Barrett et al. began by looking at the Witmer and Keller (1942) study, noting that "thirty percent of the cases came from the court and twenty percent from physicians. At the time, both of these sources requested only diagnostic service, suggesting that the children were not seriously impaired. If so, they were hardly a representative sample of disturbed children on which to form an 'improvement' actuary" (p. 414). Moreover, the authors noted that (1) the children and their families received extensive evaluation, and that such involvement oftentimes results in improvement of presenting problems, and (2) "there is reason to question whether it is best to classify the reported interventions as 'psychotherapy'" (p. 415). Barrett et al. found fewer problems with the second study used to define a comparative base rate, namely, a study conducted by Lehrman, Sirluck, Black, and Glick (1949). They did note that evaluation at the 1-year follow-up point showed the treated group to have a better quality of improvement than the control group. In fact, they quote the Lehrman et al. conclusions to the effect that their study "leaves no doubt about the fact that the children in the Jewish Board of Guardians' Treatment Group fared better in the community a year after closing than the children in the Jewish Board of Guardians' Control Group" (p. 416).

Barrett et al. (1978) reviewed other criticisms of Levitt's work and his responses to them via Levitt's subsequent reviews and substantive treatment studies. Here again one finds reason to applaud Levitt's early work. For example, Levitt, Beiser, and Robertson (1959) showed that treatment defectors did not differ from treatment continuers on 61 variables pertaining to symptoms or motivation for treatment. On the other hand, their outcome study was considered substantially flawed in that most treatments were administered by students or individuals with less than a year of experience. Barrett et al. also noted that in only 10% percent of the cases was the child alone treated and that in 40% of the cases the mother was the only family member treated. All in all, the authors advise that these early studies be recognized for what quality they possessed, and that the data that they provided probably would not reveal any new knowledge by conducting to any further analyses.

Barrett et al. (1978) completed their review by reporting on newer studies of child and adolescent psychotherapy, one by one. Interestingly, they do not attempt to aggregate findings, as in the earliest reviews, and do not make *carte blanche* statements about the overall effectiveness of child treatments. They feel that the question "Does psychotherapy work?" is one that has been abandoned by adult psychotherapy research. "Today's question should be, 'Which set of procedures is effective when applied to what kind of patients with which sets of problems and practiced by which sort of therapist?' Shifting to the more appropriate question in no way simplifies our task; indeed, it complicates it" (p. 428).

They did not specify how exactly it complicates the task. However, they did highlight the significance of one study especially. This study, by Ricks (1974), compared the long-term outcome of severely disturbed children treated by one of two therapists. Here, there were clear therapist effects, with the supershrink achieving far better long-term outcomes than his counterpart. Barrett et al. (1978) present Ricks's analyses of supershrink's strategies and tactics, as garnered from the children's case records. What seems to be apparent is that the supershrink used outside programs to augment treatment, was firm and direct in working with the children's parents, worked to develop the children's autonomy, provided the children with an anchor in reality by staying in touch and responding to their full range of feelings, and finally, tried to help the children deal with real-to-life issues with real-to-life solutions. In contrast, his counterpart with the less positive outcomes tended to introduce too much anxiety or depression by extensive use of interpretations of material presented in the therapy hour, tended to remain distant, and tended to judge good therapy on the basis of the children's production of material that was of psychodynamic interest. Clearly, here is an attempt to discover something about differences in treatment processes that might affect outcomes.

Barrett et al. (1978) reviewed only three other process studies, each having to do with nondirective play therapy, and none of these studies related processes to outcomes! In 1978, 25 years after the first review of child psychotherapy studies, and after numerous calls for the relevance of process research, not merely as a check to see that the prescribed treatments are actually being delivered but more importantly to identify key therapeutic ingredients, an astonishing fact emerges from the reviews: Literally no empirically sound information about process–outcome relationships has entered into the reviewed corpus of studies on child psychotherapy. Barrett et al. can say nothing more inspiring than "with further

development, process ratings of child psychotherapy might become prac-
ticable and useful" (p. 422).

In 1980, Michael Tramontana published a review of research on
psychotherapy outcome with adolescents. The review included 35 studies
published from 1967 to 1977. To be included, the studies had to report
some quantifiable description of outcome, had to focus exclusively on
adolescents who were from 12 to 18 years old, and could not be in case
study form. Interestingly, 18 of the studies were uncontrolled; that is, they
did not randomly assign clients to treatment and control conditions. Of
these studies, over half concerned delinquents and most investigated some
form of group therapy. Besides lacking random assignment, these studies
typically included only one outcome measure often of questionable psychometric quality, failed to specify therapist characteristics, and failed to
control for other treatments concurrently being administered. Although
most reported positive outcomes, "their findings do not constitute convincing evidence of effectiveness" (p. 434).

For the studies that used some form of random assignment, again over
half concerned delinquents, and little attention was given to the study of
either hospitalized or nonhospitalized adolescents with other psychiatric
disorders. Most therapies were administered in a group format. Therapy
versus no-therapy control groups were compared in 10 studies. In three
studies, the author reported that results were equivocal as to the superiority
of the treated groups because of some feature of the analyses or because
improvement applied only at a certain juncture of the therapy regimen.
Results of the seven other studies seemed to point consistently to the
benefits of treatment. However, the author noted that "methodological
problems in four of them seriously limit the number of valid conclusions
that one can make" (p. 440). In other words, if we add the seven controlled
studies of poor methodological quality to the 18 uncontrolled studies, we
must conclude that the majority of research on the benefits of psychotherapy for adolescents is hardly useful. Five of the experimental studies
compared types of treatment, and here the results were not definitive for
the superiority of any given brand name of therapy, as is typically the case.

In trying to summarize the studies, Tramontana (1980), reverts to the
comparison of the percent of improved adolescents in treatment conditions versus the percent improved adolescents in the untreated control
conditions. He reports that roughly 73% improve with treatment as compared to 29% with no treatment. He tells us not to take these comparisons
too seriously, not only because of methodological flaws, but also because

> a major problem with simply comparing the overall rates of positive
> outcome for treated and untreated adolescents is that it tells us nothing
> about the process of change in either case. Simply noting that about

75% of all adolescents receiving psychotherapy show a positive outcome
in no way contributes to an understanding of the specific therapeutic
conditions that lead to specific kinds of change for specific kinds of
adolescents. (p. 440)

Similarly, and with equal force, Tramontana (1980) points out that
"there has been little systematic research on the patient factors related to
psychotherapy outcome for adolescents. Consequently, one is presently left
with having to rely almost entirely on clinical judgment in predicting what
the response to psychotherapy will be for different adolescents exhibiting
different types of disturbance" (p. 444). Only severity and chronicity seem
to have been studied. What this means is that we have as little knowledge
of the psychogenic factors leading to particular (sub)types of adolescent
dysfunction as we have of the treatment processes that might best serve to
remediate them! As the author concluded himself, as of 1980, "There is
presently lacking an empirical base on which to specify particular therapeutic conditions that will lead to particular types of change for particular
types of adolescents" (p. 446).

A review focusing exclusively on the effectiveness of play therapy was
published by Phillips in 1985. He noted that in the pool of over 300 articles
published on play therapy, "case studies, anecdotal narratives, and theoretical reflections have predominated even in the professional literature.
The discrepancy between empirical understanding and ubiquitous clinical
practice raises questions regarding the interface of child-oriented research
and clinical enterprise" (p. 752). This disparity between what happens to
be the focus of research and what happens to be the most frequently
reported therapeutic practices will emerge as a major theme in the reviews
of the 1990s. In fact, Phillips was able to note that "the dearth of research
contradicts the fact that play therapy has been widely used, and in fact,
seems to have increased over the last twenty-five years (Boutte, 1971;
Filmer-Bennet & Hillson, 1959; Koocher & Pedulla, 1977)" (p. 752).

Interestingly, Phillips (1985) begins his review by focusing on process
research, an enduring interest of nondirective play therapy researchers,
defining its domains of interest by listing several of its key orienting
questions: "What does the therapist do? What does the client do? What
play occurs in the course of treatment? What is said, and by whom? What
are the therapist–child interactional contingencies, if any?" (p. 753). However, from his review, one gets the impression that very little research has
actually made any empirical progress in answering the orienting questions.
For example, roughly a half-dozen studies are cited that have attempted to
develop measurement tools for application in process studies, usually gross
category systems for the coding of verbal responses, or rating scales to
measure such constructs as empathy, unconditional positive regard, and

genuineness. He reported no studies in which measured components of process were predictive of measured increments in outcome. Instead, we find out that disturbed children more frequently express negative attitudes than nondisturbed children, that highly aggressive and younger children tend to be more expressive than less aggressive and older children, and that those children seen by therapists high in empathy, unconditional positive regard, and genuineness tend to express more positive feelings for themselves, insight, and aggression in therapy than children seen by therapists rated low on the Rogerian triad.

Outcome research is reviewed by problem type, but there is little attempt to systematically aggregate outcome findings within categories or across categories. The problems used to organize the review are the following: academic and intellectual achievement; mental retardation; anxiety associated with hospitalization; autistic and psychotic children; specific behavioral disorders, such as separation anxiety and fear of the dark; interpersonal functioning and sociometric status, and personality adjustment. As Phillips (1985) himself concluded,

> At best, play therapy appears to have minimal impact on academic and intellectual achievement. Mildly mentally retarded children seem able to engage in play therapy, but few social, personal, or cognitive gains have been made; some diffuse improvements may obtain on measures of global developmental functioning. Play therapy in the form of puppet play seems to have a short-term, mostly preoperative effect on children's anxiety associated with surgery. More directive, structured forms of play may facilitate specific communicative and behavioral goals with psychotic and autistic children. Short-term play treatment ameliorated preschooler's separation anxiety in one study; in another, play with desensitization was unsuccessful with darkness fears in young children. Equivocal, but mostly null results are found when play therapy addresses social adjustment. The positive results that have been obtained appear unrelated to the specifics of play therapy. A similar picture of mixed results obtains in the domain of personality, with early studies finding improvements and more recent investigations showing uncertain gains. (p. 757)

Such a summary could hardly be construed as sufficient to warrant an uncritical endorsement of play therapy as an effective treatment modality for childhood disorders.

In addition to identifying types of therapist and client activities that could be considered legitimate constituents of "play therapy," Phillips (1985) clearly outlined what was needed to develop our knowledge about the effectiveness of this treatment. What is needed is "a systematic program of research that clearly sets out its hypotheses, designs well-controlled studies, carefully selects its subjects, measures meaningful outcomes, and uses appropriate and informative statistics" (p. 758). Such a systematic program had not emerged, even as late as 1985.

The Advent of Child Therapy Meta-Analysis

In 1985, Casey and Berman applied to a large corpus of studies of child (ages 3 to 15) psychotherapy the meta-analytic techniques developed and applied by Smith et al. (1980) to the study of adult psychotherapy. Casey and Berman reviewed 75 studies between 1952 and 1983, having as control groups children who were sampled from a similar population to that used for samples of treated children. They did not analyze studies focusing exclusively on academic outcomes, methods of intervention designed solely to hasten the development of normal patterns of functioning, or drug, peer, or family modes of intervention. Interestingly, 57% of the studies included school children who were not seeking treatment of any kind, 15% included volunteers from the community, and 4% included children whose status could not be determined. Only 24% of the studies included children in what would normally be considered traditional contexts in which psychotherapy would be administered by professionals; 16% used outpatients, and 8% used inpatients as subjects. Therapy was broadly defined, including interventions lasting from 1 to 37 weeks. Male children outnumbered female children by a three to two ratio. Problems, although "diagnoses were frequently difficult to determine" (p. 389), were classified as fear/anxiety (9 studies), cognitive skills (12 studies), global adjustment (14 studies), social adjustment (30 studies), achievement (13 studies), personality (9 studies), and self-concept (5 studies).

With this large data set in hand and the benefit of the Smith et al. (1980) comprehensive review to point to key outcome questions, Casey and Berman focused their review to derive empirically driven answers to four superordinate questions:

1. Is psychotherapy effective with children?
2. Are there differences in therapeutic efficacy between therapies stemming from widely divergent theoretical orientations or between different modalities?
3. Does the efficacy of psychotherapy with children seem to vary across the content focus and source of the outcome measure?
4. Is psychotherapy more effective with some childhood problems than with others?

Laudably, the authors also addressed key subsidiary questions as well, using exemplary quantitative methods and evenhanded judgment.

The answer to the first question, "Is psychotherapy effective with children?," was shocking, given the largely negative answers to the same question that had been posed in the reviews of the past 25 years. Casey and Berman's (1985) answer was a resounding "Yes!" The overall effect size was reported to be 0.71; in other words, the average child receiving treatment was found, by top-notch quantitative methods, to be over two-thirds of a standard deviation better off than the average untreated child. This finding almost matches that reported in meta-analyses focusing exclusively on adult therapy: Shapiro and Shapiro (1982) reported an effect size of 0.72 for adult treatments. Children, that neglected category of persons in terms of both research and practice, could now be shown to have benefited from psychotherapy to an extent about equal to adults, that category of persons on which most research and practice had been focused. In 1985, one could now conclude that psychotherapy, on average, was effective across the life span!

We might pause and ask how the results of Casey and Berman's (1985) study could be so discrepant with the earlier reviews, most of which lament the lack of any convincing empirical proof that child psychotherapy is more effective than spontaneous remission or developmental growth. There are perhaps several contributing factors that could be forwarded to account for this glaring discrepancy. First, from a purely statistical standpoint, the use of effect sizes allows a much more powerful analysis of treatment effects than does the use of the old box-score method, with its breakdown of outcome into only two to five nominal categories. (In fact, Levitt (1957) pointed this out, noting that improvement rates increased as the number of nominal assessment categories increased from two to five.) Second, earlier reviews do not restrict their samples of treatment groups to children only, as do Casey and Berman, thus excluding such recalcitrant adolescent problems as conduct disorder and juvenile delinquency. Moreover, it is unclear whether the meta-analytic sample included "referable" childhood problems associated with serious acting out in the schools—the category shown to improve least, according to Levitt's analyses in 1963. It should also be remembered that the earlier reviews often include types of problems (e.g., medical problems) excluded in the Casey and Berman study. Third, one has to wonder about the inclusion in the latter review of 57% of studies that include children who were not referred for any type of treatment intervention: We know that the "rich get richer"; that is, less severely impaired individuals tend to benefit to a greater extent than more severely impaired individuals receiving the same treatments. (Recall that this was one of the findings in the earlier reviews.) Fourth, the earlier reviews focus more exclusively on types of nonbehavioral interventions, such as those stemming from the client-centered and psychodynamic orientations, whereas the Casey and Berman review includes more behavioral studies than nonbehavioral studies. Fifth, as the earlier reviews point out over and over again, it is often unclear whether the control groups, or the groups used for remission or improvement base rates, used in the earliest comparative research, are appropriate. Sixth, many of the earliest reviews include studies dating back to 1931; in fact, in Hood-Williams's (1960) review, all studies had been completed before 1955. For all of these reasons, Casey and Berman's positive results differ from the negative findings reported in the previous reviews. While it is thus arguable whether Casey and Berman's findings are definitive, theirs is clearly the most rigorous review in the literature up to 1985.

Interestingly, once studies that assess outcomes on activities directly taught in therapy are eliminated as overly reactive, Casey and Berman (1985) report that there is no statistical difference between outcome effect sizes associated with behavioral and nonbehavioral treatments. Although the overall effect size is diminished to 0.46, it is still statistically significant, as are the effect sizes associated with the two different overarching forms of treatment. Similarly, there are no reported differences between treatments that did and did not include play as a constituent, between treatments administered in the group or individual format, or between treatments that did and did not include a component of parent treatment. According to Casey and Berman's review, then, there is neither demonstrated superiority of one type of treatment over another (behavioral vs. nonbehavioral) nor of one modality of treatment over another. Even though competing theories of therapy differentially proscribe and prescribe the use of specific intervention techniques, even though competing theories of modalities differentially proscribe and prescribe the use of specific intervention techniques, empirical evidence points to the brand-name and modality equivalence in the degree of outcome success. Here we see the child treatment literature to be parallel to the adult treatment literature in producing paradox.

Happily, there is some differentiation of treatment effectiveness, although it does not concern aspects of the administered treatments. Rather, some differentiation of outcome effectiveness emerges when client characteristics are taken into account and the content and source of the outcome evaluation is taken into account. Therapy was least effective for social adjustment problems (effect size = 0.55) but most effective for somatic problems (effect size = 1.66), with impulsivity/hyperactivity (effect size = 1.10) and phobia (effect size = 1.16) falling in between. Note, however, that only the effect size for social adjustment problems was reliably different from any other effect size associated with target problems. In other words, therapy was equally effective for all other target problems identified, except social adjustment.

There are more differences to be noted when assessing outcome by the content of the outcome measure and by the source from which it was gathered. Effect sizes associated with outcome measures of fear/anxiety and cognitive skills were significantly larger than those associated with outcome measures of personality and self-concept. Similar differences emerge in relation to source of outcome measure. Measures gathered from observers, therapists, parents, and child performances produced larger effect sizes than those obtained from teachers or children themselves. Casey and Berman (1985) also reported that there was no significant correlation between outcome effect size and (1) the experience or sex of the therapist, (2) the date of the research publication, or (3) the setting in which the children were studied. It did tend to matter how many males were in the treatment group, with the groups with higher percentages of males receiving lower outcome effect sizes. Finally, although Casey and Berman reported a significant negative correlation between length of treatment and outcome effect size, they explained this counterintuitive finding "by the tendency of shorter studies to use outcome measures that produced the largest effect sizes, those measures similar to the activities of therapy" (p. 392).

This review was obviously good news for child psychotherapy. Treatment is effective! However, lurking behind this veil of good news is a report that also contains some disturbing information. One might well conclude that no matter what the level of training, no matter what theoretical orientation, no matter what treatment modality, no matter what treatment setting, no matter what treatment dose delivered, no matter what decade in which services are provided, all treatments are about equal! The cynic might well begin to toy with the therapy establishment with some "empirically" driven questions: Why train graduate students at all? Why train them into some arcane theoretical orientation? Why try to differentiate strategies of treatment intervention on the basis of modalities or treatment settings? Why prescribe different courses of treatment engagement? Why look for increments of improvement in treatment effectiveness across cohorts of patients or providers? Surely, there must be something very powerful that is held in common across all deliveries of treatment, and it must be this common element that is responsible for all of this praiseworthy effectiveness. Perhaps it is just a caring touch!

The data themselves might lead to an empirically incontestable argument for this wry interpretation. For example, the client-centered approach accounted for 80% of the recognizable nonbehavioral psychotherapies. It was associated with an effect size of 0.49. The behavioral approaches that were evaluated with nonreactive outcome measures were associated with a similar effect size of only 0.55. Surely we would not expect behavioral and nonbehavioral therapists to differ substantially in their interest, care, and concern for the children that they treat. Perhaps, then, common to both groups of therapists was simply a warm and caring therapeutic demeanor; that is, these were therapists who delivered at least moderate levels of what we might call genuineness, unconditional positive regard, and accurate empathy, or who just seemed to be caring and sensitive. Alarmingly, there is virtually no evidence to counter such a provocative hypothesis derived from the review, largely because there is no information about any aspect of the therapists' in-session actual behavior or attitudes. We neither know that the prescribed therapy was actually delivered nor what aspect, what component, what constituent of all of the possible in-therapy processes was responsible for the amount of positive change observed at outcome. Although in 1985 child therapy finally has been shown to work, based on information included in this review, the processes responsible for change remain obscure.

Weisz et al. (1987) published the second meta-analysis concerned with the effectiveness of psychotherapy treatments for children. They included in their sample, however, studies that focused on children ages 4 to 12 and studies that focused on adolescents, ages 13 to 18. They included 108 articles from 1970 to 1985 that compared a treatment to a control condition for typical childhood disorders, excluding those treatment studies that were focused on children with mental retardation, with reading, writing, or other school-related specific skills, with seizure disorders, and with physically handicapping conditions. They included studies with paraprofessionals and professionals providing what seemed like psychotherapeutic or counseling services, excluding those studies focused on bibliotherapy, pharmacological treatment, and tutoring. Only 30% of the studies were included in the Casey and Berman (1985) meta-analysis.

Weisz et al. (1987) focused their review on four key questions: (1) Is the level of treatment effectiveness obtained on children similar to the level of treatment effectiveness obtained on adolescents? (2) Are there differences in effectiveness between behavioral and nonbehavioral treatments? (3) Are treatments equally effective across problem types? (4) Does effectiveness vary across levels of therapist training? As one can see, these are virtually identical to the questions addressed by Casey and Berman (1985), excepting question one. Weisz et al. advance the methodological quality of reviews, however, in that, with the very large sample of studies, they were able to conduct much more sensitive data-analytic procedures to detect, for example, interactions between client age level and therapist training or interactions between treatment orientation and problem type. Such sensitivity, as we will see, allowed them to discover important outcome information that has direct relevance for treatment and training.

Weisz et al. (1987) reported that the effectiveness of therapy differed depending on the age level of the client. The effect size (0.92) associated with treatments for children was significantly larger than the effect size for treatments with adolescents (0.58). This effect changed little when controlling for treatment type or problem type. Interestingly, this effect was qualified when also considering the level of training of the therapist. The authors reported:

> Age and effect size were uncorrelated among professionals ($N = 39$, $r = 0.11$, $p < .50$) but were negatively correlated among graduate students ($N = 43$, $r = -0.31$, $p < .05$) and paraprofessionals ($N = 26$, $r = -0.43$, $p < .05$). Trained professionals were about equally effective with all ages, but graduate students and paraprofessionals were more effective with younger than with older clients. (p. 546)

Comparing behavioral and nonbehavioral therapies led to similar findings to those reported by Casey and Berman (1985). When eliminating those studies that used highly reactive measures, there was no significant difference between the effect sizes for behavioral (effect size = 0.61) and nonbehavioral (effect size = 0.51) treatments. Interestingly, Weisz et al. (1987) questioned the appropriateness of eliminating "carefully designed studies in which measures similar to the training procedures are appropriate and necessary for a fair test of treatment success" (p. 546). They thus redid the analysis but included a subset of studies that had been eliminated according to Casey and Berman's criteria, which appeared to satisfy their own "appropriate" and "necessary" criteria. In this reanalysis, the effect size associated with behavioral treatments (effect size = 0.93) was found to be larger than that associated with nonbehavioral treatments (effect size = 0.45). They concluded,

> Our findings on therapy type do not support the often noted summary of adult psychotherapy findings that different forms of therapy work about equally well. . . . Instead, we found that behavioral methods yielded significantly larger effects than nonbehavioral methods. This finding held up across differences in age level, treated problem, and therapist experience, and it was not qualified by interactions with any of these factors. (pp. 547–548)

This finding can be further dramatized by noting that there are no significant differences found in effectiveness between general classes of behavioral therapies (operant, respondent, modeling, social skills training, cognitive/cognitive-behavioral, multiple behavioral) and between general classes of nonbehavioral therapies (client-centered, insight oriented, discussion group). Furthermore, there appear to be few differences in treatment effectiveness even between specific subtypes of these general classes of behavioral treatments. For example, as forms of operant treatment, there appears to be little difference between treatments emphasizing physical reinforcers, consultation in operant methods, social–verbal reinforcement, combined physical and verbal reinforcement, and multiple operant methods. Similarly, as forms of respondent treatment, there appears to be little difference in treatment effectiveness between systematic desensitization, relaxation, extinction, or combined respondent. Thus, we might say that any behavioral treatment (of the dozen or so analyzed in the 126 studies) is to be expected to be more effective on average than any of the nonbehavioral treatments (of the three types analyzed in the 28 studies), even though the behavioral principles and theories vary so dramatically between subtypes of behavioral treatments and even though the nonbehavioral principles and theories vary so dramatically between subtypes of nonbehavioral treatment.

Consequently, even if we accept the Weisz et al. (1987) comparison to be a valid one (see the following for some reasons why it might not be valid), we have simply pushed the equivalence paradox back one small step, only to be confronted again at the level of subtypes of treatment within overarching orientations! If we simply favor Casey and Berman's more conservative elimination of studies that utilize highly reactive outcome measures over that introduced by Weisz et al., we are again confronted with the paradox; but in its full-blown form, that encompasses all treatments, regardless of their overarching behavioral versus nonbehavioral affiliation. This cuts across presenting problem, age level of client (ages 4 to 18), and therapist experience. Such results, in either form, suggest a common process of change as the simplest explanation and one that cannot be refuted by studies linking differential in-therapy processes to different or even to similar outcomes. As with the Casey and Berman results, this is certainly grist for the cynic's mill, whichever treatment orientation is said to have won the horse race of superior effectiveness.

Weisz et al. (1987) did not report any differences in outcome effectiveness across problem type (overcontrolled vs. undercontrolled), thus lending further support to Casey and Berman's (1985) finding of little differences in effectiveness across most types of childhood problems. This finding was not qualified when controlling for client age, therapy type, or therapist training, using the usual $p < .05$ critical significance level. Just as the data seem to suggest, or at least, cannot discount, a very general but common therapist-generated active ingredient (e.g., a warm relationship) across treatment approaches to account for equivalence in outcome, these data seem to suggest a very general but common patient-generated active ingredient to account for client equivalence in responsivity to treatment. What could this general capacity be? Not only does there appear to be a uniformity of treatment in terms of outcomes but possibly a uniformity of responsivity in treatment processes. The data are just not fine-grained enough to confidently conclude otherwise.

Specialized Reviews of Child Therapy Outcome

In the early 1990s, there was a rapid increase in the number of reviews of child and adolescent psychotherapy; moreover, a number of these reviews were more fine-grained; that is, they focused on specific types of treatments, patients, or outcomes. For example, Pfeiffer and Strzelecki (1990) undertook a focused, quantitative review of inpatient treatment studies from 1975 to approximately 1990. Although Pfeiffer and Strzelecki noted that previous narrative reviews reported generally positive effects for inpatient treatments, they felt it was necessary to assess this finding more carefully by including more recent studies, by using a precise and conservative statistical approach to summarizing findings, and by excluding case reports and studies focused on developmentally disabled children. Interestingly, they also established methodological criteria that each prospective study had to meet in order to be included in analyses. Unfortunately, " . . . it was found that such stringent exclusionary criteria [such as having a control condition or quantitative outcome measures] precluded a substantial portion of the available literature" (p. 848). Only two of the 34 studies reported means and standard deviations of outcome measures.

Employing a statistical formula to assess outcome efficacy, the authors were interested in assessing what predictor variables might account for variance in outcomes. They assessed intelligence, organicity, diagnosis, symptom pattern, age at admission, sex, family functioning, treatment, length of stay, and aftercare/postdischarge environment. Interestingly, the authors found that only 4 of 34 studies investigated treatment variables. In these studies, therapeutic alliance, cognitive problem solving skills training, planned discharge, and completion of the treatment program all predicted postdischarge status. However, as with all the other variables, we have no way of knowing if these treatment variables would predict outcome after the effects of methodological rigor, symptom severity, diagnosis, and other relevant variables are statistically controlled. In a recent meta-analytic review of the effect of technique variables on outcome in the adult literature, Shapiro et al. (1994) have reported that after they controlled for methodological quality, technique factors did not account for a significant percent of outcome variance. The same question can be raised with respect to the negative findings in the current review, which were related to severity of pathology, degree of family dysfunction, extent of organicity, and extent of antisocial features.

To their credit, Pfeiffer and Strzelecki (1990) did voice a strong caution that the results they reported should not be taken as definitive. How could they be, when "most of the outcome studies reviewed had no recognizable research design beyond the modest reporting of one or more measures taken at discharge. The more sophisticated studies employed a marginally improved one-group pre-test post-test design, which is, unfortunately, plagued with numerous threats to both the internal and external validity of the study . . . " (p. 852). They concluded with a somewhat ironically understated evaluation: "The field still awaits answers to the necessary and sufficient components of successful inpatient treatment, consensus on how to define treatment success, and identification of which types of patients respond most favorably to which combinations of treatments" (p. 852).

Mann and Borduin (1991) reviewed outcome studies published between 1978 and 1988 that focused on the treatment of adolescents. Included studies had to focus on adolescents 12 to 17 years old, who had clinically significant problems. Excluded from the study were outcome investigations of psychotropic treatments, academic tutoring, bibliotherapy, case reports, and studies that could not be analyzed statistically. The authors also explicitly rated the methodological quality of studies based on a system developed by Gurman and Kniskern (1978). Studies could earn as many as 16 points of "methodological credit." They noted that of the 39 studies reviewed, 9 (23%) earned 6 or fewer points and 21 (54%) earned 10 or fewer points. Only 3 studies (fewer than 8%) earned 14 or more points. These results indicate that many, if not most, of the outcome studies of adolescent treatment suffer from multiple methodological problems.

The authors found 21 studies that focus on individually focused treatments with the adolescent. The three forms of therapy were the following: social skills–assertiveness training (10 studies with an average methodological rating of 10.2); cognitive self-instruction–problem-solving training (7 studies with an average methodological rating of 10.7); and moral reasoning training (4 studies with an average methodological rating of 9.5). Probably the moral reasoning training resembles most closely traditional psychotherapy, although some of the cognitive treatments might as well.

With respect to social skills training, the authors concluded that such treatments result in improved interpersonal behaviors in role-play situations. However, they noted that few studies evaluate whether such improvements are maintained over time and across situations. Consequently, the authors concluded that "the long term effects of social skills training on adolescent functioning outside the laboratory remain unclear" (p. 513). With respect to the cognitive self-instruction–problem-solving skills training treatments, the authors concluded that both appear to be more effective than no treatments, but that it is unclear if they are better than alternative treatments, such as psychodynamic or different forms of cognitive interventions. Little in the research recommends specific treatments for specific types of adolescent problems or disorders. With respect to moral reasoning training, evidence suggested that this treatment does increase adolescents' moral reasoning abilities. However, it is as yet unclear how these advances in moral reasoning translate into more adaptive emotional and behavioral functioning.

In terms of social system treatments, the authors located 18 studies focusing on the family or peer group. Six studies focused on family systems therapy. Results seemed to indicate that such family systems intervention helps to decrease adolescent behavioral problems and family dysfunction. These results, however, are qualified in that there were few comparative studies with alternative treatments and infrequent use of observational measures to assess outcomes. Five studies assessed behavioral–communication skills family therapy. It, too, seemed to decrease adolescent problem behaviors and self-reported conflict at home. The authors again noted the absence of observational methods, lack of use with severe forms of adolescent problems, and lack of assessment of the relationship between improved family communication, family conflict, and adolescent behavior problems. With respect to peer group interventions, the authors reported finding only two studies. Both report improvements, but the authors cautioned against interpretation of these preliminary findings. Finally, five studies reported using multisystem therapy. Here, too, results were promising but too few and too flawed methodologically to recommend anything but further, better controlled, research.

Overall, the authors concluded wisely that

> studies of psychotherapy outcomes with adolescents have commonly evaluated the efficacy of specific treatments without first assessing the adolescents' needs. For example, in some studies, adolescents were taught verbal mediational skills or problem-solving methods without an initial evaluation of whether each adolescent was deficient in these areas. Pretreatment assessments of strengths and deficits are not a common practice in research because the theoretical orientations of investigators often suggest one main etiological agent for a given adolescent problem. A growing number of researchers who subscribe to integrative models of adolescent behavior, however, suggest that many adolescent problems are produced and/or maintained by a number of different factors. (Mann & Borduin, 1991, pp. 535–536)

This call for more specificity in assessment and in targeted interventions moves clinical research beyond the standard operating procedure of hinging treatment name brands to diagnoses. Instead, an assessment of psychological systems—cognitive, interpersonal, affective, behavioral—in terms of strengths and weaknesses is a prerequisite for the selection of treatment processes that could remediate or ameliorate identified problems. As Mann and Borduin (1991) remind us, if one acknowledges multiple pathways or contributions to adolescent psychopathology, even for adolescents who share the same diagnosis, then the uniform application of a treatment approach makes little sense. In other words, the selection of a treatment method hinges on the assessment of the specific pathogenic processes that contribute to the child or adolescent's maladjustment. In addition, the authors emphasize that little effort has been expended in studying what actually occurs during the therapy hour. We have seen this lapse over and over again in the history of child psychotherapy.

Another study in the same year evaluated outcomes for one type of child therapy: cognitive-behavioral therapy (Durlak, Fuhrman, & Lampman, 1991). The authors reviewed studies between 1970 and 1987. Studies had to meet several criteria to be included in the review: They had to conform to definitions of cognitive-behavioral therapy; treatment groups had to be compared to controls drawn from the same population; children had to have some degree of behavioral or social dysfunction, which excluded studies focusing exclusively on academic problems; the subjects in any treatment group had to have a mean age of 13 or younger; the child had to be the direct recipient of cognitive-behavioral therapy; and the study had to have been reported in English. Sixty-four studies were found that met these criteria. Descriptively, the modal client was a boy of a little over 9 years of age, who was seen in treatments of about 12 sessions in individual therapy in the school setting and whose assessment at outcome was on a cognitive performance variable or an unnormed measure.

Durlak et al. (1991) reviewed the studies using one of the more sophisticated approaches to meta-analysis. Overall, they found that cognitive-behavioral therapy produces statistically significant effects (effect size = 0.56). However, the authors went beyond the consideration of statistical significance and evaluated the clinical significance of cognitive-behavioral treatments. In brief, they compared the means on measures of functioning in the treatment and control groups in the treatment studies to the means on the same measures obtained from normative samples. What the authors showed is that for personality and cognitive tempo measures, children in the treated groups moved from over one standard deviation from the means of the normative groups to below the mean of the normative groups. For outcome measures assessing behavior, the treatment group mean remained over one standard deviation from the normative group mean, even though it was significantly reduced from pretreatment to posttreatment. Interestingly, all of the control groups' posttreatment scores were also reduced from pretreatment, with personality and cognitive tempo measures ending up within one standard deviation from the normative mean.

One of the main aims of this review, and a major advance over earlier meta-analyses, was to evaluate potential moderators of treatment effectiveness. Of specific interest was the role of cognitive development in children's responsiveness to cognitive-behavioral therapy, a form of therapy that relies heavily on cognitive operations. Durlak and his colleagues expected that effect sizes would be moderated by developmental level according to Piagetian theory. Since the original authors of the reviewed studies were not as developmentally oriented—that is, they did not actually include measures of the children's cognitive–developmental level—Durlak et al. had to estimate developmental level by the children's age. Their hypothesis was right: Formal operational children seemed to benefit more than concrete and preoperational children, who did not differ from each other.

Interestingly, in those studies that assessed changes in both cognitive functioning and maladaptive behavior, there was no significant correlation between effect sizes obtained across these two domains. As the authors noted, the absence of a significant relationship between changes in cognitive processes and behavior diminishes the importance of cognition in cognitive-behavioral therapy. That is, one would have expected effective treatment to modify children's cognitive processes which, in turn, would translate into behavioral improvement. The lack of such a connection raises questions about the underlying mechanism of change in cognitive-behavioral therapy. In fact, the authors concluded that cognitive-behavioral therapy, as a therapy brand name, stands for "a nonstandardized package of different treatment techniques that can be offered in many different sequences and permutations" (p. 211). Thus, "Researchers need to know which specific CBT components offered in which sequence or combination produce what types of changes in what outcome domains" (Durlak et al., 1991, p. 211). In other words, how processes in cognitive-behavioral therapy affect outcomes is still largely unknown, primarily because research has not focused on specific interventions or treatment processes. Thus, as we have seen with all the other forms of child treatment reviewed, the essential ingredients of child psychotherapy are veiled by the absence of research on process–outcome relations.

Another review of a special topic in child and adolescent treatment appeared in 1991. In this review, we find one of the only attempts to operationalize therapy process in the context of a meta-analytic review and then relate such processes to treatment outcomes. Rather than selecting studies on the basis of treatment "brands," studies were included if they contained a specific type of outcome measure, namely, measures of language functioning. Russell, Greenwald, and Shirk (1991) proposed that language functioning is pivotal to both child maladjustment and intervention. First, it is an area in which many clinic-referred children show specific developmental disorders; second, language is an integral part of the processes of self-regulation and cognitive mediation, and third, language is involved in the administration of all forms of child psychotherapy. Thus, a review of what had been discovered about language processes and outcomes in child treatment seemed clinically important.

In assessing the studies in the Weisz et al. (1987) meta-analytic review of child treatment, Russell et al. found 18 studies, including 26 treatment–control comparisons that included at least one measure of language functioning. Interestingly, studies included in the review addressed a variety of psychological problems (e.g., hyperactivity, anxiety, severe shyness, misconduct, underachievement, etc.), but no studies were included that focused on reading or writing or tutoring for specific school subjects. The children in the 18 studies had a mean age of 9.8 and most were boys (78.9%).

Language outcome measures were subdivided into two types: expressive–receptive and reading measures. In order to operationalize therapy process, the authors also assessed the type of verbal processes likely to have taken place in the treatments on the basis of descriptions of the predominant interventions in each therapy. Three types of verbal processes were identified:

> The first type is characterized by spontaneous verbal interaction in process-oriented therapy, as emphasized in traditional therapies (e.g., insight and nondirective). The second type is characterized by verbal interaction constrained by preset tasks and problem-solving goals, as in cognitive-behavioral treatments (e.g., problem-solving and self-instructional training). The third type is characterized by behavioral exchanges in which verbal interaction plays a secondary role as in operant and counterconditioning modes of treatment (e.g., behavioral parent-training, relaxation, systematic desensitization). (p. 917)

This is the first meta-analysis that attempts to describe treatment processes in terms of discourse structure and to relate such processes to outcomes on related language variables.

Russell et al. (1991) organized their review to answer four questions. The first questions asked if child therapy had any effect on the children's language proficiencies. The answer was in the affirmative, for both expressive–receptive and reading measures. Interestingly, changes in language variables and nonlanguage variables were not significantly correlated, although the absolute magnitude of the correlation was substantial ($r = .39$). This suggests that different change processes may be at work, a finding similar to that of Durlak et al. (1991) reported above, namely, that cognitive and behavioral measures did not covary. The interpretation that different change processes may be at work also received some support in the finding that length of treatment as indicated by the number of treatment sessions was correlated with the language effect sizes ($r = .45$), but not with the nonlanguage effect sizes ($r = .15$).

The authors also asked if the modality (group vs. individual) of treatment and type of presenting problem also affect outcome effect sizes on language variables. Individual therapy produced effect sizes over 10 times that of the combined other treatment modalities (1.31 vs. 0.13). This finding was corroborated across each type of treatment process (traditional verbal, cognitive problem solving, operant–relaxation). The more intensive the dialogic versus group verbal interaction, the more positive effects on the children's language proficiencies at posttreatment. There were no statistically significant differences between outcome effect sizes on language variables between children with differing presenting problems.

The most creative analyses, however, assessed effects of different types of in-therapy language interaction on language outcomes. Statistically, no significant effects were found between the traditional verbal, cognitive problem-solving, and operant–relaxation groups. There were too few studies employing each language process to obtain enough power to find even large mean differences to be statistically significant. However, treatments emphasizing spontaneous verbal-interaction processes yielded effect sizes that were over 10 times as large as those with explicit goal-oriented formats for language interaction, and over four times as large as those emphasizing behavioral rather than verbal exchanges.

Russell et al. (1991) derived three key conclusions from their study: (1) "A potentially rich and clinically significant area of child functioning has been only sporadically studied (i.e., only 17% of the 105 child outcome studies [reviewed] contained a language measure)"; (2) "Ratings or categorizations of the *in vivo* therapist and child language interaction are uniformly missing"; and (3) "This domain of functioning seems sensitive to the effects of child treatment, providing an additional, nonreactive dimension for the assessment of outcome" (p. 918). We might add that language proficiencies seem to be a key area in which pretreatment assessment, treatment interventions, and outcome measurements might all share explicit, common theoretical and methodological ground. For example, specific deficiencies, deviations or delays in pragmatic competencies (i.e., using communication skills to obtain appropriate behavioral and interpersonal goals) could be assessed at pretreatment. Likewise, interventions through pragmatic interactions with the therapist could be devised to remediate the specific pragmatic problems, and assessment of the child's posttreatment pragmatic competencies could be completed at outcome. In other words, formulation of the case, derivation of the interventions, and assessment of outcomes would take place across the same functional playing field.

The "State" of Child Psychotherapy Research

During this same period, through a series of articles, Kazdin and his colleagues (Kazdin, 1993a, 1993b; Kazdin, Bass, Ayers, & Rodgers, 1990) provided an overview of the "state" of child psychotherapy research. In a lengthy review, Kazdin et al. (1990) attempted to address three major questions: (1) To what extent does existing research address the range of factors that are related to outcome? (2) To what extent does this research address conditions that are representative of clinical practices? (3) To what extent does the extant research provide a sound, methodologically valid basis for forming inferences about treatment effectiveness, including comparative treatment effectiveness? To address these questions, the authors reviewed studies of 4- to 18-year-old children and adolescents who received some form of treatment that was compared to a control condition or to an alternative treatment. They included 218 articles that appeared in print from 1970 to 1988.

Regarding the characteristics of treated children in these studies, most studies (75.1%) focused on 6- to 11-year-olds and contained more boys than girls (mean percentage of boys was 67.3%), most studies (79.8%) did not specify the children's race, most studies (76.6%) had cases that were solicited by the investigator, and most (50.7%) included children who had acting-out symptoms. In terms of diagnoses, Kazdin, Bass, et al. (1990) reported that 37.1% of studies included children with conduct–oppositional disorders, 17.2% of the studies included children with attention-deficit/hyperactivity disorder, and 10.9% included children with anxiety disorders. Most striking was the underinvestigation of children with depression (1.8% of the studies).

Characteristics of treatment delivery were also described. For example, the median treatment lasted less than 10 weeks, with about 10 sessions. Most studies contained treatments that were delivered in groups (49.3%) versus individually (35.6%); were delivered in the schools (55%) versus the home of the child or adolescent (33.2%) or the university clinics (19.5%), and were delivered by a professional (64.5%). Over 70% of the studies examined behavioral or cognitive-behavioral treatments, with the next most common treatment being group (8.6%). Note especially that individual psychotherapy was examined in only 3.6% of the studies, and less than 1% examined psychodynamically oriented treatments.

Most studies (60.1%) compared two or more treatments, with comparisons of treatment versus no treatment (51.6%) and comparisons of treatment versus active control (39.5%) being the next most common focus. Most studies simply compared entire treatment packages versus some control condition (58.3%), with the dismantling strategy and the comparative outcome strategy being the next most common study evaluation strategy (both 26%). Note that less than 3% of the studies reviewed examined treatment processes in relation to outcome; that is, less than 10 studies in an 18-year period looked at process in relation to outcome.

In terms of methodological features of the articles, Kazdin, Bass, et al. (1990) reported that nearly 20% of the studies did not have random assignment to treatment conditions, that only 19.3% of the studies monitored or assessed ongoing treatment integrity, and that there tended to be only 12 subjects per group at posttreatment, and 10 subjects per group at follow-up, enabling researchers to detect differences between groups only when they yielded very large effect sizes. The authors also reported that direct observation or paper and pencil assessments were most common in studies (72.6% and 71.3%, respectively).

In concluding, Kazdin, Bass, et al. (1990) noted that many factors playing a significant role in treatment delivery have not been empirically studied. In fact, the relationship between specific techniques, rather than whole therapies, and treatment outcome has hardly been studied at all. Research on patterns of therapist–child interaction and its relation to outcome is virtually nonexistent. Furthermore, variables that could moderate treatment outcome, such as child and parent characteristics, have rarely been examined.

The authors also wisely pointed out that most therapy research involves little theory in guiding predictions. What has not been worked out in any respectable scientific detail are theoretical rationales for linking pathogenic processes in the client to specifically targeted interventions that are hypothesized to result in specific positive changes at outcome. As if this were not problematic enough, there is a yawning gap between the focus of empirical research and the delivery of child psychotherapy in clinical practice. Overall, clinical studies fail to be representative of child psychotherapy *as typically practiced* on a number of fronts. For example, some problems, such as adjustment disorders, are rarely studied despite being common in clinical practice. Length of treatment sharply diverges in research treatments and clinical practice; 8 to 10 weeks in studies versus 27 to 55 weeks in practice (Kazdin, Bass, et al., 1990). Studies of behavioral treatments far exceed studies of dynamic therapies, despite the fact that dynamic treatments are widely practiced. Similarly, studies often involve group treatments, whereas individual treatments are more common in practice. Such persistent problems give rise to a strong ending note of caution: "The differences between research and practice are not merely quantitative (e.g., more treatment, more severe cases), but qualitative as well (e.g., different treatments and types of cases). As the gap between research and practice increases on a given dimension, the degree of faith required to sustain clinical practice increases" (p. 739).

In order to remedy this situation, Kazdin (1990) outlined priority areas for research in a complementary review. Three areas were highlighted: clinical focus, alternative treatments, and outcome evaluation. For clinical focus, a research emphasis on the problem of comorbidity and underserved populations was recommended. As pointed out, half the children who have one psychiatric disorder also can be diagnosed as having a distinct second disorder. This may well be an underestimation, as specific developmental disorders having to do with language competencies are often unsuspected and thus not evaluated and diagnosed appropriately in clinics focused on emotional and behavioral disorders. Moreover, one can imagine how complicated it is to define treatments for children and adolescents who have comorbid conditions, especially if one considers problems with diagnostic reliability and etiological diversity within any given diagnosis. If factors are included that increase variability within diagnostic category such as race, gender, and/or ethnic background, the problem of fitting DSM-type diagnoses or their combinations to treatment-technique recommendations becomes enormous. Thus, the problem of comorbidity and within-diagnosis variability poses a significant challenge to the current research paradigm that couples brand-name treatments with diagnostic entities. Moreover, given the growing recognition that comorbidity is a relatively common phenomenon in clinic-referred samples; that is, clinic-referred children often present with a variety of problems that are not easily reduced to a single diagnosis, simple matching of treatments with diagnoses is likely to be the exception rather than the rule.

For alternative treatments, Kazdin (1990b) suggested more research on psychodynamic therapy and combined treatment modalities. The efficacy of a single technique, he points out, may not be sufficient to ameliorate a child's problem, especially if the problem manifests itself across domains with very different task demands expressed by very different social interactants. However, the problem with how to define efficacy is itself sufficiently complex to stall true progress. Thus, Kazdin recommended attending to two pressing issues: (1) assessing prosocial behavior as a powerful indicator of improvement, and (2) focusing on ways to define clinically significant and not just statistically significant change. In all of these areas (psychodynamic treatment research, multiple technique research, and investigations of clinical significance), there are plainly too few studies as yet to reach any overarching conclusions. Interestingly, even in this 1990 review, Kazdin does not include the need to assess within-therapy processes between child and therapist. Instead, the matching of brand-name therapies with specific diagnostic entities remains the focus of research.

To be fair, there is some indication in this review that the assessment of aberrant psychological processes and the evaluation of techniques targeted specifically to rectify them has gained some ground, but only on a limited scale. Kazdin (1990b) points out that cognitive problem-solving skills training draws on cognitive-developmental research to specify forms and functions of problem solving that can be expected within differing developmental levels. However, the fact remains that "little attempt [has been made] to relate specific cognitive deficits [or distortions] to particular types of clinical dysfunction" (p. 38). In addition, few studies have been guided by efforts to match specific pathogenic processes (e.g., cognitive distortions) with therapeutic procedures designed to directly address them. Given this lamentable situation, it is surprising that Kazdin falls back on recommending DSM categories or dimensional rating systems as the preferred means to specify clinical dysfunction in the future. Instead, why not recommend the specification of underlying pathogenic processes, such as cognitive, emotional, or interpersonal deficits or deviations, that contribute to the child's presenting problems, and then develop interventions that directly address these processes?

In fact, in a later review, Kazdin (1993a) appears to move toward this perspective. As he wisely points out, the lack of sound child and adolescent therapy research is not unrelated to the degree to which research on child and adolescent psychopathology has lagged behind that conducted with adults. But as Kazdin (1993b) notes, there are signs of progress. For example, he cites research on attributional biases of hostile intent that seem to lead to, or sustain aggressive behavior in children and adolescents (Dodge, Price, Bachorowski, & Newman, 1990). There is even evidence that such children misinterpret nonverbal cues on a specific dimension of behavior, dominance versus submissiveness, rather than on the positive versus the negative dimension (Russell, Stokes, Jones, Czogalik, & Rohleder, 1993). He notes also that such cognitive misattributions lead to dysfunctional aggressive behavior, which in turn leads to the social isolation of the aggressive child or adolescent. Not only is there specification of differences in cognitive, behavioral, and social functioning between aggressive and nonaggressive children and adolescents, in this example, but there is specification of the temporal relations in the pathogenic processes. In other words, not only do we get quantitative differences between forms of functioning of normal and aggressive children but also specification of a temporal cycle causally linking these differences. As Kazdin (1993b) points out, "Such research serves to identify potential points of intervention to interrupt aggressive behavior" (p. 648). We might also add that such research on basic cognitive and social processes can help to suggest the forms of intervention as well as their point of application.

For example, if it is true that aggressive boys do have nonverbal decoding biases that habitually lead them to distort the meaning of emotionally laden situations, then interventions geared to enhance the accuracy of the children's nonverbal decoding ability in non-emotionally laden situations seem to be a rather obvious choice around which to build an intervention strategy. However, the building of this strategy might also benefit from a sensitive reading of basic psychological research having to do with learning, discourse processes, and nonverbal encoding and decoding processes. In other words, in both case formulation and treatment strategy, a return to basic research in the traditional areas of psychology, especially developmental psychology, seems considerably overdue and highly warranted, particularly for those interested in upgrading the research on nonbehavioral interventions.

However, the main point of this example is that the design, development, and selection of a specific treatment depends on an understanding of the underlying processes that contribute to the child's presenting problems. To rely exclusively on diagnoses for treatment selection risks the assumption that there is a uniform pathogenic process underlying the presentation of children who share the same diagnosis. The reality of comorbidity alone raises doubts about embracing this assumption. Instead, as the foregoing example illustrates, treatment selection must be based on an assessment of the pathogenic mechanisms that contribute to the child's presenting problems.

Thus, as Kazdin (1993b) observes, progress in child therapy will go hand in hand with advances in developmental psychopathology.

CONCLUSION

We concluded the last chapter with the observation that child psychotherapy no longer involves fitting children, regardless of type of problem, to a uniform treatment, but instead requires the selection of treatment methods that hold the greatest promise for ameliorating children's specific problems. The question, then, is whether there is an empirical basis for the selection of effective treatments for specific problems? As indicated by this review, the effectiveness of child psychotherapy has been controversial for some time. However, a series of meta-analytic reviews of child and adolescent psychotherapy converge on the same conclusion, namely, that psychosocial treatments for children produce statistically, and at times, clinically significant effects. Clearly, these results should be reassuring to child practitioners or developing child clinicians, who hope to alter or modify the problems of their clients. Overall, then, child therapy appears to be useful.

However, lurking in the shadow of this brightly encouraging conclusion are a number of important caveats. First, as Weisz, Weiss, and Donenberg (1992) have shown, the relatively large treatment effects obtained in most laboratory or university-based studies of child psychotherapy have not been reproduced in actual clinical settings. After comparing laboratory-based versus clinic-based studies, these authors concluded: "Currently, we lack convincing evidence that the large and positive effects of psychotherapy demonstrated in controlled psychotherapy research, and summarized in meta-analyses, are being replicated in the clinic and community settings where most real-life interventions actually occur" (p. 1584). Obviously, there are important differences in the practice of child psychotherapy in these two contexts. In the ideal laboratory environment, youngsters are recruited for treatment, they tend to form homogeneous groups with similar types of problems, therapy is targeted to the focal problem, and therapists have received specialized training in the targeted treatment and are not overburdened by large caseloads. In the clinic, youngsters have problems that are serious or complex enough to have led to referral, children are quite heterogeneous and often evince multiple problems, therapy is typically not directed toward one focal problem, and therapists typically have not been recently trained in specific treatment procedures and are often burdened by heavy and diverse caseloads. Thus, perhaps it should not be surprising that there is a significant gap between the results of controlled child outcome studies and the results obtained from actual clinical settings.

Interestingly, the authors suggest that there may indeed be important reasons why laboratory studies of therapy produce significant effects. They suggest that such effectiveness may be related to the degree to which laboratory conditions result in the clear delineation of focal problems that will actually become the target for the technical processes of specific interventions. But, if we believe most of the previous reviews of child psychotherapy outcome, including some meta-analyses, we know that most of the reviewed studies, laboratory or not, could improve considerably in these very areas; that is, specification of focal problems in terms of pathogenic processes and specification of treatment processes rather than brand-name therapies is almost absent from the literature. If Weisz et al. (1992) are right, however, then we can surely expect more positive results from child treatment as formulations of pathogenic mechanisms and specification of treatment processes improve.

The second caveat is that empirical evidence for the effectiveness of child *psychotherapy,* in contrast to child *behavior* therapy, is less compelling, that is, closer inspection of meta-analytic results seems to indicate that the overall large effect sizes obtained in controlled research are largely attributable to various forms of behavior therapy. Given these results, the child psychotherapist, or therapist trainee, might be tempted to give up on nonbehavioral methods and convert to the practices of child behavior therapy. However, in an effort to prevent premature conversion, several factors must be considered.

First, what appear to be substantial differences between behavioral and nonbehavioral methods may be largely a function of the type of outcome measures utilized by these two approaches. In fact, when Casey and Berman (1985) eliminated reactive measures of outcome, estimates of the effectiveness of child psychotherapy and child behavior therapy were comparable. Although Weisz et al. (1987) contest this approach to the data, it remains the case that there have been an insufficient number of comparative outcome studies for comparable problems with comparable outcome measures to draw any firm conclusion about relative efficacy (Kazdin, 1990b).

A related issue to consider when weighing the relative efficacy of different treatments concerns the *clinical* significance of treatment effects. In the child therapy domain, claims for the superiority of one form of treatment over another have been based on differences in effect sizes between brand-name treatments (e.g., cognitive-behavioral vs. client-centered) relative to control or no treatment conditions. Although one may obtain statistically significant differences between effect sizes for different treatments, these differences may not be clinically significant. First, for any treatment we will want to know what percentage of the treated group actually returned to within-normal levels of functioning—say to within one standard deviation from the mean of a normative sample on an index of adaptive functioning (e.g., social competence). Treatments that are significantly different from control conditions may fail to meet this second criterion of significance. Thus, whereas one or both treatments may appear to produce statistically significant treatment effects, the outcomes may be of limited clinical value. Second, when comparing treatments, we will want to know if we are comparing treatments that are both clinically significant, neither clinically significant, or split on clinical significance. In each case, we will have to devise some principled bases to decide when a statistical difference between two treatments is clinically significant. The upshot of this perspective is that we do not yet have the theories, or the studies, to assess different child treatments in terms of clinical significance or in terms of comparative significance. Without such a framework, the meaning of apparent differences in treatment effects between forms of child psychotherapy and child behavior therapy remains ambiguous.

A second major problem with drawing conclusions from the existing child therapy outcome literature is that nonbehavioral forms of child psychotherapy have been underinvestigated. Furthermore, existing studies of child psychotherapy fail to represent treatments that are actually used in clinical practice (Shirk & Russell, 1992). In our review of nonbehavioral treatment studies, the reported rates of treatment were compared with the frequencies of treatments in a meta-analytic sample. There was a large disparity between the two.

> Among practicing child psychiatrists, 88.7% rated psychodynamic therapy as useful most or all of the time, but only 7.2% rated client-centered therapy useful most or all of the time. A similar pattern holds for practicing child psychologists, 50.3% and 22.7% respectively. Yet there

were over three times as many client-centered compared to psychodynamic studies in the meta-analytic sample of nonbehavioral treatments.
(Shirk & Russell, 1992, p. 706)

This nonrepresentativeness was evident in other areas as well. For
example, group treatments were predominant in the meta-analytic sample
but seldom preferred or practiced by child psychotherapists. Moreover, the
treatments in the research sample were short—over 20% had fewer than 10
sessions. In practice, the average length of treatment is around 30 sessions
for psychiatrists and 21 sessions for child psychologists (Kazdin, Bass, et
al., 1990). Thus, it is not clear that child *psychotherapy*, as it has been
theoretically conceived, has been evaluated empirically.

Compounding this problem is the fact that the methodological quality
of research on child psychotherapy is painfully poor. For example, Barrnett,
Docherty, and Frommelt (1991) reexamined evidence for the effectiveness
of child psychotherapy that had accumulated since 1963. Barrnett et al.
(1991) broke down their review into six areas: treatments versus no
treatments, individual versus family, individual versus group, and studies
dealing explicitly with therapist, client, or therapy variables. Whereas they
report box scores for each area, study by study, their overall conclusion
remains invariant: In each area and as a whole, the methodological quality
of the studies is so poor as to obviate any scientifically respectable conclusion about the effectiveness of child psychotherapy. In this regard their
conclusion, presented in 1991, differs little from those who responded
soberly to Levitt's initial assertions that child psychotherapy is ineffective.

The authors do make an important contribution. Instead of just
lamenting the poor methodological quality of the research in general, they
actually report specific lapses, study by study, within each content area and
also present a summary of the frequencies of the flaws in the set of 43
studies taken as a whole. The picture Barrnett et al. (1991) paint is not very
pretty; in fact, it might better be described as a wasteland. Forty out of the
43 studies have poorly specified inclusion and exclusion criteria; 40 out of
the 43 studies have poorly specified treatments at the level of actual
interventions, therapist characteristics at the level of experience and
gender, and treatment course in terms of checks on the delivery of the
putative treatments. In other words, in over 93% of the studies we do not
know in adequate scientific detail who was treated, who delivered the
treatments, or what treatments were delivered—and that is just the start. In
36 of the 43 studies, the equivalence of the control groups on key
pretreatment variables was questionable. They make the very important
but often overlooked point that random assignment of small numbers of
subjects to treatment groups does not ensure their equivalence on critical
variables. Moreover, in 25 of the 43 studies, poor measurements were used,

or inadequate outcome assessments were done. Obviously, if the assessment of the authors is true, then we have a very poor knowledge base with which to conclude anything about the effectiveness of child psychotherapy; and if there were any room to doubt this sobering conclusion, the authors ask us to fathom the fact that over half of the reviewed studies suffered not from two or three but from all four methodological flaws simultaneously.

There is also evidence that poor design quality affects estimates of treatment effectiveness. In our review of the nonbehavioral treatments included in the meta-analysis by Weisz and colleagues (1987), we (Shirk & Russell, 1992) evaluated each study on eight methodological characteristics (i.e., lack of random assignment, lack of fidelity checks, etc.). A full 62% of the reviewed studies had three or more methodological flaws. The effect size associated with the nine studies with the poorest methodological quality (0.31) was only half as large as the effect size (0.63) of the nine studies at the top third of the distribution of methodological quality. Such results are consistent with the findings of Weiss and Weisz (1990), which show that methodological shortcomings have an impact on effect size estimates, namely, that better designed studies tend to produce larger effects.

Given these results, we hypothesized that the superior showing of behavioral treatments in meta-analytic comparisons could reflect the superior design quality of behavioral outcome studies rather than differences in treatment effectiveness; that is, differences in effect sizes between behavioral and nonbehavioral treatments might be confounded with differences in design quality in their respective samples of outcome studies. Weiss and Weisz (1995) tested this hypothesis by utilizing two methods for assessing methodological quality. Surprisingly, their results indicated that nonbehavioral outcome studies were marginally better than behavioral studies in terms of design quality. Moreover, when design quality was statistically controlled, the magnitude of the difference in treatment effects remained relatively stable. One interpretation for their findings, then, is that the existing sample of behavioral outcome studies appears to be as flawed methodologically as the sample of nonbehavioral studies, and that statistical control for design problems accounts for little change in estimates of relative effectiveness. This is certainly a worrisome conclusion given recurrent evidence for the overall poor quality of the nonbehavioral outcome literature. In essence, the findings of Weiss and Weisz (1995) raise the fundamental question of whether we can make valid comparisons from a sample of methodologically flawed studies—even when we control for design quality. At what point do we simply say that these studies are so flawed individually, they are not worth summarizing collectively? (Shirk & Russell, 1995). This point is addressed by Greenwald and Russell (1991), who argue for a more critical appraisal of the fitness of individual studies for inclusion in meta-analytic comparisons.

We propose that the most valid meta-analytic comparison of child treatments would include only those studies that pass methodological muster at the level of the individual study (Shirk & Russell, 1995). In other words, if one wishes to conduct a "horse race" between types of treatments, only thoroughbreds should be entered. Unfortunately, this would mean that many of the already limited number of child psychotherapy outcome studies would be disqualified.

With these caveats in mind, reasons remain for cautious optimism about the effectiveness of child psychotherapy. Meta-analytic results indicate that client-centered and cognitively oriented treatments produce statistically significant treatment effects. Unfortunately, there have been so few studies of insight-oriented or dynamic child treatment that it is difficult to draw any firm conclusions about its utility. However, a recent series of studies from the Anna Freud Center provide new evidence for the potential impact of such treatment on child psychopathology. In these studies, data derived from chart reviews indicated that psychodynamic child treatment can be clinically useful, especially for young children (Fonagy & Target, 1994; Target & Fonagy, 1994). Nevertheless, well-designed, controlled outcome studies of child psychodynamic therapy have yet to be conducted.

Overall then, despite promising results, the child psychotherapy outcome literature provides a very fragile framework for the selection of specific treatments for different childhood disorders. The heart of the problem, quite simply, is the absence of a sufficient number of studies of adequate methodological quality that compare outcomes for children with different types of problems. In brief, the dearth of research on child psychotherapy undermines any effort to prescribe treatments on the basis of their known efficacy for particular problems.

There are other, perhaps deeper, problems as well. The preponderance of studies has employed designs that compare treatment brands (i.e., whole treatments) with each other or control conditions. Yet most treatment approaches comprise many different processes and techniques that can be offered in various combinations and sequences. Thus, the focus on treatment packages or brands is unlikely to shed light on the essential ingredients of child psychotherapy. To accomplish such an aim, researchers will have to redirect attention to what actually occurs within therapy sessions, that is, by focusing on the delivery of specific techniques or on interactions between child and therapist, and then relating these processes to treatment outcome. But as Kazdin, Bass, and colleagues (1990) have reported, less than 3% of all studies of child therapy have employed a process analysis strategy. Some may argue that such an approach is premature at this point and must await compelling evidence that treatment packages, as a whole, produce significant effects. We contend that the absence of process analyses severely limits our ability to understand what truly accounts for change in child treatment and undermines our ability to design effective interventions.

In essence, little effort seems to have been expended in studying what actually occurs during the therapy hour. We have seen this lapse over and over again in the history of child psychotherapy research. To put it all together, we might conclude with a statement such as the following: Treatment processes are neither connected theoretically to types of individual deficits, distortions, or conflicts in specific areas of individual functioning prior to treatment, nor are they connected in research to the gains or losses produced by treatment at outcome or follow-up. This lapse in bridging the presenting psychological problems to their demonstrable remediation at outcome through a careful analysis of treatment processes, the active and inactive ingredients of therapy, has been the most glaring lapse in the history of child psychotherapy research.

The primary challenge seems almost too simple to recommend. We can no longer be satisfied with knowing so little about what goes on in the therapy hour, and how what goes on in the therapy hour is related to changes at outcome. Developments in the analyses of in-therapy processes are rapidly appearing in the adult psychotherapy literature and desperately need to be applied to child psychotherapy.

It is important to note, however, that there is a very rich tradition already established that takes as its object of study what people say to each other. Psychologists wishing to study treatment should consider this extensive basic research literature that has explored discourse and conversation, including conversations between parents and children. What we need to know is how to construct our conversations in a way that targets the deficits or deviations uncovered in the initial evaluation of the child's problems. The same could be said of supportive interpersonal interactions. Here again, a substantial developmental literature has focused on the relationship between supportive processes and psychological well-being. Such knowledge must be imported to the domain of child psychotherapy if we are to understand the process of change.

In brief, psychologists wanting to study therapeutic treatments should remember that they are psychologists first. The phenomena relevant to understanding therapy are not very different from the phenomena that psychologists study in other systematic areas of the field. Interpersonal, emotional, cognitive, and developmental processes, in their abnormal and normal manifestations, are the focus of therapy in one way or another. Just because we are dealing with abnormalities and treatment processes does not mean that they are less relevant. In fact, a major aim of this book is to link basic research on such processes with the complex interactions that constitute child psychotherapy.

A similar argument can be made about the specification of childhood problems. Child psychotherapy is geared toward the remediation or alteration of psychological processes that contribute to the child's presenting problems. These processes are largely interpersonal, emotional, or cognitive in nature. Thus, the focus of treatment is not the child's manifest problems, as captured by a DSM diagnosis or behavior rating scale, but the pathogenic processes that underlie such problems. Interventions, then, are designed or selected on the basis of an understanding of the pathogenic processes that contribute to the child's focal problems. Our descriptions of such processes can be both formal, as in characterizing biases in cognitive attributions among aggressive children, and temporal, as in characterizing recurrent cycles of affect dysregulation in bulimics. Obviously, the task of specifying the pathogenic processes that contribute to child maladjustment is a formidable one, perhaps more challenging than establishing a reliable diagnostic system for categorizing patterns of manifest problems. However, as is already apparent to some, the selection of treatments on the basis of diagnoses is just not adequate (Beutler, 1989).

It is our contention that the problem with the traditional approach, that is, matching treatment brands with diagnostic entities, is that it fails to conceptualize both treatments and disorders in terms of component psychological processes. As a result, formulation of the case and derivation of the treatment method lack common conceptual ground. Thus, the task for child psychotherapy research is to identify the essential psychological processes that constitute both therapeutic interventions and variations in childhood maladjustment. We believe that identification of these essential ingredients will provide the link between clinical problems and clinical interventions.

3

⌒

The Process
of Child Psychotherapy:
Process Research

T HE EXISTING outcome research on child psychotherapy, limited in scope and marred by numerous methodological flaws, provides an unstable foundation for the selection of effective treatments for different childhood problems. But of equal importance, the existing outcome literature has rarely focused on the delivery of specific techniques or patterns of therapist–child interaction that could be systematically related to therapeutic change. Instead, much of the research has focused on the comparative effectiveness of brand-name therapies for groups of children who are frequently poorly defined in terms of patient characteristics. This has led some to conclude that we need new, methodologically improved comparative outcome studies to establish a firm foundation for prescriptive treatments. However, comparisons of treatment brands will offer little insight into the processes that contribute to therapeutic change. As we have argued, treatment brands, such as cognitive-behavioral or psychodynamic therapy, are umbrella terms for complex sets of techniques and patterns of therapeutic interaction. Thus, we simply cannot turn to more or even better outcome research to identify the processes responsible for change. Instead, we need to actually look at what is done in the therapy hour, and to connect significant therapeutic events in sessions, comprised of aspects of therapist–child interaction, to changes that may occur in the pathogenic processes or structures that led to the child's referral. Through changes in these pathogenic processes or structures, it can be expected that the child will attain better adaptive levels of functioning at outcome. This, of course, is a basic premise of child psychotherapy, that one needs to change some internal process or structure in order to facilitate therapeutic progress.

To put it another more empirically driven way, an essential task confronting the field of child psychotherapy is to describe and measure whatever it is that actually happens between the therapist and the child in the hour in which they interact. Such descriptions and measurements would help us formulate answers to the very simple question: Of what is child therapy essentially and inessentially comprised? Having a good grasp of what comprises child therapy would then enable us to relate levels and kinds of essential therapeutic ingredients to changes in the child's affect, interpersonal behavior, or cognitions. Such is the study of therapy process and its relation to outcome, an area of focus every bit as time-honored as the more common comparative outcome study.

But what in the protean complexities of therapist–child interaction should be considered *figural*, that is, of essential importance to the process of change, and what should be considered *ground*, that is, of only inessential or incidental import or consequence? Without knowing how to partition all of that which comprises the therapist–child interaction into active change-causing ingredients, on the one hand, or inactive, causally inert ingredients, on the other, how can researchers come to choose one set of behaviors or dimensions of interactions over others as the focus of their studies? Obviously, choices as to what is considered figure or ground will be related to the researcher's theory of change and, we hope, to the body of accumulating research evidence. Theories about what is essential or inessential in the therapeutic process must guide the choice of research variables, just as it guides the formulation of intervention strategies in actual practice.

In reviewing studies of the process of child psychotherapy, we will be aiming to derive guidance, some empirical and some theoretical, about what kinds of treatment processes make sense to study empirically and to continue to implement in clinical practice. Perhaps even more important, we aim to properly and meaningfully formulate the essential intervention strategies, their instantiated processes, and causal mechanisms of change. This last point should not be underrated. The careful explication of essential strategies, processes, and change mechanisms for process research or for clinical treatment should be considered requisite for both the science and practice of child psychotherapy.

Child therapy process researchers, despite much current debunking, even by us, have in fact established a tradition that spans nearly half a century. For example, Table 3.1 presents the bulk of studies on child therapy processes. As can be seen, we located 22 studies, with the first study

TABLE 3.1. Published Process Studies of Child Treatment, 1946–1993

Authors	Publication year	Comparative, process, process–outcome	Descriptive, hypothesis testing	Segment of therapy used in analysis
			Type of study	
1940s–1950s				
Landisberg & Snyder	1946	Process	Descriptive	100%
Lebo	1952	Comparative–process	Descriptive	10%
Lebo	1955	Comparative–process	Descriptive	10%
Moustakas	1955	Comparative–process	Hypothesis testing	100%
Moustakas & Schalock	1955	Comparative–process	Descriptive	100%
Lebo	1956	Comparative–process	Hypothesis testing	100%
Moustakas, Sigel, & Schalock	1956	Comparative–process	Descriptive	16 minutes
Lebo & Lebo	1957	Process	Hypothesis testing	3%
1960s				
Guerney, Burton, Silverberg, & Shapiro	1965	Process	Hypothesis testing	100%
Dana & Dana	1969	Comparative–process	Descriptive	100%

(continued)

TABLE 3.1. *(continued)*

Authors	Publication year	Comparative, process, process–outcome	Type of study	
			Descriptive, hypothesis testing	Segment of therapy used in analysis
		1970s–1980s		
Boll	1971	Comparative–process	Descriptive	Unspecified
Siegel	1972	Comparative–process	Descriptive	4 minutes
Wright, Truax, & Mitchell	1972	Comparative–process	Descriptive	15 minutes
Truax, Altman, Wright, & Mitchell	1973	Comparative–process–outcome	Hypothesis testing	15 minutes
Truax & Wittmer	1973	Comparative–process–outcome	Descriptive	"363 samples"
Howe & Silvern	1981	Process	Descriptive	12 minutes
Mook	1982a	Comparative–process	Descriptive	4 minutes
Mook	1982b	Comparative–process	Descriptive	4 minutes
		1990s		
Russell, Greenwald, & Shirk	1991	Meta-analytic, comparative, process	Descriptive	100%
Smith-Acuna, Durlak, & Kaspar	1991	Comparative–process	Descriptive	100%
Russell, van den Broeck, Adams, Rosenberger, & Essig	1993	Process	Descriptive	16 child stories 16 therapist stories

appearing in 1946, almost a full half-century ago, and the last studies appearing in print in 1993, with a suggestion of more to come. There is evidence of some accumulation of knowledge, as well, with later studies building critically on some of the earlier studies. Moreover, at least a few researchers seemed to have embarked on programmatic investigations, and did not simply take one shot at a problem and then give up and go on to something else. This is, by way of a forecast, some of the good news.

But from some of the same facts, we can derive some of the bad news. For example, the rate of production of studies that might pinpoint mechanisms of change in child therapy has "progressed" at a slumbering pace— less than one study every 2 years! As noteworthy, over one-third of the studies appeared before 1960, over one-half either before 1960 or after 1990! Reviewing this small set of studies in some detail could easily convince the reader of how little we know about the critical processes of child psychotherapy, of how little cumulative progress is observable in the literature and, of course, of how much can and should be done in the future.

But these studies should not be dismissed en masse, as is often done. There are some important lessons to be learned from them, both methodologically and substantively. Consequently, we will focus in some detail on each study, not simply because we believe it is only through process research that mechanisms of therapeutic change will be best identified and assessed in relation to outcomes, but because collectively this set of studies reveals what the field has already endorsed, at least implicitly, as the figural areas in which potential mechanisms for positive change can be found and, furthermore, this tradition suggests, through detailed demonstrations, how best to study them. We also embark on this detailed review because we have some confidence in one of the conclusions drawn from the outcome literature, namely, that the more scientific-like the control and care surrounding the delivery of treatment, the stronger the positive treatment outcomes; and being knowledgeable about the scientific work of one's predecessors is part and parcel of this scientific-like care and control. Admittedly, we will not obtain definite empirically derived answers from this literature about what causes therapeutic change; but with some care, its analytic distillation will produce more than a thimbleful of guiding wisdom. This wisdom, we hope, will help guide the theoretical task of formulating essential intervention strategies, of isolating processes of positive change in the therapist–child interaction, and of specifying causal mechanisms of change.

The review will proceed by decades, with the 1940s and 1950s combined. Enough detail about the studies will be provided to give the reader a sense of the research problems, methods, and findings that comprise each study. Enough criticism will be leveled at each study to indicate its limitations to contributing to our knowledge about change processes in child psychotherapy. Following each decade, a brief recapitulation will be given. The chapter will end with overall conclusions that we feel can be drawn from this literature.

THE 1940s AND 1950s

In the first published study, conducted by Landisberg and Snyder (1946), the authors asked one basic question: "What actually takes place in this type of [i.e., nondirective] play therapy?" (p. 203). To this they added several more pointed questions, such as, "Is the nondirective relationship or something else responsible for change?," or "How do therapists' verbal behaviors affect client responses?" They studied four cases of three different counselors, coding each of the counselor's statements or actions into one of five major categories and coding each of the clients' statements or actions into one of eight major categories. The clients were all 5 or 6 years old and represented different types and levels of psychopathology, with three cases being described as successful and one as unsuccessful or incomplete. Unfortunately, it is unclear from the article just how many sessions were included in a course of treatment, how many sessions were coded, and what the absolute number of coded actions or utterances were for each client/case.

The authors reported a cluster of interesting descriptive findings. Clients produced three-fifths of all codable behavior. Thirty percent of all behaviors in the interviews were nondirective therapist statements, 25% were clients giving information, and 24% were clients taking some positive play action. Several times, dependent findings were reported as well. For example, at the level of exchanges, the authors reported that client giving of information or taking some positive action most often followed therapist reflection of feeling. At the level-of-treatment phase, the authors reported that during the second fifth of therapy, therapists' recognition of feeling significantly decreased from the first fifth, whereas at the same time therapists' restatement of content increased from the first fifth of treatment, before both returned to their previous levels for the rest of therapy. The authors explain this "phase" phenomenon by suggesting that child clients might regress somewhat in therapy before presenting feeling-toned material that the therapist can reflect in the latter three-fifths of therapy. On the client side, marked increases in physical action, accompanied by expressions of feelings, were noted over the course of therapy; and this is explained by suggesting that levels of therapeutic catharsis increased over the later phases of treatment. Interestingly, when client expression of feelings was dichotomized into positive and negative feelings, a number of findings emerged. First, positive feelings were more often expressed in the first two-fifths of therapy than negative feelings. Second, it was negative feelings that showed an increase over the last three-fifths of therapy, with positive feelings remaining at about the same level. When the expression of feelings was partitioned according to their target, the authors reported that the child clients' expressions of feelings about themselves and about their counselors remained at about the same low level throughout therapy. It was only expressions of feelings toward others and external situations that increased over the course of therapy. Finally, the authors reported that there was nothing in the client cases that could be categorized as insight.

We can see that in this first study the authors were more interested in documenting what went on in nondirective play therapy than in testing a priori hypotheses about treatment processes or change mechanisms and their relation to outcomes. It is also difficult to know how such findings might contribute to strong hypothesis-testing research about processes. Except for the reciprocal drop in reflection of feelings and increases in restatement of content during the second fifth of therapy, the therapists' behavior seems remarkably constant, a finding that seems intuitively hard to believe, but consistent with nondirective principles (Russell, 1984). Such principles basically recommend that the provision of the therapist conditions (e.g., warmth, genuineness, and empathy) be constant throughout the therapy engagement. In point of fact, this nonintuitive finding may well have to do with the gross categorization of the therapists' verbal and other behavior (Russell, 1984). On the client side, the increase in cathartic behavior seems consistent with nondirective theory, especially the increasing release of negative feelings over the course of therapy. Confronted with a consistently safe, supportive environment and consistently warm, accepting therapists, the children allow themselves to express unhappiness and anger at their caregivers and/or life situation.

In the second study, Lebo (1952) criticized Landisberg and Snyder's research on two key points: (1) The categories they used had been developed for the description and investigation of nondirective adult therapy, and (2) the small sample of children in the study was remarkably homogeneous as regards their age, and presumably their developmental status on important dimensions of behavior. To rectify this situation, Lebo sought to investigate five age groups (4-, 6-, 8-, 10-, and 12-year-olds), each with four children, and he used categories deemed more applicable to child play therapy than that used in the earlier study by Landisberg and Snyder. Interestingly, he recruited children who were "normal" in terms of their social adjustment and "treated" them in a "therapy" lasting three sessions. In other words, this may have been the first analogue study of the process of child therapy. He categorized a randomly selected 10% of the verbal behavior of the children, presumably assuming that important types and changes in the children's verbal participation would not be systematically "bunched up" in discrete segments of interaction.

Lebo (1952) found that the most prevalent speech category across all ages is simple descriptions and comments about play and information and stories about the family, school, pets, teacher, play room, and self, that is, objective information about in- and extratherapy circumstances. Such objective information giving and storytelling accounted for between 29% to 40% of the children's utterances. This study was clearly the first to provide some empirical evidence that storytelling in therapy is so prevalent.

Interestingly, there were very strong age trends. As the age of the children increased, they told the therapist fewer of their decisions, explored therapeutic limits less, made fewer attempts at forming a relationship with the therapist, and decreased their number of requests for information. At the same time, the children increased statements of their likes and dislikes, made more information statements, and increased their unclassifiable utterances. Lebo interpreted these results to indicate that as children grow older, they become more independent of the play therapy situation. Interestingly, children at all ages failed to verbalize insight. This is explained by the author as possibly resulting from the children's normal status, whereas insight is typically developed in therapy with maladjusted individuals.

Like the first study, Lebo's (1952) is basically descriptive. However, in his study there is little concern with client and therapist dependencies or with changes over time points or phases of treatment. In fact, we do not know how many therapists were involved or who the therapists were, what level of training, what gender, and so on, although it is suspected that Lebo himself was the therapist. We obviously cannot be sure they were exposed to nondirective play therapy, as no "checks" on therapist behavior are reported. Given the analogue character of the study, it is difficult to know what could be generalized to nondirective therapy with disturbed clients in realistic courses of treatment. What seems clear is that children's speech behavior varies as a function of their age, which, as a matter of fact, should not be surprising. What would be surprising would be to find normal 12-year-olds talking like normal 4-year-olds! As in the first study in this tradition, Lebo did find that giving information was an important component in the speech of the children at every age, a finding that dovetails with what we know about adult speech in therapy (Czogalik & Russell, 1994a, 1994b).

In an attempt to improve the categories he used in the 1952 study, Lebo (1955) published a new set of categories with some significant revisions and additions. In the first study, two categories had to be collapsed into one, because the coders could not reliably distinguish between them. In the new category scheme, the two categories were redefined. The categories were (1) simple descriptions, information, and comments about play and playroom (e.g., "This is an army"; "These are prisoners"; "More marbles"; "The room's different"), and (2) straight information and stories about the family, school, pets, teacher, self, and so on (e.g., "We have a big house"; "I went to the park yesterday"; "I have a sister"; "I was waiting for you"; "I thought you were my mother"). With these new definitions of basically objective information-giving or storytelling categories, the coders reanalyzed the corpus used in the 1952 study, and Lebo reported that "the new definitions [of the two categories] have been found to be successful in differentiating the statements made by children in play therapy" (Lebo, 1955, p. 376).

Perhaps more interestingly, Lebo also added several categories having to do with vocalizations rather than verbalizations because, first,

> they should serve to emphasize differences in speech habits between younger (e.g., 4-year-olds) and older children. Second, they should call the play therapist's attention to the fact that the significance of speech as an expressive medium varies from one age level to another. Third, the vocalizations represented by these categories (e.g., sound effects such as cluckings, sirens, machine gunning, explosions and mumblings or talking to the self in a voice that is too low to be heard) seem to be as much a part of emotional expression as do the other categories. (p. 376)

Although no new empirical findings about processes were reported by Lebo (1955), this study emphasizes how much importance these early child therapy process researchers placed on obtaining just the right set of developmentally sensitive descriptive categories. This focus on measure development will be a recurrent theme in the following decades, but at times, without the corresponding developmental sensitivity. Moreover, the absence of systematic efforts to link therapy processes, no matter how well measured, with treatment outcomes will also persist over time.

Moustakas (1955) presented a detailed hypothesis-testing study of differences between normal and disturbed children's expressions of negative attitudes in play therapy. Negative attitudes were defined as "any behavior accompanied by definite expression of feelings not socially acceptable, or not constructive, or evasive" (p. 315). Nine aggressive and nine nonaggressive 4-year-olds (IQs ranging between 105 and 145!) were seen in "at least" four 40-minute sessions of nondirective play therapy conducted by a male therapist, who may or may not have been blind to the clients' status (disturbed vs. normal). From the first and third interviews, two raters identified 241 negative attitudes and rated them in terms of their intensity on a 3-point scale (minor, moderate, and severe). Types of negative attitudes were subclassified and compared across the groups as well.

Moustakas (1955) reported findings that support his hypotheses. Disturbed children expressed negative attitudes more frequently than did nondisturbed children. Basically, the disturbed children expressed on average about eight negative attitudes per session, whereas the nondisturbed children expressed about five negative attitudes per session. The differences collapsed across sessions were statistically significant. The intensity of the expression of the negative attitudes also differed across the groups. As expected, the disturbed children expressed their negative attitudes with significantly more intensity than did the nondisturbed children. Interestingly, there were also significant differences between the groups in the proportions of types of negative attitudes expressed. Disturbed children's proportion of negative attitudes that involved diffuse hostility, hostility toward home and family, cleanliness anxiety, orderliness anxiety, and regression in development were significantly greater than those of the nondisturbed children. The nondisturbed children expressed a greater proportion of hostility toward siblings than did their nondisturbed counterparts, but with less intensity. Finally, it was found that the disturbed children expressed negative attitudes in a diffuse and generalized way, whereas the nondisturbed children expressed their negative attitudes more directly or in a focused manner.

We see that in this study, again, only the children's speech is subjected to analysis. There is no analysis of contingencies between therapist and child verbal behaviors, and there is no analysis of changes in the children's speech over the sessions sampled. In some ways, it should come as no surprise that aggressive children express more and higher levels of intensity of hostility, anxiety, and regression in development than do nondisturbed children—whether they are in the beginning stages of therapy or not. It would be odd, given the descriptions of their disorders, if this were not the case. In concluding, however, Moustakas (1955) did suggest an interesting hypothesis about the developmental course of nondirective therapy: "It is possible, as this study suggests, that as therapy progresses the negative attitudes of the disturbed child may become similar to those of well-adjusted children, expressed more clearly and directly, less frequently, and with mild or moderate intensity of feeling" (p. 325). We would only add that nothing in this cross-sectional study of 18 4-year-olds suggests such a development. What is very interesting about this study, however, is that it does employ nondisturbed children's verbal behavior in the counseling session for purposes of comparison. This may be the first study, in the child or adult literature, that uses the speech of nondisturbed subjects as a possible processive outcome criterion for assessing disturbed patients' deviations, and, as per Moustakas's suggestions, for assessing, through social comparison, their return to normal levels of speech interaction in therapy.

In the same year, Moustakas and Schalock (1955) published a study specifically focused on the therapist–child and child–therapist interaction, as well as their separate characteristic modes of participation in play therapy. The set of descriptive categories that they employed to code therapist and child behavior were quite comprehensive, comprised of some 82 adult categories and 72 child categories (a summarization of the published report follows). The categories were constructed "on the assumption that adult–child interaction involves reciprocal stimulation: that the child's behavior is potentially as significant in influencing the adult's behavior as the converse" (p. 143). In addition, an anxiety and a hostility rating were made, along with the categorization of the adult's or the child's behavior at every 5-second interval.

Moustakas and Schalock (1955) recruited five emotionally disturbed and five normal 4-year-olds from the Merrill–Palmer Nursery School. Each was seen for two 40-minute play therapy sessions conducted by the same nondirective male therapist, Moustakas himself. As many as 1,000 therapist and child behaviors were recorded per session. The master tables of the frequencies of therapist and child behavior are not presented in their research report; instead they summarize their data with respect to a set of specific questions. The questions they asked focus on both the client and the therapist's behavior and their contingencies in both the disturbed and normal groups of children.

With respect to the therapist's overall behavior, Moustakas and Schalock (1955) reported that five categories of therapist behavior accounted for 85% of their interaction, of which 9,084 instances were recorded. In descending frequency, these categories were the following: (1) Attentive Observation, (2) Recognition of Stimulation (e.g., "Um Hm. I see"), (3) Giving Information Verbally, (4) Interpretation by Restating Verbalized Feelings, and (5) Seeking Information of an Impersonal Nature. Examples of seldom or never used categories included (1) Restriction with an Explanation, (2) Enthusiastic Cooperation, (3) Reassurance, (4) Directing with a Threat, (5) Seeking Personal Information, (6) Seeking Permission, (7) Giving Qualified Permission, (8) Seeking Help, (9) Seeking Reassurance, (10) Seeking Reward, (11) Orienting Roles by Use of Status and Power, (12) Criticism, (13) Disciplinary Action, and most restricting and forbidding categories.

Surprisingly, the authors noted that there are few differences in the therapist's behavior across the disturbed and nondisturbed groups of children. Out of an unreported number of comparisons of categories, Moustakas and Schalock (1955) report that there was only one significant difference among the five most prevalent categories, and it pertained to Attentive Observation, with the therapist showing relatively more Attentive Observation with the disturbed (62%) than with the nondisturbed group

(57%). However, the rank order of the therapist's use of the different categories with the two groups was high. The authors interpret these findings to mean that the primary emphasis of this therapist's behavior was on "being there" with both groups, a stance made manifest in his attentive observing, listening, and statements of recognition.

With respect to the children's overall behavior, seven categories accounted for approximately 95% of their interaction behavior, of which 9,544 were recorded, 4,610 instances for nondisturbed and 4,934 for disturbed children. The seven categories, in descending relative frequency were the following: (1) Nonattention, (2) Attentive Observation, (3) Statement of Condition or Action, (4) Seeking Information, (5) Giving Information Verbally, (6) Recognition of Stimulation, and (7) Nonrecognition of Stimulation. The authors reported only one significant difference between the two groups of children, namely that the disturbed group showed more Nonattention (47%) than the nondisturbed group (33%). They also noted a trend for the nondisturbed group to evince more frequently behaviors such as (1) Joint Participation in Activity, (2) Seeking Help, (3) Orienting the Role of Therapist in Play, (4) Directing by Suggestion, (5) Seeking Permission, and (6) Rejection by Changing the Subject and by Denying the Validity of the Therapist's Statement. In other words, there was a trend for the nondisturbed group to be more fully oriented to interacting with the therapist than the disturbed group. The authors also reported that there was a large difference in the expression of hostility between the two groups. The disordered group had 418 episodes in which some hostility was expressed, as compared to only 23 in the nondisturbed group, a finding similar to that reported by Moustakas (1955).

Moustakas and Schalock (1955) concluded that their most striking finding was that there seemed to be more similarity than differences between the two groups of children. In fact, a rank-order correlation of the frequencies of the groups' use of the categories was substantial (.69). The differences that emerged boiled down to dimensions of Attentiveness, Interactiveness, and Hostility, with the first two categories being somewhat related and tied to the degree of verbal interactive behavior. The authors noted that both groups did spend considerable time playing alone, asserting that such a finding "seems to emphasize the value to children of being free to operate on their own in the therapy setting" (p. 149). They also noted that had they coded only verbal behavior, 47% of the behavior of the disturbed group and 33% of the normal group would have been overlooked. This also suggests that the disturbed group acted out rather than verbalized their experiences more than the nondisturbed group. Most surprisingly, the data were interpreted to mean that "such approaches as reward, praise, affection, giving reassurance, and so on have been overemphasized in such interaction. In the nearly ten thousand observations made in this study, the children did not once seek reward or affection" (p. 150).

In looking at 1,882 interaction sequences initiated by the therapist, Moustakas and Schalock (1955) reported that to the therapist's offered verbal information ($N = 688$), children responded with five major categories: (1) Attentive Observation, (2) Statement of Condition or Action, (3) Seeking Information, (4) Recognition of Stimulation, or (5) Rejection by Ignoring or Evading of Stimulation. There were no real differences between the disturbed and nondisturbed groups' responses to this therapist behavior. To six subcategories of Therapist Interpretation ($N = 963$), three types of child responses were dominant: (1) Statement of Condition or Action, (2) Recognition, or (3) Rejection by Nonrecognition of Stimulation. Surprisingly, few differences between the disturbed and nondisturbed children surfaced here, with acceptance being the most frequent response. Similarly, to the therapist's statements orienting the child in time ($N = 51$), half of the children's responses accepted and half rejected the orientation, with the disturbed children expressing more hostility. Therapist Suggestions were well accepted by both groups, with Cooperation being the predominant child category.

Therapist responses to children's initiating behaviors ($N = 771$) were also analyzed. To the children's Seeking Information, the therapist responded 13% of the time with Attentive Observation, 73% with Giving Information, and 14% with Seeking Information. There were no significant differences in his responses across the two groups of children. To the children's Directing by Suggestion, and Directing by Command, the therapist's predominant response was Straightforward Cooperation.

This was a most intensive process study, indeed. Its limitations, however, are severe. First, it concerns only 10 4-year-olds seen by one nonblind researcher–therapist in an analogue course of nondirective play therapy. Second, there is no analysis of changes in the process over even the very short course of analogue therapy. Third, we have no real idea of what diagnostic category or underlying pathogenic process characterizes the children described as disturbed. Fourth, we have no idea how many actual analyses were done, so that what was reported as "significant" differences may have been more the result of chance findings among many null findings than of systematic reliable differences. In addition, because the same therapist saw both groups of children, it is questionable whether standard statistical procedures are appropriate to use in the first place.

Besides these points, we learn that this therapist varied his behavior very little across groups and that these nondisturbed and disturbed children behaved very similarly with this therapist. Even the contingencies between the therapist's and children's behavior, taken both ways, varied little across groups. That the disturbed children had relatively more hostility and noninteractive behavior than the nondisturbed children seems entirely consistent with their description as disturbed in conduct generally, and a study of therapy process was hardly needed to confirm this point. Similarly, it can be argued that this therapist provided a consistently therapeutic, nondirective verbal approach to both groups of children. However, it can just as easily be pointed out that there seemed to be very little that was unique in his use of techniques with the disturbed children. In other words, we can ask whether he was providing therapy at all, or at least, whether he was attuning his interventions individually to each client. In a nutshell, this study may have been able to provide clues as to general base rates of interactional behavior for these children with this therapist, and thus provide hints on ways to better focus future research studies.

In 1956, Moustakas, Sigel, and Schalock published their categories for the analysis of child–adult interaction. What they wanted to provide was a procedure and a method for objectively describing adult–child interaction. They wanted their system to be comprehensive, to have relevance and to be meaningful, and to include behaviors that would be easy to identify. They also wanted to develop a system that would be of use to researchers of differing theoretical orientations. In assessing their categories, they applied them to three adult–child types of interaction: therapist–child and mother–child in a laboratory playroom, and mother–child at home. The overall reliability of the categories was well within the acceptable range across all situations.

Of particular concern here was the therapist–child interaction. One therapist, who saw two anxious and withdrawn children in 45-minute sessions, was employed. The description of the therapist's behavior was much the same as in the earlier study by Moustakas and Schalock: "Approximately 93% of the therapist's behavior consisted of attentively observing the child; that is, his most frequent response was in the nature of *being there*, watching and listening. Interpretation and Orientation were the only other approaches used to any considerable extent by the therapist" (p. 131). So too, the children's behavior was quite limited in range: Approximately 95% of their time was spent in solitary behavior. "Nonrecognition or rejection of the therapist by ignoring or evading the therapist's stimulations was the most frequent interactive behavior, accounting for about 37% of the child's total behavior" (p. 131).

Interestingly, the children's style of interaction was different with the mother, in both the play situation and at home, with each being far more interactive than with the therapist. This study suggests (but only suggests) that the therapist's style of interaction differed from the mothers', and that the children responded differentially to them. It also suggests what might be expected: a natural suppression of a child's basic response rates with a stranger in a strange situation. One can thus wonder how representative the behavior of a couple of children is when it takes place in one or two meetings with a stranger who must seem interactively odd as compared with their primary caregiver. Moustakas and colleagues' work may thus be indicative only of very early therapeutic interactions with very young children, if indicative at all (for it may still be something about the individual therapist, or setting, that accounts for the children's behavior). More generally, the findings suggest that the category system does allow for differentiation of therapy play talk from play talk with the mother in the laboratory, and of the latter from talk with the mother at home in familiar surroundings. The findings may also suggest that "being there" may be a consistent structure of nondirective play therapy. Obviously, a better formulation of the structure of "being there" is needed, one that is richer both theoretically and empirically (i.e., tied to actual sets of behaviors).

The next year Lebo (1956) published another study, this time assessing the suitability of play therapy for children of differing ages. He hypothesizes that play therapy may not be well suited to the pubescent 12-year-old group. Suitability in this study was indexed by the number of verbalizations of the child: "The amount of verbal productivity of the child in relation to the length of the therapist's speech is often regarded as indicative of therapeutic success. If the child speaks little, it is felt that successful communication has not been established and that therapy is headed for failure" (p. 233). Lebo again chose normal children, four at each of five age levels (4, 6, 8, 10, and 12), and recorded their speech in three 1-hour therapy sessions conducted by the same play therapist. Total number of statements, statements made while playing with recommended and non-recommended toys, and while not playing with toys, were calculated.

Lebo (1956) reported that there were 4,092 statements made by the 20 children in the three sessions, which translates into roughly 68 child statements per session, if they were evenly distributed. Apparently, they were not. Lebo reports that 1,131, 863, 891, 759, and 448 statements were made by 4-, 6-, 8-, 10-, and 12-year-olds, respectively. There were 2,579 statements made when playing with a recommended toy, only about 8% of which were made by the twelve year olds; other age groups made between roughly 20% and 28%. This was the most striking difference between the 12-year-olds and the other age groups. There were only 581 statements made while playing with nonrecommended toys. Here again, the 12-year-olds only accounted for about 12% of these statements whereas 4-year-olds accounted for 26%, and 8-year-olds another 34%. Lebo concluded from this data that "toys do not adversely affect the frequency of verbalizations at age levels four through ten. However, the recommended toys seem to sharply lose their effectiveness at the twelve-year age level. The unpopularity of recommended toys is not a gradually developing process. It seems to appear suddenly" (p. 236).

This study was hypothesis-testing in character. Once again, however, there is no attention to contingencies between therapist and child behavior or to changes or developments in the process of therapy. Most striking, despite Lebo's explicit hypothesis, there is no effort to relate processes to actual outcomes. The study focuses on normal children being seen in an artificially shortened course of "therapy" by one, and only one, therapist. Obviously, generalizations from this study to actual therapy with actual clients with different therapists are impossible. One can certainly wonder if 12-year-old disturbed, rather than nondisturbed, children might not in fact behave similarly to their chronologically younger nondisturbed counterparts on some dimensions, including rate of verbalizations, with recommended and nonrecommended toys. The current study does little to help answer this question.

There is a further problem with this study that clearly stands out. The analyses that Lebo (1956) conducted do not control for the overall frequency of statements made by each group. For example, it is true that 12-year-olds only made 7.79% of all statements made when children are playing with toys, and 4-year-olds made 28.34%. However, of the 448 statements of the 12-year-olds, 201 of them were made when they were playing with toys, 44.8%. Of the 1,131 statements of the 4-year-olds, 731 of them were made when playing with toys, 64.6%. So there is still a difference, but now one of 50% and not a huge 400%! The strongest conclusion to make from this study is that exposure to a play therapy room full of toys and a nondirective therapist is associated with a reduction in normal children's verbal output as their age increases from 4 to 12.

Lebo and Lebo (1957) published a more comprehensive study of aggression and age in relation to verbal expression in nondirective play therapy. These authors formulated and tested eleven hypotheses. Briefly, with respect to aggression, they hypothesized that aggressive children would show more aggressive types of verbal behavior, tell more stories, show more interactive interest in the counselor, show less dependent behavior in their speech, and be less polite than nonaggressive children. With respect to age trends, they hypothesized that 4- and 6-year-olds' aggressive and assertive speech would be more prominent and that they would test the playroom rules more frequently, would interest themselves in the counselor more readily, and would be less polite than the 9- and 12-year-olds. It was also hypothesized that 6-year-old children would tell the most stories, more than 4-year-olds, who lack some forms of storytelling competence, and more than 9- and 12-year-olds, who have been socialized away from storytelling per se as an interactive or solitary play strategy.

Children's aggressiveness was assessed by their scores on teacher-rated scales focusing on aggression and dominance. Groups of children were formed by application of cutoff scores that had been used previously in the literature. There were between 20 and 24 children in each of the four age groups and between 26 and 36 children in each of the three levels of aggression. Children were seen in three 1-hour nondirective play-therapy sessions by the same therapist, the senior author. Three percent of the "verbatim style records" were randomly selected and scored with Lebo's (1955) revised 24-category system. Analyses were done both on frequencies and proportions, using nonparametric procedures. Only the results from the analyses of the proportions will be presented, for reasons mentioned earlier.

The authors reported that there were significant differences between the groups of aggressive children on 11 of the 24 categories, and differences between the age groups on 10 of the 24 categories. Eight of the same categories are involved in the significant differences in both analyses. The authors summarized the results as follows:

> 1. The speech of the aggressive children contained significantly more comments about their play, aggressive statements, story units, definite decisions, explorations of the limits, evidences of interest in the counselor, attempts to establish a relationship with the counselor, negative statements about the self, positive statements about the self, and significantly more exclamations that did the nonaggressive children. 2. The speech of the aggressive children contained fewer unclassifiable remarks (Yes, Hello, OK) than the speech of the nonaggressive group. 3. The speech of the younger children (those ages four or six, and sometimes also those aged nine), contained significantly more aggressive statements, story units, explorations of the limits, evidences of interest in the counselor, attempts to establish a relationship with the counselor, negative statements about the self, positive statements about the self, comments pertaining to time, sound effects, and significantly more statements which could not be heard than did the children aged twelve. 4. The speech of the younger children contained significantly fewer unclassifiable remarks (Yes, Hello, OK) than did that of the twelve year olds. (p. 10)

Lebo and Lebo (1957) concluded that the process of nondirective play therapy is different for children of differing levels of aggression and age and suggested that theory and research on nondirective play therapy needs to incorporate such knowledge in the future.

Findings in this report seem to corroborate Lebo's earlier work on aggression in play therapy. The generalizability of these findings remains problematic, however, due to several severe limitations. Again, we have only one therapist, Lebo himself, who obviously must have been aware of the children's general age level, and perhaps even their likely membership in one of the aggression groups. We have no analysis of developing processes in the course of therapy. We have no analysis of contingencies between the therapist and the children's verbal behavior. From the data, one can infer an interaction between age group and aggression group, but no direct analyses were undertaken to assess this possibility. Besides the teacher ratings on an objective rating system, which represents an advance over simple teacher nominations, there is no diagnostic assessment of the children or classification of type of psychogenic process giving rise to their aggressiveness. Such limitations mandate that the results of this study are merely suggestive and need further corroboration in better designed studies.

Summary

In the first two decades of child psychotherapy process research, each of the eight studies focused on client-centered play therapy. With respect to the clients, four of the eight empirical studies included children 6 years old or younger, and no study included children older than age 12. Children were either nondisturbed or had problems with aggressive conduct or anxiety. There were a total of 134 children studied in the 1940s and 1950s. In terms of the therapist and therapies, only one study may have included courses of therapy lasting over four sessions. As best as we could determine, there were a total of five different therapists involved in the eight empirical studies. In fact, it is possible that two therapists, Moustakas and Lebo, treated all but four of the 134 children in the studies. Both therapists would be considered highly experienced.

In terms of the aims of, and methods used in, the studies, all were focused as assessing some aspect of the in-session process of client-centered play therapy, and none of the studies attempted to relate processes to outcomes. Each study used verbal and nonverbal coding systems to assess client and therapist behavior in the sessions. Only one study assessed changes over time points or phases of therapy, and only three studies looked at dependencies between therapist and child behavior, and this was done using contingent relative frequencies (i.e., percentages of types of utterances following a certain criterion utterance), rather than more systematic methods of analyses (e.g., those based on conditional probabilities or cross-correlations). Several studies assessed differences in involvement in therapy processes as a function of age and level of psychological disturbance (basically normal children vs. disturbed children). Anyone looking critically at any given study, however, could find multiple serious threats to its validity—internal, external, and statistical conclusion validity.

In terms of findings, however, several deserve mention. First, these authors did demonstrate fairly convincingly that verbal and some aspects of nonverbal behavior of therapist–client interaction could be reliably coded. Second, at least some of the categories of description could be useful in discriminating the in-session behavior of children of differing ages and the in-session behavior of aggressive versus normal children.

There are other more substantive findings as well. For example, the exchange of objective information through the seeking and responsive giving of information, about events in and outside of the sessions, seems to be a constituent of the client-centered therapy process. Whether it contains active change producing potential was, however, a question that was not addressed. Similarly, therapist behaviors indicating recognition, attentive concern, and a focus on the client experience (restating or reflecting clients' feelings) also seem to be a constituent of the client-centered therapy process, which should come as no surprise. The question of how such relationship factors, which were remarkably constant across groups of clients, come to be involved in client change is not answered empirically in any of these studies. The closest we came to an answer to this question is in the very first study, where we find that most of the children's responding followed therapist nondirective statements, and that the children's expression of negative feelings increased over time (in the context of a stable level of positive feelings), but this is hardly strong evidence! Be that as it may, this finding does seem to suggest that there was a demonstrable relationship between the theory of client-centered technique and what these therapists actually did in the sessions.

In conclusion, if we were to speculate about where to locate change processes from this set of studies, something like the following might be reasonable. First, there may be something corrective about therapists' behaviors that emphasize and highlight an attentive and concerned stance of "being there" or "being with" the client. There is even some suggestion that this stance should be instantiated differently—at least across the 4- to 12-year-old age levels. Second, there may be something corrective in therapists' behaviors that formulate, emphasize, and highlight the clients' moods, or feelings, or affects as these create the subjective contexts through which "objective" events are understood. In other words, and not surprisingly, from these studies we might conjecture that intervention strategies focused on the relationship and on the affective dimensions of interaction will have something essential to do with securing positive client change.

THE 1960s

Guerney, Burton, Silverberg, and Shapiro (1965) developed a coding system to be applied to tape recordings, rather than direct observation, of children's play-therapy sessions. They used four content categories (Positive and Negative Feeling, Dependence, and Leadership) in addition to two "leftover" categories (Not Applicable and Inaudible). The authors were particularly interested in two questions: (1) Could the categories be reliably applied, and (2) could the adult verbal responses in nondirective play sessions be used to understand children's corresponding in-session behavior? Roughly 200 fifteen-second segments from six different tapes of child play sessions were coded. The authors reported that all categories were reliably coded and that there was nearly a perfect rank-order correlation between the adults' and the children's category usage. The authors concluded, on the basis of their analyses and on the basis of "their qualitative observation, [that] when the adult is taking a client-centered role, his responses seem to provide a valid picture of the behavior of the child" (p. 616).

Although the data may provide some evidence of the categories' reliable application, there is little that should convince us that we get an accurate picture of the children's behavior from the therapists' behavior. There could be a near perfect rank-order correlation between the adult and the child categories without there being any contingency between them! Furthermore, we really do not know what samples were looked at from what part of therapy, and so on. Consequently, this study fits in the tradition of child process studies in terms of its emphasis on measure development.

Similarly, Dana and Dana (1969) reported a study of the systematic observation of children's behavior in two types of group therapy, one Rogerian and one more dynamic. Five groups of three to five children (ages 3 to 8) of various diagnoses (we are not told what they are) were seen for 15 to 19 sessions by two therapists. Six categories were used to code behavior in the sessions: (1) Watching, (2) Movement, (3) Play While Alone, (4) Play with Child, (5) Vocalization, (6) Speaks to Child and Speaks to Therapist. The authors reported no statistical analyses in their paper but claimed that

> inspection of these results suggested that, while all groups increased in frequency of movement, the Rogerian aegis seemed to produce some general inhibition of play, vocalization, and speech. Relatively less change was noted for "conventional" therapy groups, although there was some increase in amount of speech directed toward the therapist. (p. 134)

Like many studies during this period, the primary focus of this work is on the development of reliable coding procedures for in-session child behavior. And although the study fails to report even the most rudimentary statistical analyses, attention is directed toward comparisons of treatment process across types of child therapy.

Summary

Although very small in scale and brief in report, these two studies from the 1960s marked some eventful changes. First, recordings were now being further explored as a means by which to secure process data, and it was shown that categories of therapist and child responses could be reliably coded from such recordings. Second, the study by Guerney and colleagues (1965) seemed to pose a new question about the mirroring or tracking quality of interaction in play therapy, although the rank-order analyses fell short of revealing the type of dependent relationships one would need to describe such phenomena in detail. Third, the study by Dana and Dana (1969) presents the first comparative process study, one that looks at changes in in-therapy behavior over the course of treatment as a function of "brands" of treatment, client-centered versus psychodynamic. One may also note that now several therapists are studied, rather than a single one, as in many studies in the 1950s. Fourth, actual clients in real courses of group therapy are now being studied.

Admittedly, both of these studies are crude, to say the least, and in themselves offer little by way of substantive findings about the process of child psychotherapy. They perhaps can be seen as marking a transition from an exclusive focus on client-centered therapy to comparative treatments, and from a focus on relative frequencies to a more comprehensive way of studying the relationship between what the therapist does and what the client does.

THE 1970s

In the 1970s, five studies continued the trends initiated during the previous decade. Boll (1971) attempted to duplicate Dana and Dana's (1969) study, only he focused on children 8 to 11 years old rather than 3 to 8 years old. It is unclear from the published report who were the therapists. Interestingly, the 15–20 sessions with the four or five children were divided into early (Weeks 1 through 5) versus late (Weeks 6 through 10) periods. Again no statistical analyses were reported, but the authors note that the children treated by an active therapist did not increase their activity levels, whereas the children treated by the nondirective therapist "increased their amount of play, vocalization, speech and movement markedly" (p. 26), just the opposite of the findings of Dana and Dana (1969). The nondirective group was also described as more hostile and aggressive than the directive group.

Again, this study begins to look at type of therapy by time phase of treatment. The "look" is again rather crude, and we really do not have enough information to assess its contribution. For example, there is no information in the report about diagnostic or other characteristics of the clients, except for their ages. The authors themselves suggest that future studies can use systematic observation of in-therapy events to begin to assess the effects of therapist, age of patient, concurrent other treatments, as well as therapeutic orientation.

Wright, Truax, and Mitchell (1972) sought to assess the applicability to child therapy of three scales that had been frequently used in adult process research, namely, accurate empathy, nonpossessive warmth, and genuineness. Because these scales had been tied to adult verbal expression and because child therapy was thought to rely often on nonverbal behaviors, the authors felt that their suitability in child therapy research should be assessed rather than presumed. The first question to be addressed was whether they could be reliably applied by raters to child therapy data.

To assess their reliability, three 5-minute segments from two sessions of therapy conducted by 16 different therapists were rated on the three scales by three trained observers. Reliabilities for accurate empathy, nonpossessive warmth, and genuineness were reported to be .72, .53, and .34 respectively, all significantly different from chance. The authors also reported a significant correlation between accurate empathy and nonpossessive warmth ($r = .50$). Appropriately, they concluded that although statistically significant, the reliabilities for nonpossessive warmth and genuineness were lower than what had been typically obtained with adult therapists. For this reason, they suggested that these adult scales be revised in order to be more suitable for assessment of the therapist-offered conditions in child therapy, ones that may be offered more nonverbally than in adult treatment. One can see that this study falls right in line with those concerned with measure development and with attunement to the special needs of child therapy.

Like the Boll (1971) study and the earlier Dana and Dana (1969) investigation, changes in play therapy over time were also a focus of Siegel's (1972) study, but with therapist-offered conditions added as another factor. In this study, 16 children in grades two through four were seen by 16 play therapists. Four-minute excerpts from Sessions 3, 8, 12, and 16 were coded on the 24-category system used by Lebo (1955) and on the Accurate Empathy, Unconditional Positive Regard, and Genuineness Scales. These scales all obtained adequate reliabilities (.81, .70, .84, respectively), qualifying Wright, Truax, and Mitchell's earlier findings and suggestions.

The four children receiving the highest therapeutic conditions were compared with the four children receiving the lowest therapist-offered conditions. The authors reported some very suggestive results. There were no statistical differences between the groups on their use of the 24 language categories in Session 3. However, group differences were found in later sessions. In Session 8, the high-conditions group showed more positive statements about themselves than the group that received low therapist-offered conditions. In the 12th session, the high condition group showed more aggressive statements and insight statements. In the 16th session, the same group showed more positive statements about themselves and more insight than the low therapist-offered condition group.

This study is notable in that it attempted to study a hypothesized change process—therapist-offered conditions—and to record its impact at various levels over several time points in therapy with real clients and real therapists. It also is the first study we have seen in which insight statements are actually recorded and presumably made by the children in the treatment session. Unfortunately, we are not provided with the data or with within-group analyses to see if trends over time existed in the use of the process categories. We also have no way of knowing if there might have been a diagnostic category × conditions interaction, or psychopathogenic process × levels of offered conditions interaction. It should also be pointed out that if each and every one of the 24 Lebo (1955) categories was compared at each time point across the two groups, then 96 comparisons would have been made and only five differences found—hardly different from what might have been expected by chance. Obviously, there are a host of alternative competing explanations for the findings, even if they were statistically robust. For example, it could very well be that there is some other therapist trait correlated with level of therapist-offered conditions that might have been responsible for the process difference. Nevertheless, we can see some development in the sophistication of the questions being asked, and we can see some continuity in the fledgling tradition of process research on child therapy—even if it boils down simply to the use of the same descriptive category system!

In 1973, Truax, Altmann, Wright, and Mitchell published the substantive findings of their reliability study of therapist-offered conditions. This article contains by far the most thorough reporting of subject and therapist characteristics, as well as data collection and analyses, to date. For example, we learn that the 16 therapists consisted of four Ph.D.-level clinical child psychologists, six were child psychiatry residents in their third year of training, and six were clinical psychology interns. The psychiatric interns were in psychodynamically oriented training, and the psychologists, Ph.D.'s and interns, were described at basically eclectic in orientation. The 16 patients were on average 9 years and 3 months in age, and were described as having mild emotional problems, considered to be primarily neurotic or character disordered in nature.

We receive precise information on what samples of interaction were studied: "Three 5-minute samples were taken from each of two regularly scheduled therapy sessions one week apart for each case. The 5-minute video tape samples were taken at the 20th to 25th minute, the 30th to 35th minute, and the 40th to 45th minute of each session" (p. 313). These 96 segments were rated on their level of accurate empathy, nonpossessive warmth, and genuineness by separate groups of three raters each. The most outstanding feature of this study, however, was its attempt to relate process differences in levels of therapist-offered conditions, not to process differences emerging in later sessions as had been done before, but to outcome differences—the very first in the literature! A host of child *and* adult outcome measures were used: Therapists evaluated the children early and late in therapy on the Current Adjustment Rating Scale and on a five-item follow-up questionnaire; parents filled out the Item Rating Scale early and late; and a psychometrist administered the adult-based Psychiatric Status Schedule.

The authors reported that the psychometrist ratings on the Psychiatric Status scales indicated that the children improved from early to late in therapy on three items (out of an unreported number of analyses): amount of change in last year, relationships with friends and family, and children's satisfaction with their own adjustment). There were, however, no significant differences between the children receiving the high versus the low therapist-offered conditions. Several important differences did emerge in the therapist- and in the parent-reported outcome data. The children showed improvement on 8 of the 13 nonredundant items on the Current Adjustment Scale: (1) Overall function, (2) Change in past year, (3) Relations with friends and relatives, (4) School adjustment, (5) Own satisfaction with adjustment, (6) Attaining school potential, (7) Attaining potential as a person, (8) Friends' satisfaction with their relationship with the child. Additionally, on three items—(1) Overall function, (2) Overall change in past year, and (3) Relationship with friends and relatives—there was superior improvement reported for the children who received the high therapeutic conditions than the low conditions.

Similarly, the parents reported that children changed significantly on the following 8 of 31 items on the Item Rating Scale: (1) Likes teacher more, (2) Talks less hatefully, (3) Less emotionally disturbed, (4) Fears have decreased, (5) Laughs more, (6) More sociable, (7) Respects adults more, and (8) Enjoys playing with other children. On nine items—(1) Overall score, (2) Less emotionally disturbed, (3) Fears have decreased, (4) Laughs more, (5) More sociable, (6) More controllable, (7) Needs less tranquilizing medicine, 8) Develops fewer bad habits, and (9) More able to express feelings—the children receiving high therapist-offered conditions improved more than the children receiving low conditions. On most significant items, the improvement in the high conditions group was two points greater than that of the low conditions group on the 9-point scales used in the study. The authors also reported for the first time deterioration effects:

"Children seen by therapists in the lower half on therapeutic conditions showed deterioration on five times as many measures as children seen in the upper half on conditions" (p. 317).

The authors concluded that "high therapeutic conditions produced positive change while low therapeutic conditions produced negative change, suggesting that child therapy can be a two-edged sword: Depending upon the therapist's level of interpersonal skill, it can be for better or for worse" (p. 317). They underscored this point by noting that the average score for the accurate empathy and nonpossessive warmth was higher for the low therapy conditions than that reported in other studies using the same split-half methodology. Moreover, the therapists in the study were mostly eclectic and psychodynamic in training, not expert client-centered counselors, showing that the importance of these conditions cuts across therapy orientation.

Here was one of the first process–outcome studies in child psychotherapy, one that even incorporates multiple outcome measures from three different sources. Obviously, many things could be improved in this study: Samples were small; reliabilities of two of the process measures probably attenuated the results to some degree; there may well have been a confound of therapy orientation, race or gender of the therapists with levels of therapist-offered conditions; and the statistical procedures could certainly have been handled better. We should, of course, be worried about the lack of random assignment of children to therapists: perhaps there were some children to whom therapists could offer the therapeutic conditions more easily, and these children were not distributed evenly across the high and low groups. Even with these faults, this study seems to shine in comparison to those published previously. It does offer some evidence of a process–outcome relationship between an hypothesized key "process" element that cuts across brand-name therapies.

Another notable feature of the Truax et al. (1973) study is how the construction of scales is so painstakingly tied to a theory of the "necessary and sufficient" conditions of therapy, that is, how yoked the scales are to the conceptualization of a therapeutic condition provided by therapists. One should be careful here, for these conditions are often talked about as though they are processes. In fact, according to client-centered theory, it is the constant and stable provision of high levels of these conditions provided throughout the course of therapy that is thought to provide the type of environment in which processes of client growth could occur. The difference between stable conditions or constant structures and their variable quantitative or qualitative processes can be seen more sharply in other studies in the 1980s and 1990s, which use more sophisticated data-analytic techniques.

Truax and Wittmer (1973) published another process–outcome study, this time focusing on a different population, a different modality of treatment (i.e., group therapy), and on a different potential therapist provided mechanism of change. In this study, 73 delinquents, 14 to 18 years old, half females in residential treatment, were assigned to eight therapy groups on a random basis. Six therapists, one psychoanalytic, two client centered, and three eclectic, who were all relatively experienced, provided group sessions roughly twice a week for a total of 24 sessions. The study's purpose was to evaluate the relationship "between the therapist's confronting clients with their defense mechanisms and therapeutic outcome" (p. 201).

Over 350 samples, two from each session, were reliably rated by two experienced clinicians on a 5-point Likert-type scale assessing the degree of therapist confrontation of the adolescent defense mechanisms. Groups were dichotomized into relatively high and relatively low levels of defense confrontation, and the two groups differed significantly. Change scores (pretherapy scores minus posttherapy scores) were compared across groups on numerous dependent measures ($N = 20$), with the pretherapy scores serving also as a covariate. The authors reported that "in virtually all measures of outcome, those patients who were confronted with defense mechanisms showed the greatest therapeutic gain. . . . Overall, then, the findings support the psychoanalytic and learning theory orientations toward utilizing confrontation of defense mechanisms" (p. 203).

This study actually begins to examine the relation between a pathogenic target (defense mechanisms) and a technique (confrontation) that is aimed at altering it, albeit both elaborated in only the broadest fashion. We are not dealing with diagnoses or brands of therapy comparatively assessed, but specified, problematic psychological structures and interventions specifically aimed to bring about their change. Unfortunately, we do not find out how the interventions are delivered over the course of treatment, or how the defense mechanisms change (e.g., in qualitative leaps, by incremental softening, or by transformation). Moreover, we learn little about their processive interaction, the contingencies between the children's defense utilization and the therapists' confrontation. In the 1980s and 1990s there is greater emphasis on these issues and how best to examine the content and form of child therapy. However, this study reflects a dramatic shift in focus; *pathogenic mechanisms and therapist interventions now constitute the essential processes under investigation.*

Summary

This could be called the first decade in child psychotherapy process research when comparative studies reign supreme. Of the four nonmeasurement development studies, two are comparative process studies and two are comparative process–outcome studies. But there are more significant developments as well. First, all of the studies concern children with real problems, who are treated by practicing clinicians in realistic courses of therapy from a variety of brand-name perspectives (client-centered, psychodynamic, eclectic). Second, three of the four studies concern, not traditional comparisons of brand-name therapies, but comparisons of levels of component therapist processes (provision of therapist conditions or confrontation) that are thought to cut across orientations and to be causally related to both client in-session changes and to outcomes. Third, one study actually pinpoints a plausible pathogenic structure (clients' use of defense mechanisms) as a target for the therapists' interventions. Fourth, multiple measures and multiple perspectives are used to assess outcomes. Fifth, the quality of the studies, the size of the samples of the therapists and the clients, and the statistical techniques all seem to have improved over those found in the previous decade. Sixth, for the first time, studies include adolescents, rather than mostly very young children (3- and 4-year-olds); and seventh, there is evidence that not only emotional or interpersonal changes occur in the client during sessions, but also cognitive changes, as measured by insight and levels of self-evaluation.

We find out that therapist-offered conditions can be reliably coded from recordings of child psychotherapy and that such reliability can vary across research labs. We find that in all three studies that assess a therapist-offered condition or a therapist-offered intervention strategy (confronting children's defenses), that higher levels lead to more positive client change both in the course of therapy itself and at outcome. In fact, the outcome data, although significant across three different sources of evaluation (therapist, parent, and psychometrist), were still less dramatic than they might have been had the results not been attenuated by the relatively low reliabilities in the Wright et al. (1972) study.

Summarizing the substantive findings in the most general way, the studies in the 1970s suggest that interpersonal processes, or the therapist-offered relationship, can affect both in-session client changes and post-therapy outcomes. Moreover, therapist implementation of an intervention strategy specifically targeted at a pathogenic process can also affect positive change at outcome, even in group therapy that is generally known to result in less substantial gains than individual therapy.

There are obvious limitations to these studies, methodologically and conceptually. One glaring problem methodologically is the lack of control for therapist effects or effects of orientation. It could very well be that differences in therapist-offered conditions were not what caused the process or outcome differences, but some other therapist characteristic. Since therapists were not randomly assigned, and since key therapist factors were not controlled, we cannot rule out alternative explanations focusing on differences between therapists comprising the high and low therapist conditions groups. The same argument is relevant when considering the mix of orientations in the high and low groups.

Another problem has to do with the use of single item scales for such complex constructs as accurate empathy, unconditional positive regard, and genuineness, or even "confrontation of defenses" and the generally low levels achieved on these scales for even the group designated as "high." Moreover, there are other problems with construct validity, reliability, and predictive validity. As Mitchell, Bozarth, and Krauft (1977) conclude in a reappraisal of the therapeutic effectiveness of these interpersonal conditions, "The mass of data neither supports or rejects the overriding influence of such variables as empathy, warmth, and genuineness in all cases" (p. 483).

There is another sort of limitation as well. Although mechanisms of defense were used as targets for therapist confrontations, it can be expected that different sorts of predominant defenses could lead to the same diagnostic outcome (juvenile delinquency) in different individuals. For example, isolation of affect may enable one teenager to act cruelly to others without feeling remorse, just as projection may provoke another teenager to act cruelly to others because they seem to deserve punishment. We can speculate that the very positive findings for levels of confrontations could have been even more substantial had the juveniles been assessed for their predominant defense and confrontations individually targeted. In other words, although the study has the virtue of focusing on a pathogenic mechanism and a therapist intervention, understanding the process of change will require greater specification of both components.

THE 1980s

Howe and Silvern (1981) presented a study focused on the development of a research instrument to be used in collecting observations of children in play therapy. Interestingly, this study was the first in the literature to propose criteria, substantive *and* quantitative, that any observational system for play therapy should satisfy and then used them in a critical review of past observational systems. The six criteria are worth mentioning:

1. Behaviors relevant to major schools of play therapy should be included.
2. Behaviors relevant to psychodiagnosis, therapy process, and outcome should be included.
3. Dimensions of behavior whose interrelationships are considered controversial in the literature should be measured separately.
4. Reliability must be demonstrated.

5. Subsets of related behaviors must be shown to empirically cohere and thus reflect underlying dimensions of a construct.
6. Such clusters should be shown to be stable.

In reviewing a subset of the extant coding systems, Howe and Silvern (1981) found it seriously lacking. Problems cited included the confounding of behaviors that might be relevant to different underlying dimensions of children behavior (e.g., overt and fantasy aggression coded into the same category); categories of behavior clearly relevant to clinical theories were routinely omitted (e.g., style of coping strategies); inclusion of categories relevant to only one theoretical perspective (mostly client-centered); and basing the construction of category systems on

> a methodological rationale which ruled out the possibility of assessing playroom behavior in terms of theory-related concepts of individual differences linked to theoretical controversies. The strategy underlying these research efforts (Lebo, 1952; Moustakas & Schalock, 1955) was to construct a list of categories capable of classifying every child behavior or comment, regardless of its purported significance for diagnosis or therapy process. (Howe & Silvern, 1981, p. 169)

The authors criticized the previous research efforts on three other grounds: They used mutually exclusive categories, which ruled out finding underlying dimensions of behavior; they failed to assess the stability of the behavioral ratings; and the previous authors often presented overall percent agreement between ratings on all of the categories, so it was impossible to determine which specific categories in the system were reliable by more appropriate means (agreements corrected for chance, correlations, etc.).

Howe and Silvern (1981) then reviewed the theoretical and empirical literatures that form the basis for the selection of the four content domains—(1) Emotional discomfort, (2) Competency, (3) Coping strategies, and (4) Fantasy play—to be assessed. For each content domain or dimension of behavior, the authors formulated a set of "more narrow, behavioral a priori categories thought to be conceptually linked to the dimension in question" (p. 170). Significantly, the authors leave to empirical study the question of whether the specific selected behaviors actually reflect the proposed dimensions.

Two raters were trained in the use of the 31 items. After training was completed, they scored 76 12-minute segments of therapy drawn from two consecutive sessions of treatment with ten 4- to 12-year-old children of widely different pathologies (psychotic to borderline to neurotic). Therapists were either doctoral or postdoctoral students. Analyses revealed that adequate reliabilities were obtained on only 13 of the 31 items (intraclass correlation .45 and percent agreement within a point of 80% across the 76 segments).

Factor analysis of the 13 items and analyses of their interrelationships were used, rather than their a priori groupings, to form multiitem scales. The authors reported three nonredundant scales—(1) Emotional Discomfort Scale, (2) Fantasy Play Scale, and (3) Social Inadequacy Scale—defined by five, four, and four items, respectively. Items defining the Emotional Discomfort Scale were (1) Talks about worries and troublesome events, (2) Inappropriate aggression at the therapist, (3) Conflicted play, (4) Quality and intensity of affect, and (5) Play disruption. Items defining the Fantasy Play Scale were (1) Variations in fantasy story scenes, (2) Qualitatively different fantasy roles, (3) Abrupt fluctuations between fantasy and reality, and (4) Time spent concentrating play on characters rather than things. It should be pointed out that Item 3 correlates negatively (-.73) with the scale. Items defining the Social Inadequacy Scale were (1) Body stiffness, (2) Incoherent or bizarre content, (3) Therapist not included in the activities, and (4) Therapist interventions met with hostility or withdrawal. The authors also reported a fourth Maladjustment Scale, comprised of all of the items on the Emotional Discomfort and Social Inadequacy Scales (which were significantly correlated, $r = .51$), except the frequency-of-talk-about-worries item. Each scale was stable across segments within sessions and across the two sessions sampled from each treatment.

This study is notable for its attempt to use theory to guide the development of measures of underlying dimensions of therapy process and for its relative methodological sophistication. This study attempts to locate essential processes to study, based on clinical and developmental theory, and does not purport to be interested in everything that happens in the therapy hour. Its findings, too, add something to our knowledge of the structure of child participation in play therapy. For instance, whereas most previous studies had included single, mutually exclusive categories pertaining to separable aspects of emotion/feelings, aggression, interactive quality of interaction, and fantasy play, the current study makes a significant step forward in identifying the underlying dimensions that these individual items seem to index. The analysis of stability was especially instructive, in that it showcased one way to assess whether the proposed measures of process could provide an adequate basis for investigating individual differences—without stability, differences may be due to measurement errors.

As the authors acknowledged themselves, the study has significant limitations. First, we should note that at most, it provides some information on how the child's participation in play therapy was structured and how the structures seemed to be interrelated. There is no investigation of changes, qualitative or quantitative, in these structures over time, and there

is no investigation of the relationship between these structures of participation and outcome. Second, there is no investigation of how the identified
structures of participation might have varied across the children in the
sample. One would have expected significantly different scale scores across
children of such disparate diagnostic classes. Thus, we find out little about
process differences that might be predicted by type of pathology. Third,
we must note that there is no investigation of the therapists' behavior or
differences in orientation and their relationship to the children's participation or diagnosis. In other words, we learn very little about process. As
the authors conclude, "In the context of a current absence of empirical
research concerning play therapy and related diagnostic procedures, the
value of the present study was primarily in the demonstration of some
degree of success in developing a methodology for reliable, clinically
relevant observations of children's play therapy" (p. 181).

Mook (1982a, 1982b) published two articles focused on therapist and
client verbal participation, respectively, in a series of therapy sessions with
two child clients. Procedures and analyses were similar in both papers,
although different coding systems were employed. In the study of the
therapists' participation, Mook employed three systems to assess the
therapists' verbal behavior: a category system to code the type of verbal-re-
sponse mode the therapist used (e.g., interpretation, approval–reassurance, information, reflection, etc.); the Carkhuff scales for empathic
understanding and respect; and a system of "grammatical" categories for
assessing the nature of the verbal inquiry (affirmative, negative, and
questioning), tenses (e.g., present, past, future), the nature of subject
(client, therapist, or other) and the nature of the object (person, thing,
none). The speech of two female graduate students was transcribed and
coded. They each saw a female child client, one 8 and one 12 years old,
biweekly over a 6-month period, and were supervised in an integrative
humanistic and dynamic model of treatment. Five audiotapes were transcribed for one therapist and four for the other, one session being sampled
from each of the last five months of therapy.

Like many of the early studies of process, Mook focused on the
applicability of "adult" measures to therapist behaviors. However, his most
innovative analyses employed a version of factor analysis developed by
Cattell in the 1940s and applied by Cattell and Luborsky (1950) and others
in the study of psychotherapy processes in adult treatment. Basically, this
version of factor analysis, called P-technique (see Russell, 1995) is applied
to a single subject's scores on a set of variables measured repeatedly over
time. The results of the analyses reveal which variables in the set covary
with each other over time, thus revealing underlying patterns or structures
of processes. Mook (1982a) applied this technique to each of the therapist's
scores on the 28 variables making up the empathy scales, the verbal-re-
sponse scores, and the grammatical categories, across the 221 repeated

measurements for Therapist A and the 163 repeated measurements for Therapist B.

Unfortunately, Mook (1982a) did not report the details of the factor analyses (e.g., decision rules for the retention of the factors, amount of total variance each factor accounts for, reliability or stability of the factors, or the equivalence of factors across the two therapists). She did report loadings and interpretations for six factors for each of the therapists. We are told that Therapist A's first three factors account for 60% of the variance. They are described as (1) Client is questioned about herself and others by means of restatement, reflection, and open questions; (2) Therapist encourages and affirms the client in the present; (3) Therapist affirms, approves, and guides present client activity. Factors 4–6 account for another 23% of the variance; (4) Therapist talks about herself and gives information; (5) Therapist questions client about others and things; and (6) Therapist communicates empathy and respect and uses interpretation.

In contrast, the six factors for Therapist B together accounted for 53% of the variance. The six factors are described as follows: (1) Therapist affirms client in present and talks about others, situations, the client, and herself by means of interpretation, minimal encouragement, and restatement; (2) Therapist uses confrontation, self-disclosure, and interpretation with respect; (3) Therapist respectfully questions through open questions and reflections; (4) Therapist gives information, questions about situations through closed questions, and uses direct guidance; (5) Therapist talks in the past tense and uses approval and reassurance; and (6) Therapist talks about herself by means of self-disclosure.

There are obvious parallels and differences between the patternings in the two therapists' speech. Due to the lack of information on the factor analyses, and some obvious problems in the interpretation of the loadings (e.g., Therapist B has bipolar factors that are interpreted as if they were not), it is perhaps best to see this first application of P-technique to child therapists' behavior as an exploration of the feasibility of the method, that is, exactly as the author intended it to be seen. As we will see, improvements in the application of this method can lead to the collection of important information about both the structure and change in the therapist's participation in child treatment. It has the potential of identifying key structures of engagement, as well as paradigmatic types of changes, both qualitative and quantitative, that may illuminate how therapy works. We should point out that even these novice therapists' patterns of participation, taken at a very abstract level, include in their first three factors information seeking, technical work (interpretation, confrontation), and the provision of affirming encouragement—perhaps the triadic heart of therapeutic engagement!

Use of the P-technique with the child data revealed six factors of client participation for each of the girls. Again the details of the analyses are missing. Basically, Mook (1982b) described the first three factors of Client A as accounting for 50% of the variance in her verbal participation. Factor 1 was basically a grammatical category indicating that the child's speech is oriented in the affirmative in the present tense and is concerned, not with herself or therapist, but other subjects. Factor 2 described the client's speech as concerned with her problems and self-exploration, that is, the work of therapy seen from the client's side. Factor 3 described an information-seeking pattern of discourse. Factor 4 was a play factor oriented to the formulation of plans, and Factors 5 and 6 basically described friendly discussions or talk about things unrelated to the client's problems.

The first two factors of Client B's speech concerned reminiscing in the affirmative about events unrelated to her problems and therapeutic work, that is, self-exploration, statements of her problems and feelings, and understanding and insight. These two factors accounted for 45% of the variance in her speech. The remaining four factors, accounting for an additional 38% of the variance, concerned statements of her problems in the affirmative, simple agreement or cooperation, information and advice seeking, and friendly discussions.

There were commonalities and differences in the organization of the two girls' verbal participation in their therapies. The most striking differences concerned the presence of a play factor oriented to future planning in the younger and not in the older client's speech, and conversely, the presence of insight and understanding in the older but not in the younger child's therapeutic work factor. Also, the older child's speech was temporally oriented to events in the past to a greater degree than the younger child's speech, which was more present, and through play, future oriented. Commonalities included the high degree to which both girls' verbal participation is oriented to concerns not related to their problems, and factors describing therapeutic work, and information and structure seeking.

From both of Mook's (1982a, 1982b) studies, there is very little that we can learn about how or when the underlying organization of the children's or the therapists' speech changes over time or as a function of their interaction—the very substance of process. We do get recurring hints of age differences in the style of participation in play therapy, and we get hints about what might be stable structures of the verbal participation of children in play therapy. But "hints" are really all we get. These were graduate students in training and a mere two clients with only vaguely specified disorders—learning disorders with emotional difficulties. We also do not know what relation any of the so-called processes have to outcomes—considered at the end of therapy or even at a session level. Like the studies before it, this one delivers a promissory note: Here is a method that probably could be used in the future with further refinements to study the process of child psychotherapy in some detail.

Summary

If the 1970s can be considered the decade of the comparative study, then the 1980s can be considered the decade of multi-item scale development. Both a priori and empirical means are employed to develop process scales especially suited to the study of child psychotherapy. Moreover, all three studies can be seen to be concerned with stability: In the Howe and Silvern (1981) study, the stability of children's participation in play therapy is assessed within sessions and across sessions. In the Mook (1982a, 1982b) studies, stability is indirectly examined by the nature of the analytic technique itself: P-technique reveals which variables covary together over time within a client's and therapist's speech.

In addition to refocusing attention on measure development, the studies also place techniques, interpersonal skills, and orientations in time and valence (positive, negative, question) on an even playing field, and ask the empirical question of how they covary. Previously, levels of one dimensions were used to block therapists to study levels of the other variables. Although these methods of research are not unrelated, the studies in the 1980s use much more powerful techniques to reveal interrelationships among processes in child therapy.

Substantively, this set of three studies provides only hints about significant within-session processes, as none of the studies relates its process findings to outcomes. In fact, none of the in-session processes is related to diagnostic dimensions or pathogenic processes. Be that as it may, they still provide useful information, when seen in the context of the other extant process studies.

For example, one key conclusion to be derived from the Mook (1982a) study is that there are empirically demonstrable differences between the processes, in both a structural and temporal sense, instantiated by training therapists who are supervised in one and the same type of therapy. Although one might be tempted to attribute such variability to the therapists' level of experience, Mook's results suggest that treatment types are composed of patterns of therapist behaviors and that there may be substantial variation in their implementation to specific cases. Again this finding underscores the importance of analyzing the actual processes that are implemented in specific cases, and then evaluating how variations in these processes are related to treatment outcome.

There are a number of comparable findings across these studies. For example, we have seen how verbalization of problems and emotions has figured significantly in the descriptions of client participation in child therapy. In the three studies in the 1980s, such verbalizations are not only noted, but also form relatively stable structures in the interactions of the clients. This has been a thread that has woven its way through most of the studies in this tradition. Uncovering conflicts and feelings that are internal through verbalization rather than action is a major emphasis in most child psychotherapies. Interestingly, in all three studies such verbalization is also related to other behaviors constitutive of therapeutic work: attaining insight and understanding, and increasing levels of self-exploration (in Mook, 1982b), and to levels of interpersonal relatedness (in Howe & Silvern, 1981). There is also a lot of process that seems to be "fill" or unrelated to the task of therapy.

With respect to findings concerning therapist structures of participation, we have only the data from the two therapists in the Mook (1982a) study, but here, too, we find some familiar themes. Seeking and giving information and guidance seems a stable structure of therapist participation. Moreover, providing a warm, caring relationship also appears to be another factor of participation—the relationship or interpersonal factor. Finally, an interpretive or cognitive work factor also emerges, with its emphasis on confrontation and interpretation.

These studies all have major flaws that curtail their generalizability. In fact, they were not conceived to provide rock-bottom substantive findings; instead they are indications of how sophisticated studies could and should be conducted in the future. In the 1990s, some of these suggestions have indeed been implemented, at least in terms of further measure development.

THE 1990s

A rash of new efforts at method development have taken place in the early 1990s. In the first study, Smith-Acuna, Durlak, and Kaspar (1991) attempted to develop an all-purpose set of child psychotherapy process scales that could be used to assess therapist and client perceptions of treatment. They used as their sample referred clients ($N = 20$, mean age = 8.9), about equally divided in terms of broad type of disorder (internalizers and externalizers), and who received long-term psychodynamically oriented therapy from 15 graduate students in their beginning years of training. Therapists and clients provided ratings for six sessions that occurred within a 3-month period of treatment. Therapists filled out questionnaires after the completion of sessions, and independent examiners administered the scales to children after the same sessions.

For the therapist, the authors focused on four dimensions: (1) Therapist's positive (12 items) and negative (20 items) affect, (2) Therapist's perception of his or her levels of acceptance (5 items), warmth (4 items), and structuring (3 items), (3) Therapist's perception of children's positive (12 items) and negative (20 items) affect, and (4) Therapist's goals as measured by the degree to which the therapist sought insight (2 items), catharsis (3 items), or independence (4 items). For the parallel child form, only the affect and behavior scales were useful: child's positive (6 items) and negative (8 items) affect; child's perception of therapist's positive (6 items) and negative (8) affect; and child's perception of the therapist's warmth (6 items), acceptance (4 items), and structure (8 items).

The authors reported Cronbach's alphas and item–total correlations for each of the 17 subscales making up their therapist and child report, dropping items from scales that had correlated below .2 with the total score. Sixteen of the original 85 items in the therapist scale were dropped, resulting in internal consistencies ranging between .61 for therapist's warmth to .88 for therapist's perception of child's negative affect. Seven of the original 46 items in the child scale were dropped, resulting in internal consistencies ranging between .68 for child's perception of the therapist's provision of structure to .86 for child's perception of therapist's positive affect. The authors reported that there are no correlations between the therapist and child scales.

In their discussion, Smith-Acuna et al. (1991) noted that, "the scales on both measures either closely paralleled or were identical to those produced in adult studies (Orlinsky & Howard, 1975), suggesting that the basic psychotherapeutic process may be broadly similar for both adults and children" (p. 128), and that their scales were more reliable than the subscales used in the parallel adult instruments. These conclusions seem somewhat speculative and premature, given that (1) items for the scales were basically derived from the adult form, (2) factor analyses were not performed to assess the empirical distinctiveness of the subscales, and (3) no analyses were done to assess if there were any reliable differences in the levels of internal consistency reported for the adult versus the child forms. Similarly, the authors argued, based on the "better" reliability of the child versus the adult forms, child therapists and child clients may have more uniform or less complicated perceptions of the process than their adult counterparts. Again, such a conclusion seems rather speculative, given the data analyses performed, since the perceptions of both therapists and children could have varied quite extensively while the reliability of the raters remains quite good.

This study does break new ground in attempting to assess the perceptions of both participants in the therapy and in attempting to identify "universal" processes in treatment, as judged from the participants' perspectives. It chooses what are by now familiar aspects of session processes for study: affect, interpersonal orientation, and cognitive insight, with an additional focus on independence. Unfortunately, there is little theoretical rationale for these dimensions other than their appearance in an adult process measure. Moreover, like most of the measure development studies reviewed, there is little focus on the in-therapy interaction or on the development of processes over time. The authors do reiterate that "it is important to obtain process data from a perspective independent of both therapists and clients. Independent raters working from audiotapes or videotapes could provide useful information regarding how client and therapist perceptions are anchored behaviorally to events occurring during treatment" (Smith-Acuna et al., 1991, p. 129).

In the same year, Russell, Greenwald, and Shirk (1991) attempted to relate different types of in-session conversational interaction or verbal process to changes in child clients' language achievement and other speech-related outcome measures. The authors used as their database 18 previously published outcome studies that contained pre- and posttherapy measures of language proficiency. Coders rated the therapies provided in each study in terms of their predominant mode of verbal process. Three types of verbal process were distinguished. The first type was characterized by spontaneous verbal interaction. The second type of verbal process was constrained by preset tasks and goals related to specific problems. The third type of process was predominantly characterized by an emphasis on behavior and only secondarily on language (such as in counterconditioning treatments and relaxation).

The authors reported some interesting results. Increments in positive change were over 10 times as large for treatments using spontaneous verbal interaction than those constrained by preset tasks and over four times as large as those deemphasizing language interaction. Such increments were obtained for both individual and group therapies. Although not statistically reliable, the difference in the magnitude of these effects suggests a possibly fertile ground for future process research. This may be especially important in that analyses show that changes in language- and nonlanguage-based measures are not significantly correlated and that the magnitude of change in language- but not nonlanguage-based measures correlates with number of sessions. These tentative findings suggest that different change processes may be at work for these two domains of functioning.

This article is notable in that it draws attention to a key area of functioning, especially for school children, namely, language proficiencies. It attempts to connect outcomes in this domain to treatment processes and to differentiate them from outcomes in other domains. Nevertheless, this study hardly tells us anything specific about types of verbal processes that function as change mechanisms, or how such mechanisms are instantiated over the course of therapy. In fact, there is little in it that helps us relate processes to disorders or to more specific characterizations of the children's dysfunction.

In the next year, Shirk and Saiz (1992) published a report describing the development of a measure of the therapeutic alliance specifically constructed for children. In the tradition of the more theoretically driven attempts to develop measures of child process (e.g., Howe & Silvern, 1991; Wright, Truax, & Mitchell, 1972), Shirk and Saiz adopted and adapted Bordin's (1979) analysis of the therapy alliance and attempted to tie it to a developmental perspective on alliance formation, rooted firmly in attachment theory and social cognition. Like Bordin, they differentiated between the affective quality of the relationship and collaboration with more concrete tasks of therapy.

Based on pilot empirical studies, Shirk and Saiz (1992) divided affective orientation into two multi-item ($N = 8$) scales, bond and negativity. They gave one example of a bond item ("I like spending time with my doctor") and one example of a negativity item ("When I am with my doctor, I want the session to end quickly"). The parallel form for the therapists asked basically the same question of the clinicians (e.g., "The child likes spending time with you, the therapist"). Note that as in the Smith-Acuna et al. scales (1991), the therapist is asked to evaluate the subjective experiences of the child. Shirk and Saiz also included a scale for the degree of collaboration on a therapeutic task, namely, degree of verbalization of problems, and the four-item Menninger Collaboration Scale (Allen, Newsom, Gabbard, & Coyne, 1984).

To assess the psychometric properties of the scales and their interrelationships, a sample of 62 hospitalized children, 7 to 12 years old, with elevated scores on both internalizing and externalizing scales of the Child Behavior Checklist (Achenbach & Edelbrock, 1983), were administered the scales by a hospital staff person during their third week of treatment. Therapists, who were mostly psychodynamic in orientation and who saw the children in treatment about three times a week, completed the parallel form as well. The authors reported that the internal consistency of the scales ranges from acceptable to excellent for all of the scales (alphas ranged from .67 to .88). As theorized, the quality of the affective relationship, as measured by the bond and negativity scales, was significantly related to the degree of task involvement, for both the therapists and the clients. In addition, therapist ratings of bond and negativity were correlated with scores on the Menninger scales. There were even moderate relationships between the therapists and children's ratings of the quality of the therapeutic alliance, but not for ratings of the children's task involvement. The authors concluded that further use and development of these scales should be undertaken to help researchers and clinicians understand the process of child therapy.

This measure development study has obvious strengths. First, it is driven by theory and focuses on a single parameter of treatment, rather than on every verbal utterance or action, as in earlier studies. Second, it uses clearly disturbed clients in real therapy with practicing clinicians. Third, it is the only study that assesses the internal consistency of piloted multiple-item scales dealing with the therapeutic alliance, using a sample drawn from a single time point; this is not true of the Smith-Acuna et al. (1991) study or the Estrada, Russell, McGlinchey, and Hoffman (1993) scales reviewed later. Consequently, internal consistency and test–retest reliabilities are not confounded. Fourth, it sets out clear lines for future research, stressing developmental and social-cognitive factors that may mediate alliance formation in child therapy.

Like other measure development studies, however, there is still little focus on an investigation of process per se; after all, we get a view of only one time point. In addition, it is not clear how many different therapists were involved with the treatments, and what specific pathogenic processes led to each child's hospitalization. We also learn nothing about the relationship between the strength of the alliance or the extent of client verbalization and treatment outcome. Finally, we can wonder about the relationship between the subjective ratings of the client and therapist and the actual events in therapy. As with other studies in this tradition, multiple sources of assessments (participant report, expert judgments, codings or ratings of actual behavior) are not used in the same study. In 1992, we still lacked any study that incorporated them all!

Russell, van den Broek, Adams, Rosenberger, and Essig (1993) presented a study of one "supershrink's" (Richard Gardner) specific intervention technique, the mutual storytelling technique, with mildly disturbed children. They were interested in assessing whether the children's prompted stories are transformed in Gardner's putatively therapeutic retellings. The narrow focus on narrative was justified by these investigators because "narratives are a) deemed essential for our functioning as human beings, b) considered theoretically important by psychotherapy theorists, c) used routinely in standard assessment batteries, d) recognized by practicing psychologists as useful [in their clinical work], and e) incorporated into the clinical treatment armamentarium" (p. 339). We have also seen, in our review of previous studies, that stories are among the most frequently used types of response of children in nondirective types of therapy.

Russell, van den Broek, et al. (1993) focused on three clinically relevant dimensions of narrative: their structural connectedness (e.g., to what degree events are connected causally and temporally), the degree to which the psychological interior of action is made manifest (e.g., to what degree the protagonists in the story evince perspective taking and their own psychological or motivational perspective on the events they talk about or enact), and their linguistic complexity (e.g., number of words per segment). The authors felt that if the therapist's narrative was to be reparative or therapeutic, then it should model or illustrate how events are tied together causally and temporally, how events are linked to subjective perspectives, and to achieve such repair through language that is not too disparate from the child's in terms of its complexity.

The authors sampled 16 child stories and their contiguous versions retold by Gardner from *Gardner's Therapeutic Communication with Children* (1971). The stories had to be at least three sentences long, and they were told by children described as having low self-esteem, impulse control problems, familial difficulties, and/or attention deficits. Each story was assessed by several coders, who demonstrated adequate levels of reliability along the connectedness (two measures), subjectivity (four measures), and complexity (two measures) dimensions. Scores on the eight variables were compared across the children's and therapist's stories.

As expected, Gardner's stories were more structurally connected and manifested more subjectivity than the children's stories. Surprisingly, his stories contained more conceptual redundancy than the children's, perhaps indicating that he paid special attention to the relation between the introduction of new material and the need to rehash it in ways that would promote child uptake. Descriptively, these were not small differences. The means of his scores were all one or more standard deviations different from the children's, except on the measure of conceptual redundancy, which was 0.88 standard deviations different. It was also noteworthy that clauses that contained the most causal connections in the therapist's stories also contained more markers of subjectivity than clauses with less subjectivity. This finding suggested that the therapist may have been attempting to repair, foster, or augment the children's intentionalist theory of mind (roughly, that humans have important psychological interiors) by demonstrating that its features (wants, desires, hopes, motives, etc.) are causally connected to what transpires in action. There was little difference between the degree of subjectivity in clauses with high or low causal connections in the children's speech.

One finding on the relationship between child and therapist narratives was especially interesting. If the children's narrative had relatively little structural connectedness, representation of subjectivity, and elaboration/complexity, then the difference between the therapist and children's narratives was relatively large, and vice versa. The principle here seemed to be: "Provide a lot relative to where there is little, or provide little relative to where there is a lot, without regard to the current level of [the child's] narrative proficiency" (p. 354).

Russell, van den Broek, et al. (1993) concluded that narratives could, in fact, be an object of process study, and that, at least for one "supershrink," there were demonstrable differences between children's stories in therapy and the therapist's retellings. The authors also concluded that the uncovered differences made good clinical sense. Imparting a more complete picture of the causal and subjective worlds of action in a simple language seems to be a goal of almost all therapies. The authors noted that future studies with more therapists and clients would need to be conducted and that such narrative techniques, to be considered worthwhile, would have to be linked to changes in the children's storytelling in therapy and to the children's actions in everyday life. Moreover, the narrative transformations found in the therapist's speech would have to be shown to be different from those that any adult speaker would make, in order to be considered uniquely therapeutic.

This study has several strengths in that it appears to have been theoretically motivated, focused on clinically relevant but yet linguistically sophisticated measures, and was concerned with both the structure and sequence of one common form of intervention found in child treatment. Perhaps the suggestion of several critical dimensions for the study of narrative processes is its strongest contribution; but apart from measure development and the suggestion of how to proceed in future studies, this study provides little valid knowledge about a tried and true mechanism of change.

In the next year, Estrada and Russell (1994a, 1994b) and their colleagues attempted two types of studies that had yet to be done in the child process research tradition. In the first study, they developed a measure of child and child therapist participation in therapy called the Loyola Child and Child Therapist Psychotherapy Scales. Unlike previous scales in the literature (Shirk & Saiz, 1992; Smith-Acuna et al., 1991), the authors attempted to develop scales that objective raters could apply to ongoing or recorded child therapy sessions. Modeled after the adult Vanderbilt Psychotherapy Process Scales (Strupp, Hartley, & Blackwood, 1974), the Loyola scales attempt to assess both positive and negative aspects of the participants' involvement in therapy. The items in the scales were written to cover a broad range of therapist and child behaviors and attitudes, so that they would be applicable in assessing most therapies and could be used across child and adolescent developmental levels of functioning. Each item attempted to focus on a single behavior or attitude and to minimize the level of inference needed by judges.

The scales consist of 31 items in a 5-point Likert format with 14 child and 17 therapist items. To assess reliability, 117 segments of therapy were rated by three independent coders. Segments were roughly 15 minutes in length, and were sampled from 39 therapy sessions, drawn from 13 different therapies. Therapists in this study were graduate students in training, who were supervised in the delivery of predominantly psychodynamic treatment, and clients were moderately to severely disturbed children, ranging in age from 6 to 16, all with some kind of externalizing disorder. Overall reliability of the child items was .85. Overall reliability of the therapist items was .72.

Estrada et al. (1994) conducted a principal components analysis of the child and child therapist scales. Three participatory factors emerged for the child items. The first factor was dubbed Therapeutic Relationship (or bond) with high loadings on items assessing Trust, Openness, and high negative loadings on Negative Reaction and Noncompliance. The second factor was labeled Therapeutic Work because of high loadings on items assessing Productivity, Understanding, Exploration, Feelings, and Engagement. The third factor was labeled Therapeutic Readiness because of high loadings on items assessing Activity, and Motivation, and high negative loadings on an item taping Lack of Interest. These scales together accounted for 73.4% of the total variance (47.3%, 18.2%, and 7.5% for the first, second, and third factors, respectively).

For the therapist scales, three factors also emerged. The first factor was dubbed Technical Work because of high positive loadings on items assessing Productivity, Integration, Feelings, Planfulness, Guidance, Suggestions, Understanding, and Active Participation, and high negative loadings on an item assessing Distractibility. It accounted for 42.3% of the total variance. The second factor, accounting for 16.9% of the total variance, was labeled Therapeutic Relationship because of high positive loadings on items assessing Relationship, Warmth/Friendliness, and Empathy, and high negative loadings on an item assessing Difficult Interactions. The third factor was labeled Technical Lapse because of high positive loadings of Passivity and Inappropriateness, and high negative loadings on Limit Setting. The third factor accounted for 7.5% of the total variance.

The authors related these findings to those obtained when the therapists and the children were asked to evaluate their sessions (e.g., Shirk & Saiz, 1992; Smith-Acuna et al., 1991). Basically, on the child side, the findings in each of the studies seemed to point to the child bond or relationship, technical work or tasks focused on cognitive or emotional dimensions and, as conjectured in the Shirk and Saiz piece, to the child's readiness or willingness to engage in the process of therapy as essential ingredients in the psychotherapy. For therapists too, technical work or tasks again focused on cognitive and affective material, and provision of a "therapeutic" relationship figured as key in the process of therapy.

Interestingly, in both the child and the therapist scales, bipolar factors were common. The higher the levels of child trust and openness, the lower the levels of child negative reactions and noncompliance. The higher the levels of child motivation and activity, the lower the levels of child lack of interest. Patterns were similar for the therapist: the higher the levels of therapist technical work, the lower the levels of therapist distractibility; the higher the levels of therapist provision of a relationship, the lower the levels of difficult interactions; and the higher the levels of passivity and inappropriateness, the lower the levels of therapist limit setting. These factors and their bipolar organization suggest not only three ways (for the children and for the therapists) in which the process of child therapy is structured but also dynamic inverse relationships between the processes making up the stable structures.

In a second series of studies, Estrada and Russell and their colleagues (Estrada, Russell, Durlak, Elling, Piette, & Jones, 1994a, 1994b, 1994c) applied a complex 19-category language analysis system to child therapy sessions that had been independently rated using the Loyola child and child-therapist psychotherapy process scales. Six sessions are selected from the 18 that had been rated previously on the Loyola scales and represented the three best and three worst sessions. The six clients were school-aged (6 to 10 years old), and exhibited moderate to severe externalizing behavioral problems. Therapists were trainees with between 2 and 3 years of experience. Over 4,000 utterances were coded on some 19 categories.

Like Mook (1982a, 1982b) the authors applied P-technique to the language data, separately chaining the therapist and client data from the six sessions. Application of the P-technique revealed four client and four therapist factors. Factors of participation identified for the child were the following: (1) Objective Information Exchange, (2) Negative Affect–Directing Fantasy Play, (3) Forecasting about Significant Others, and (4) Expression of Affect. Factors of participation identified for the therapists were (1) Seeking and Acknowledging Information, (2) Talking about the Child's Significant Others–Fantasy Play, (3) Self-involving Disclosure, and (4) Technical Work. Good sessions were shown to differ from poor sessions in expected directions on many of the factors.

Although the authors reported their findings for the child and therapist separately in two articles, their most creative findings concern the patterning or structure of interaction between the clients and therapists and how such patterning of processes differ across the good and poor sessions. In order to obtain data on the client and therapist interaction, the authors (Estrada et al., 1994a) assigned the four relevant factor scores to each client and therapist utterance. From these scores, correlations were calculated across two therapist–client exchanges, resulting in a 16×16 correlation matrix. This matrix was submitted to principal components analysis, revealing six structures of therapist and client interaction.

The six structures of interaction were labeled to reflect the factors of therapist and child participation that loaded highly on them across the two exchanges. Factor 1 (Contested Play–Therapeutic Work) describes a somewhat contested interactional process in which the therapists talk about significant others or engage in fantasy play and, reciprocally, the children answer with negative affect or attempt to direct the fantasy play. Analyses revealed that this interaction pattern typically extended over at least two exchanges (therapist–child, child–therapist), and that good sessions had significantly higher levels of Contested Play–Therapeutic Work than poor sessions.

The second factor was dubbed Therapist Disclosing–Questioning due to its loading highly on the first and on the second exchange. None of the child factors loaded heavily on either the first or second exchange, indicating a lack of systematic responding to the therapists' disclosing or questioning behavior over at least two turns of talk. Poor sessions demonstrated significantly higher levels of this factor as compared to good sessions. It is as if the therapists are attempting to get the child to engage with him or her through disclosing and questioning, but not having much success.

Factor 3 was called Child Emoting, reflecting high-positive loadings on Child Expression of Affect on the first exchange, and again on the second exchange. The third factor describes the children's expressions of affect in the absence of therapists' responses over at least two exchanges. Significantly higher levels of this interactional process were found in poor sessions than in good sessions. This finding, that novice therapists avoid engaging high levels of client affect, that is, retreat or turn passive, has been reported in several previous studies of adult therapy, and seems to indicate an area in which training can focus.

Factor 4 was termed Child Forecasting about Significant Others, because of high positive loadings on Child Talking about Significant Others in the Future on the first exchange, and high negative loadings on Therapist Seeking and Acknowledging Information, and high positive loadings on Child Talking about Significant Others in the Future on the second exchange. This factor describes a clear pattern of interaction, one in which the children's discussions of significant others with a future orientation is prompted by therapists' information seeking, and continues more or less on its own. This is a factor that describes child planning or consequential thinking in the context of therapist questioning. Good and poor sessions did not differ significantly on this factor.

Factor 5 was named Sustained Therapist Work, due to high positive loadings on Therapist Seeking and Acknowledging Information and on Therapist Technical Work on the first exchange, and high positive loadings on the latter on the second exchange. Factor 5 identifies another pattern in which the therapist sustains therapeutic work through seeking, acknowledging, and appraising therapy material despite limited or no input from the child. Although levels of seeking and acknowledging information decline on the second exchange, the therapists continue to appraise cognitively the material without input from the children. Significantly higher levels of this factor were found in poor sessions than in good sessions. This may indicate a lack of client responsiveness or it could be an indication of the tendency for novice therapists to do too much interpretive work in the absence of clear indications of the children's comprehension, acknowledgement, and so on.

Finally, Factor 6 was called Objective Information Exchange, reflecting high negative loadings on Therapist Seeking and Acknowledging

Information and high positive loadings on Child Objective Information Exchange on the first exchange, and again on the second exchange. This factor describes a sustained focus on the exchange of "facts," from the child to the therapist. This is a basic structure in adult therapies as well (Czogalik & Russell, 1995). The good sessions and the poor sessions were about equivalent on this factor.

This study is the first in the child process tradition to combine perspectives (i.e., objective raters' perspective of in-session child and therapist behavior and objective coding/ratings of utterance-by-utterance in-session interaction) and to determine and compare multivariate structures of interaction sequences across good and poor sessions. In addition, this study can be read to provide evidence of discriminative validity for the Loyola Child and Child Therapist Psychotherapy Process Scales. Sessions that differed on these scales were shown to differ at the level of child and therapist interaction sequences. The study also suggests substantive results on two levels: (1) It provides some tentative answers to the question of what the *structure* of child–therapist interaction is like; and (2) it provides some tentative answers to the question of how good and poor sessions differ from each other at the level of therapist–child interaction sequences. Obviously, the answers to both of these questions must be considered "tentative": The therapists were trainees, the samples were small, there are high-level statistical issues, and there is a lack of focus on process–outcome relationships that all compromise the findings' generality. Moreover, it is possible that these findings, based on objective assessments, may not dovetail with assessments based on client and therapist subjective reports.

What we can say in a general way, however, is that interactional sequences focused on processes comprised of emotional and cognitive work differ quantitatively in good and poor sessions that have themselves been differentiated at a global level in terms of the therapists' and children's interpersonal relationship, therapeutic work, and emotional expressiveness. In a sense, this last study begins to close in on the focal-process question from a more or less inductive, quantitative point of view. It gives us results that can be read as candidates for locating key processive change mechanisms. Its most glaring shortcomings can seen in this light: The study is not theory driven in terms of its conceptualization of key change mechanisms, and the latter are not conceptually linked to presenting problems formulated in terms of each child's specific underlying pathogenic processes.

Summary

The 1990s can be viewed as the decade in which studies in child psychotherapy process embrace a broader range of methodological techniques and begin to look more closely at structures of interaction or intervention strategies through the use of multi-item scales and multivariate techniques of analysis. With respect to methodologies, we can see that the 1990s pushed in two very different directions. For instance, for the first time, instruments were devised and assessed that used the participants themselves to gain the subjective, phenomenological evaluations of their multidimensional experience of therapy process. At the same time, instruments were devised and assessed that used expert raters for evaluations of the client and therapist's participation in the therapy process. These raters were not coding sentences or utterances into discrete categories, but assessing the interaction of the child and therapist on Likert-type scales whose content clearly reflected a focus on clinical material. Similarly, more than ever before, studies went to extremes in terms of the units of interaction they studied: On the one hand, single sentences were subjected to ratings on over thirty categories; on the other hand, whole narratives, spanning more than a dozen sentences, were taken as the units of analyses, or even larger, discourse orientations, as in the Russell (1991) meta-analysis. Note that such units seem far more theoretically motivated than simple time sampling, as had often been the case in the past. Last, for the first time, there are findings organized at the level of child–therapist interaction.

The field also seemed to settle, either theoretically or empirically, on a few select dimensions or processes as the essential ones. For therapists, the therapeutic relationship or alliance, technical work or tasks, and emotional focus or processes seem to arise in most studies as the underlying organizing constructs in the therapists' experience or participation in therapy. Moreover, relationships between these processes or foci were explored, through correlational and factor-analytic methods, across subjective participant and objective observer points of view. In addition, specific targets in the child client's interaction were isolated and analyzed in relation to the therapists' intervention strategies. For example, repairing the child's narrative picture of the causal and temporal interrelationships between actions and imparting a more thoroughly consistent "theory of mind" with its focus on internal intentions and motives and attitudes seemed to be an aim in Gardner's mutual storytelling technique. Finally, the field also moved beyond evaluating processive or treatment outcomes of therapists who were blocked on the basis of some single characteristic (i.e., level of therapist offered conditions) to evaluating differences in microinteractional processes in sessions deemed good or poor through multidimensional objective ratings.

With respect to the investigation of child clients' participation in the process of psychotherapy, many similar developments can be noted. The question of whether children's subjective experience of psychotherapy can be studied fruitfully has certainly been answered, at least for school-aged children—and we would presume for adolescents as well. Whether studied through self-report or objective observer ratings, we also see a narrowing of focus on some key areas in which change processes are likely to occur. The interpersonal relationship with the therapist, in its positive and negative aspects, appears to be a key constituent of child therapy and, as in studies of adult therapy, its management seems to be related to levels of engagement in the other often more narrowly focused *tasks* of treatment.

These therapeutic tasks also seem to have been narrowed down through theory and research. Not only is emotional processing relevant in relation to the therapist (and, in fact, most previous studies of child therapy process in the tradition we have been reviewing indicate that there is very little direct relationship–talk between therapist and child), but placing objective events within the subjective horizon of feelings and attitudes seems to be an essential ingredient in the child's participation in therapy. Finally, the child's cognitive processing of information—through insight, understanding, planning, or perspective taking—also appears to be key in understanding the child's participation. In fact, the seemingly simple process of formulating and exchanging objective information about one's life experience, which shows itself as a predominant constituent over and over in the study of child and adult therapy, may in itself help provide a cognitive framework that is essential to understanding both the social and the interior world, not to mention securing gains on such usually resistant-to-change assessment instruments as language proficiency tests!

This was also the first decade in which structures of interactional processes of participation in therapy were investigated. What this means is that for the first time the field has a tentative picture of how the client and therapist organize their interactive discourse over the course of sessions and what levels of such organization are associated with good and bad sessions. Generally, we see that poor sessions have higher levels of unresponsive interaction (i.e., therapists do not respond in specific ways to what happens in the child's turn at talk, and children do not respond in specific ways to what happens in the therapist's turn at talk) than good sessions. Good sessions, in contrast, have higher levels of interactive and alternating exchanges concerning significant others and productive play.

Similar types of flaws plague most of the studies reviewed. We might boil them all down to one key problem: the enormous expense of securing enough patients and therapists, and the research facilities and personnel necessary to conduct psychometrically sound and meticulously focused process studies. For example, most studies that assessed the internal consistency of their process scales were forced through low participation rates to confound it with test–retest reliability or to confound it because of the nonindependence of the scores (i.e., the same therapists were used with different clients). Similarly, most studies had only small samples of therapists and clients, even if their many actual interaction sequences were the focus of intensive study. These were not studies whose levels of statistical power raised questions about the magnitude or clinical significance of the significant effects. These studies, as had many before them, seem to have been conducted on shoestring budgets, and to suffer therefrom, not in vision or importance, but in fundamental psychometric quality.

CONCLUSION

It would be easy to land a devastating broadside of methodological criticisms at this set of process studies. Suffice it to say that there is much room for improvement in almost every area of research reviewed, even if we do see steady improvement in the form of the questions asked and the choice of methods used to answer them. Given low budgets, the general neglect of the study of child treatment, and a specific disinterest in process, one should see this set of studies, not as easily dismissible *en masse,* but as providing a fairly rich collective basis on which to build creatively and with more rigor in the future.

In what direction do these initial studies point us? First, we should note that the study of process in child therapy has not been typically linked to comparative studies of therapy outcomes, as in the adult literature. That has meant that there are roughly as many comparative process studies as comparative process–outcome studies. More significantly, diagnostic categories of children have not, in the main, been compared across types of therapy, which has been and is currently the practice in most adult and child outcome research, research that has not bothered very much about looking at what happens within the clinical hour. From our reading of the process studies, we should neither lament the absence of this practice nor aim to duplicate it in the future. Instead, the studies themselves provide both theoretical and empirical grounds for pursuing an alternative approach.

On the empirical side, children have been shown to respond differentially over sessions of treatment and at outcome to different levels of therapist-offered conditions and to different levels of an intervention strategy, namely confrontation, in two of the best designed studies in this tradition. Nothing compares to them in the "treatment brand by diagnosis" studies of child treatment reviewed earlier. These findings, in fact, seem to cut across brand-name therapies, which, ironically, are never instantiated in the treatment interaction anyway. From an empirical point of view, the constituents of therapy seem to boil down to certain essential structures or strategies of interaction, and these seem to cut through the packaging needed to tout a recognizable treatment brand.

This should make good psychological sense and should not be surprising even to those devoted to theories of psychotherapy. If we delve deeper than brand-name descriptions of processes, should we be surprised to find general structures of participation, or a focus on essential modes of relating and meaning making, that dovetail with our psychological and developmental understanding of human interaction more generally? We think not and, in fact, view the field of child therapy and its research at its best as an application and adaptation of the systematic knowledge accrued in the traditional areas of psychology.

However, children of different developmental levels respond differently even to the same therapeutic intervention strategies. At the grossest level, it may be a simple fact of development that 6-year-olds will be more interested in toys in the therapeutic playroom than teenagers! It may very well be that the number and composition of the essential interactional structures may vary across developmental levels. Indeed, it would be surprising if they did not. Although there is some significant overlap in the interactional structures of child therapy reported by Estrada et al. (1994) with those reported by Czogalik and Russell (1995) in adult therapy, there are noteworthy differences. For example, there are four structures around which the adult therapy interaction seems to be organized, whereas there are six in the child therapy interaction. The seemingly greater complexity for the children is partly related to the dual plane of interaction found in some child treatments, namely, play and discourse.

From another angle, we found that therapists being supervised in the same brand of therapy differed quantitatively on stable structures of participation that, on the face of it, have only a weak inferential link with their therapeutic orientations, and a stronger link to systematic processes at work in most occasions of adult–child interaction. This finding emerges in the child process literature partly because some of the linguistic and quantitative tools of analysis that have been applied are, in fact, far more sophisticated than those associated with most comparisons of processes across treatment brands in the adult literature (see Czogalik & Russell, 1994b, for a demonstration of this point).

From the theoretical–methodological side, two points made in several studies should be highlighted. One suggestion is simply this: We should study pathological processes, processes involved in their remediation, and processes that reflect increased adjustment or well-being as if they are cut from the same cloth. We would add that the same should be true of our treatments. It should seem rather odd that a well-related child doing well in school but with night terrors would be referred for therapy emphasizing interpersonal issues or levels of attachment and assessed at outcome on peer nominations and school achievement measures. Rather, our formulation of the pathogenic process leading this child to night terrors should dovetail with our treatment intervention strategy, which should be framed in terms of what would count as positive processive and posttreatment outcomes.

The second point is more theoretical, but related to the first. Formulations of cases and formulations of treatment processes, which aim at specifiable targets and projected adaptive goals, should antedate and provide the context in which treatments are both administered and assessed. What is needed, then, is systematic theorizing, guided by psychological research, about basic therapeutic change processes. The existing process literature is suggestive about what therapeutic processes might be important for the treatment of children. But this literature is only suggestive, in part because it is so sparse, but also because so many of the studies have not been guided by theoretically derived conceptualizations of change processes. Instead, many of the studies are descriptive accounts of child or therapist behaviors, largely uninformed by conceptual models of change. In order for child psychotherapy process research to advance, we cannot be satisfied with our current characterization of treatments by theoretical labels (e.g., psychodynamic or client-centered). Instead, an explication of the putative change processes that constitute treatments, either uniquely or across well-known therapeutic approaches, is needed in order to focus process-oriented investigations of child psychotherapy. Such a shift in focus is also likely to be beneficial to practitioners who are regularly confronted with decisions about how to respond to the behavior of children in actual sessions.

Finally, it is our contention that the explication of basic change processes in child treatment will be enhanced by viewing them in the context of a body of research whose central concern is the *analysis of change,* namely, research on developmental processes. In fact, we propose that many therapeutic interventions represent formalized variations on basic developmental change mechanisms. Thus, we believe that a review of developmental models can augment our understanding of therapeutic change processes.

In the next chapter, we will summarize the results of our theoretical and empirical reviews and propose an alternative approach to understanding the process of child psychotherapy. At the heart of our proposal is the simple idea that both childhood disorders and the methods aimed at changing them should be conceptualized in terms of basic psychological processes. This is hardly a radical idea, but it most assuredly points in a different direction than the current orientation to child psychotherapy research, with its focus on brand-name treatments and diagnostic entities. In many ways, it involves recovering the insights of the child-therapy practitioner and formalizing them as an integrated model of child-therapy research and practice.

4

~

Conceptual Interlude:
Essential Ingredients
for Revitalizing
Child Psychotherapy

Our reviews of the theoretical and empirical literature on child psychotherapy have, on the one hand, opened a vast domain of therapeutic interventions for children, but on the other, have failed to provide a compass for navigating this empirically uncharted terrain. With regard to theory, we have identified three major approaches to child psychotherapy that share the assumption that internal psychological processes mediate emotional and behavioral problems and constitute the principle focus of therapeutic intervention. Within each of these major approaches—psychodynamic, client-centered, and cognitive—we have also discovered considerable variation in the types of interventions and patterns of therapist–child interactions prescribed by each approach. In other words, each brand of therapy is composed of multiple interventions and patterns of interaction that could be applied in various combinations to children presenting with different types of emotional or behavioral problems. The pressing question, then, is how to select the most promising method for a particular child. Unfortunately, our review of the empirical literature revealed precious few answers to this question. Thus, to this point, psychotherapy researchers have largely failed to provide child clinicians with either a map or a compass for directing their clinical practice.

THE EQUIVALENCE PROBLEM
IN CHILD PSYCHOTHERAPY

Perhaps it should not be surprising that existing research on child psychotherapy has produced equivocal results regarding differential treatment effectiveness. A substantially more intensive effort in the adult psychotherapy field has yielded similar results. Psychotherapy has been shown to be better than no treatment, but evidence for the clear superiority of a particular approach remains unconvincing or controversial (Beutler, 1991; Stiles et al., 1986). Given the paucity of research on child psychotherapy, it may be premature to hope for a set of empirical guidelines for matching treatments with categories of clinical problems. As Casey and Berman (1985, p. 395) note, even when child treatment approaches are lumped into two broad categories, behavioral and nonbehavioral, the "two classes of therapy tended to study children with different problems and to use different measures of treatment efficacy." Eight years later, this view is echoed by Kazdin (1993a) who asserts that "classes of treatment (e.g., behavioral vs. nonbehavioral) and individual treatment techniques within a given class of treatments do not consistently vary in effectiveness" (p. 134).

Within the more narrow domain of child psychotherapy, treatment comparisons are even more difficult to make. Here one finds some treatment approaches almost unexamined (e.g., psychodynamic), and some modalities poorly represented (e.g., individual psychotherapy; Shirk & Russell, 1992). In brief, there simply have been too few comparative outcome studies to rule out the null hypothesis, namely that different child psychotherapies produce similar effects, or as Luborsky, Singer, and Luborsky (1975) put it, "All have won, and all must have prizes" (p. 995). Moreover, process research, particularly research that links process variables with treatment outcomes, has been so limited that the identification of key techniques and patterns of interactions is, at best, in a nascent state. Consequently, child psychotherapists have little empirical evidence to support the implementation of specific interventions for children with specific types of problems.

Faced with unconvincing evidence for the differential effectiveness of various treatment methods, child psychotherapists might reasonably reach a number of conclusions. The first might be that child psychotherapy research is so underdeveloped that the application of virtually any conceptually coherent therapeutic approach to a wide range of childhood disorders remains acceptable in the absence of counterevidence. Here one might argue that operating within a single theoretical orientation provides the practitioner with an internally consistent set of guidelines and expectations for directing therapeutic practice (Rice & Greenberg, 1984). One advantage of the application of interventions derived from a coherent therapeutic orientation is that it prevents the practitioner from combining incompatible techniques that could cancel each other's intended effects. Clinical practice based on allegiance to a therapeutic orientation is justified on the basis of theoretical coherence and remains defensible until the limits of the approach are demonstrated.

Alternatively, in the absence of empirically validated treatment guidelines, one might conclude that most forms of child psychotherapy have something to offer, and that an eclectic solution to treatment planning is the most reasonable approach. This conclusion is congruent with the perspective that therapy is essentially idiographic in character, and much more of an art than a science. Accordingly, unique combinations of methods and techniques tailored to the needs of specific children represent the "craft" of the skillful child therapist. Unfortunately, such a conclusion can also lead to the application of an amalgam of techniques and methods with no evidence for effectiveness. Moreover, not all techniques may be equally compatible. Such "improvisational" therapy represents the principal hazard of an atheoretical, eclectic approach.

A third conclusion might be that child therapies are not so different after all; that is, despite their apparent theoretical differences, child therapies seem to produce relatively similar effects. In essence, child psychotherapists have been deceived by the *illusion* of diversity. Apparent differences in child therapy *theory* are not significant when transformed into actual clinical *practice.*

The illusion of diversity can be understood in several ways. The first might be framed as a methodological interpretation. Theories of child treatment both prescribe and proscribe sets of actions by child therapists. For example, nondirective, client-centered therapy cautions against the use of interpretation while calling for the reflection of expressed emotion. In contrast, psychodynamic child therapy, with its emphasis on insight and self-understanding, prescribes the use of interpretation. In practice, then, one would expect that child therapy conducted by practitioners of these two orientations would differ significantly. Unfortunately, unlike the adult literature, no research has been conducted to determine whether therapists who profess different therapeutic orientations *actually* conduct therapy sessions in different ways; that is, it is possible that once the door closes and the therapy session actually begins, therapists behave quite similarly despite their divergent theoretical orientations. For example, a child with a particular type of disorder, such as an undercontrolled conduct problem, may elicit a relatively narrow range of behaviors from therapists of widely different theoretical persuasions. Consequently, theoretical orientation may not translate into significant differences in therapeutic practice. Viewed from this perspective, different approaches to child therapy produce relatively equivalent effects because, in practice, they are actually quite similar. Diversity is an illusion, because differences in theory do not lead to variation in practice.

This view is plausible, given the relative lack of concern with treatment fidelity in the child psychotherapy literature. Among the existing studies of child psychotherapy, few use treatment manuals to ensure that therapies are delivered as prescribed by theory (Shirk & Russell, 1992). When taken in conjunction with the fact that many treatments in this research literature are delivered by nonprofessionals or professionals-in-training, there is good reason to be concerned with the unintentional homogenization of child psychotherapies. Given these methodological constraints, perhaps it should not be surprising that theoretical diversity does not readily yield evidence for differential effectiveness.

In contrast to the interpretation that differences in the actual practice of child therapy have been overestimated, a second view acknowledges differences in practice but minimizes their importance. This view rests on the dichotomization of psychotherapy process into two broad categories, typically labelled "specific" and "nonspecific" factors. The former refers to specific *techniques* that constitute the unique features of a treatment approach. The latter, by contrast, refers to shared features that are common to all forms of psychotherapy. According to this point of view, the features shared by diverse psychotherapies override differences in specific technique. Thus, the apparent equivalence of psychotherapies can be attributed to the shared, or nonspecific, factors. Differential rates of interpretation versus reflection of feelings, each corresponding to a particular theoretical orientation, are essentially epiphenomena of the essential mechanisms of change. Instead, factors such as hope, expectation of change, or an emotional relationship—common ingredients in all "good" therapy—account for the lion's share of the therapeutic effect.

Among some of the most promising findings from the child-therapy process literature are results indicating that therapist-offered conditions—warmth, empathy, and regard—are related to positive changes in children's emotional and behavioral problems. However, these results must be viewed cautiously, because there have been so few studies of therapist characteristics and behaviors in the child literature. The absence of research in this area is perplexing. First, an early study by Ricks (1974)—the frequently cited "supershrink" study—reveals that therapists who operate from the same theoretical orientation and who treat comparable child clients do not produce equivalent outcomes. Instead, therapist characteristics rather than technical differences appear to be responsible for outcome differences. Similarly, we found that in each study that focused on therapist-offered conditions, both processive outcomes (changes in therapy interaction) and posttreatment outcomes are related to the degree to which warmth, empathy, and regard are evinced by the therapist.

One might expect that such findings would have stimulated research on child therapist characteristics and their relation to treatment outcome. Instead, the field has restricted its focus to outcome designs that attempt to minimize variation across therapists within a particular theoretical orientation. Consequently, the contribution of therapist characteristics and variations in therapy process has been neglected in the child psychotherapy literature.

Alternatively, the lack of clear evidence for treatment superiority might not be due to therapist factors that cut across theoretical orientations but rather to a common core of child patient processes. Again, the limited child therapy research literature has tended to focus on comparisons of whole therapies or treatment brands. This approach appears to be based on the assumption that change is largely the result of something done by the therapist. However, as Rice and Greenberg (1984, p. 14) remind us, "It is the client who changes." This view is underscored by Strupp (1973, p. 1) who notes that one essential ingredient of psychotherapy is "a client who has the capacity and the willingness to profit from the experience." Interestingly, despite the fact that children rarely refer themselves for treatment, very little attention has been directed to the characteristics of child clients or to their performances in therapy that may be related to outcome. Although it has been surprisingly difficult to identify consistent relationships between specific client behaviors and therapy outcome among adults (Stiles et al., 1986), a growing body of evidence suggests that a client's overall involvement in treatment, as reflected in constructs such as positive participation (Gomes-Schwartz, 1978) and the therapeutic alliance (Horvath & Luborsky, 1993), is a consistent predictor of outcome. This finding seems particularly relevant for treatments applied to "reluctant consumers," such as many child clients. Given the fact that children usually do not seek treatment for themselves and that others are often more distressed than the child (Shirk & Saiz, 1992), the degree to which a child engages in the process of therapy may be a more powerful predictor of outcome than the particular type of treatment applied. In fact, there is emerging evidence in the child process literature for common structures of child participation that define "good" sessions. For example, emotional experiencing and interpersonal relatedness with the therapist have been provisionally identified as key elements of children's involvement in therapy.

Both of the foregoing interpretations of the illusion of diversity represent challenges to the importance of therapeutic orientation as an organizing heuristic for understanding child psychotherapy. In the first case, diversity is more apparent than real, because theoretical differences do not translate into practical differences. In the second, differences associated with therapeutic orientation are "illusory" because they are relatively inconsequential compared to the nonspecific factors that cut across theoretical orientations and represent the critical mechanisms of therapeutic change. Although both of these arguments are plausible, a more challenging proposal emerges from our review of the history of child psychotherapy research. Put simply, the absence of compelling evidence for differential treatment effectiveness, and consequently, the lack of a clear framework for treatment selection, follow from a flawed formula of the essential ingredients of child psychotherapy.

REVITALIZING CHILD PSYCHOTHERAPY: ESSENTIAL INGREDIENTS REVISITED

Current approaches to differential effectiveness assume that evidence in the form of *treatment type* by *problem type* interactions will accumulate with a sufficient number of studies. The hope has been that various therapeutic orientations—what we have called "brand-name" therapies—will prove to be differentially effective with children presenting with different disorders. For example, cognitive therapies may be more useful with impulsive children; nondirective treatments more effective with traumatized children; and psychodynamic therapy more successful with overcontrolled children. Unfortunately, the limited body of child psychotherapy research has not produced consistent patterns of treatment brand by diagnostic group interactions. Although one might argue that the failure to find the desired results is largely due to the nascent state of child psychotherapy research, for example, to the limited number of direct comparisons of treatments for the same diagnostic groups (Kazdin, 1993a) or to other methodological problems, such as sample heterogeneity (Shirk & Russell, 1992), it is also possible that this approach to uncovering the differential effectiveness of treatments is destined to produce unconvincing results. In fact, we propose that the current approach to the problem of comparative effectiveness is conceptually misguided on two fronts.

The Problem of "Brand-Name" Treatments

Children in treatment do not respond to the therapeutic orientation of their therapist any more than a vulnerable child responds to his or her parent's diagnosis of depression or schizophrenia. In its early days, research on risk and resilience tended to compare children raised by parents with various diagnoses with those raised by "healthy" parents. This research revealed a variety of deleterious effects of growing up with a disturbed parent (cf. Watt, Anthony, Wynne, & Rolf, 1984). However, such an approach provided very little insight into the processes that produced the deleterious effects. In order to address this critical problem, it became necessary for developmental psychopathologists to move beyond comparisons of parents with different diagnostic labels to an analysis of interactional processes. In the area of developmental psychopathology the question shifted: What about a parent with a specific disorder affects the child?

Analogously, child clients are not directly affected by their therapist's treatment orientation but by the organization of the therapist's behavior in relation to them. Just as a disturbed parent's diagnosis may be associated with certain interactional processes, a therapist's orientation presumably prescribes a pattern of behavior in relation to child clients. However, it would be foolish to assume that there is an invariant relationship between therapeutic orientation and therapist behavior. Most therapeutic orientations prescribe a range of possible interventions with children; that is, treatments often involve multiple components. As Durlak et al. (1991) have demonstrated, most treatment approaches, such as cognitive-behavioral therapy, involve a "package of treatment techniques that can be offered in many sequences and permutations," and across studies of the "same" treatment "there was no systematic combination of the components" (p. 211). Moreover, therapists operating within a specific therapeutic orientation typically individualize treatments based on an assessment of their client's problems (Persons, 1991). Consequently, knowing, for example, that a therapist is psychodynamically oriented does not necessarily mean that he or she will emphasize interpretation in treatment. Instead, for a particular child, the psychodynamic therapist may choose to emphasize supportive techniques as the primary method of intervention.

It is also the case that there is overlap in techniques and patterns of therapeutic interaction across treatment brands. For example, both client-centered and psychodynamic therapists support the expression of thematic or emotionally charged play with child clients. Thus, instead of comparing different "brand-name" therapies and assuming that knowledge of therapist orientation is equivalent to knowledge of treatment process, it seems more useful to identify and compare variations in the application of specific techniques or variations in patterns of therapist–child interaction. If one is to understand the differential effects of treatment, the processes that constitute the treatments represent the appropriate unit of analysis.

The Problem of Diagnostic Grouping

The hope of finding evidence for "treatment type by problem type" interactions has been based on the assumption that current diagnostic categories are meaningfully related to differences in the effectiveness of various psychosocial interventions. For example, children with oppositional defiant disorder may be less responsive to client-centered therapy than children diagnosed with dysthymic disorder. Similarly, psychodynamic therapy may be effective for separation anxiety disorder but not for attention-deficit/hyperactivity disorder. But as Beutler (1989) has pointed out, the descriptive dimensions found in the current diagnostic system for mental disorders lack a clear relationship with treatment selection. In other words, a psychiatric diagnosis typically provides little information about the relative value of different forms of psychosocial treatment. Instead, as Beutler notes, patients are likely to receive the type of therapy "in which the therapist is most experienced, trained, or devoted" (p. 272).

The unbridged gap between diagnosis and treatment for psychological problems is rather perplexing. Why doesn't diagnosis entail clear treatment strategies? The heart of the problem seems to follow from incompatible conceptual frameworks in diagnostic and psychotherapeutic theories. The current approach to diagnosis (DSM-IV), like its earlier version (DSM-III-R), attempts to establish diagnostic categories that can be objectively described, operationally defined, and of use to clinicians of different theoretical orientations. Given the emphasis on reliability and transtheoretical utility, references to underlying, inferred, pathogenic mechanisms that are tied to specific etiological theories largely have been purged from the diagnostic criteria. Instead, the system focuses on observable patterns of symptoms. Problems are classified at the symptom level, not at the level of underlying pathogenic mechanisms. For example, the diagnosis of conduct disorder requires the observation of symptoms such as running away from home, deliberate destruction of others' property, forced sexual activity, cruelty to animals, or truancy from school. In essence, the diagnosis can be made without reference to the underlying source of the problem or inferences about etiology. This approach to diagnosis stands in sharp contrast to theories of psychotherapy (Persons, 1991).

Unlike the current diagnostic system, theories of child psychotherapy are closely tied to etiological models and conceptualizations of underlying pathogenic processes. Prescriptions for therapeutic action are derived from formulations of underlying pathogenic mechanisms. However, in the current diagnostic system, the connection between classification and pathogenic process has been broken. In brief, a conceptualization of underlying psychological processes, essential to psychotherapeutic models, is missing in the current approach to diagnosis. Consequently, the conceptual link between diagnosis and treatment—the pathogenic formulation—has been lost.

Given the medical origins of psychiatric diagnosis, the dissociation of diagnosis from pathogenic process is somewhat surprising. As Persons (1991, p. 100) has observed, "In medicine, diagnoses are intended to reflect underlying pathogenic mechanisms." Fever, body aches, and lack of energy, though frequently co-occurring, are insufficient to constitute a diagnostic syndrome. This familiar cluster of symptoms could result from either a viral or bacterial infection, or could be associated with other pathogenic processes. The diagnosis and, in turn, the treatment, depends on the determination of the underlying process (Persons, 1991).

Thus, when overt symptoms and not underlying processes are the primary focus of diagnostic classification, one can encounter serious problems in differential treatment selection. Strayhorn (1988) has pointed out that it is quite common to find children who share the same clinical diagnosis but who require very different psychotherapeutic interventions. Extending his example, imagine three children who share the diagnosis of dysthymic disorder. The first child presents with a rather unremarkable family history; however, the child's mother reports that her son slapped himself on the face after he received a "B" on a math quiz. She notes that although she and her husband value school achievement, their son seems driven to perform and is devastated when he fails to meet his self-imposed high standards. The parents become increasingly concerned when their son seems to lose his usual zest and appears more moody and detached. In interview, the boy seems agitated and comments: "If I don't get the best grade, it proves I'm nothing but a loser." In contrast to this youngster, a second depressed child sits alone in the waiting room. The fact that her aunt has dropped her off at the clinic reflects a rather remarkable family history. We learn from intake materials that the child lost her mother at an early age. When her father remarried, her stepmother wanted a "fresh start," and she urged her husband to send his daughter to live with extended family. Although the plan was to be temporary, the child has continued to live with a series of relatives for nearly 3 years. Contact with the father remains episodic and rarely planned. In the initial interview, the child draws a picture of her family but omits herself saying, "There's no room for me." Finally, a third youngster presents with all the signs of depressed mood. He sits lifelessly in a chair with his eyes nearly closed. When asked to join his therapist, he lumbers down the hall at an incredibly slow pace. His fatigue is palpable. He shows little interest in the games or toys in the office. When the therapist comments on how "down" he seems, the boy begins to cry. However, he is unable to tell his therapist much about what is making him feel so sad. Although his verbal output is quite sparse, several comments are worth noting. He briefly talks about spending time alone watching television. When asked about friends, he manages only a short comment, saying, "Who needs them; they just put you down anyway."

In turn, these three children present the clinician with significantly different concerns. Self-criticism, loss and parental rejection, and social isolation represent core issues, but not in equal measure for each child. All three present with depressed mood and some combination of low self-esteem, low energy or fatigue, feelings of hopelessness, poor concentration, and eating or sleeping problems. Although all three children meet the diagnostic criteria for dysthymic disorder, their cases are marked by important differences in family history and focal concerns. Would our choice of therapy and treatment plan be the same for each child, given their shared diagnosis? As is evident from these minicase presentations, effective treatment strategies would not be based on formal diagnosis, but on a formulation of the pathogenic processes. For example, with the highly self-critical child, we might attempt to promote insight into the nature and origins of the child's self-evaluative standards, whereas therapy with the "abandoned" child might emphasize supportive processes and efforts to restructure family relations. These examples clearly illustrate the level of analysis typically found in clinical practice. Formulations of pathogenic processes are linked with corrective therapeutic actions. As Persons (1991) has pointed out, in practice, therapeutic interventions are not based on diagnosis; but instead, treatment plans and corresponding interventions follow a pattern of hypothesis testing about the underlying mechanisms that contribute to the patient's difficulties.

To summarize, the hope of finding evidence for differential treatment effectiveness has been based on the assumption that *treatment types (brands)* and *diagnostic entities (disorders)* represent the appropriate units for analysis. In essence, these components currently constitute the essential ingredients of child psychotherapy research. The expectation has been that "brand-name" therapies will be differentially effective with various diagnostic syndromes. Although this perspective represents an advance over the uniformity principle, that treatments can be applied equally to all disorders, or the allegiance principle, that treatment selection is based on therapist loyalty to an orientation, this interactional perspective fails to conceptualize both treatments and problems at the appropriate level of analysis. Treatment orientations typically involve multiple components such that knowledge of therapist orientation is not equivalent to knowledge of therapy process. Moreover, child clients do not respond to the orientation of their therapist, but to the therapist's behavior in sessions. On the treatment side of the interaction, it seems more fruitful to consider the actions of the therapist in therapy than the therapist's theoretical orientation. On the problem side, diagnosis rather than formulation has been the preferred unit of analysis. Yet children with the same diagnosis can require significantly different treatment plans and procedures, in large measure due to important differences in underlying pathogenic processes. Because diagnosis has been detached from formulations of pathogenic process, the conceptual connection between diagnosis and treatment planning has been severed. If the goal is to selectively apply interventions to child problems, then the case formulation must be restored.

ESSENTIAL INGREDIENTS REDEFINED

It thus appears that child psychotherapy is in need of an alternative conceptual formula. At the heart of our proposal is the notion that progress in the field of child psychotherapy hinges on a redefinition of the essential ingredients in terms of basic psychological processes. The current formula, with its emphasis on treatment packages and diagnostic entities, fails to conceptualize both treatments and disorders in terms of component psychological processes. Consequently, case descriptions and treatment interventions lack a common conceptual framework. Therefore, the major task for child psychotherapy researchers is to identify the essential psychological processes that constitute both therapeutic interventions and variations in childhood maladjustment.

Viewed from one perspective, our proposal is quite modest, and, in fact, rather conservative. In simplest terms, it involves reestablishing the link between treatment planning and case formulation. Like the current interactional model that seeks to match treatments with disorders, we assume that some forms of therapy are better suited to certain problems than others. Child therapy based on the uniformity assumption or allegiance to a specific orientation is explicitly rejected. However, unlike the current interactional model, the interaction terms of *treatment type* by *problem type* are reformulated.

On the side of treatments, if one is to understand the differential effects of child therapies, then the processes that constitute the treatments represent the appropriate unit of analysis. On the side of problems, current diagnostic groupings lack the conceptual dimensions to guide treatment. Instead, in clinical practice, the selection of interventions is based on the case formulation (Persons, 1991). And although case formulations may seem far too idiographic to be useful as a heuristic for guiding treatment selection, case formulations are essential in the actual conduct of psychotherapy (Persons, 1991), and typically are not idiosyncratic. To take this a step further, we propose that classes of cases, even cases with diverse manifest symptomatology, can be formulated in similar ways because of shared pathogenic processes. In turn, the choice of an intervention will be based on the "goodness of fit" between the psychological processes that constitute the intervention and the formulation of the underlying pathogenic process.

Judgments of treatment efficacy, then, must be based on an analysis of the effects of specific treatment processes for children with shared pathogenic mechanisms. Although such a model must ultimately be judged in light of empirical evidence, this approach has the virtue of conceptual coherence. Both interventions and problems are conceptualized in terms of component psychological processes. Treatment processes are linked to problems through a formulation of underlying pathogenic mechanisms. As such, intervention strategies are closely tied to models of developmental psychology. *A basic tenet of this approach is that therapeutic interventions for children cannot be dissociated from models of developmental psychopathology, and that formulations of pathogenic processes are integral in the design and selection of effective treatments.*

It is noteworthy that our review of the theoretical literature on child psychotherapy revealed multiple models of pathogenic process. Often the existence of multiple models are framed as rival formulations for the same pathological phenomenon. An alternative perspective, congruent with current thinking in developmental psychopathology, is that there are multiple pathways to childhood maladjustment, including similar forms of maladjustment. As Kazdin and Kagan (1994) have argued, the assumption of a single pathway to a specific disorder, although popular, is unwarranted. Instead, multiple paths or pathogenic processes may lead to a given outcome. As indicated in our review, existing psychotherapeutic models tend to emphasize a limited set of pathogenic pathways and corresponding sets of intervention strategies. In the extreme, some theories (e.g., client-centered child therapy) fail to establish the boundary conditions that constitute the limits of the model. In other words, a single pathogenic process is hypothesized to underlie multiple forms of child psychopathology. A comprehensive approach to child psychotherapy must account for multiple pathogenic pathways and embrace a wide range of treatment processes that could offset pathological development. This means that it is unlikely that any single therapeutic approach (treatment brand) is sufficiently comprehensive to account for the diversity of pathogenic mechanisms that contribute to child psychopathology.

This perspective appears to be consistent with the contemporary emphasis in clinical practice on multimodal or eclectic approaches to treatment (Kazdin, Siegel, & Bass, 1990; Snow & Paternite, 1986). Certainly "systematic" eclecticism has emphasized the "goodness of fit" of therapeutic procedures with clinical problems. And like technical eclecticism, one assumption of our approach is that therapeutic processes can be identified in, and lifted from, their theories of origin. Of course, the danger in this strategy is that once removed from their theories of origin, therapeutic procedures will be arbitrarily applied. Technical eclecticism without a model of psychopathology runs the risk of degenerating into unsystematic eclecticism, in which therapeutic decisions are guided by subjective impression or current fads.

In contrast, we propose that the selection of therapeutic strategies must be closely tied to formulations of underlying pathogenic processes. For example, if a child's problem is formulated in terms of obstructed affect expression, then the treatment of choice would emphasize expressive processes. However, rather than assuming that the myriad forms of child psychopathology invariably entail problems with the expression of feelings, a critical component of a formulation-based approach is a careful *assessment* of the goodness of fit of a particular pathogenic model with a specific case. Thus, before embarking on a therapeutic intervention that emphasizes the expression of feelings, the child clinician must ask: What evidence do I have that this child has difficulty expressing feelings? In essence, the formulation-based approach also restores the link between psychological assessment and treatment, a connection frequently broken in studies of psychotherapy outcome (Persons, 1991).

Redefining the essential ingredients of child psychotherapy in terms of *change processes* and *case formulations* establishes the principal tasks, and major challenges, for the remainder of this volume. Three questions will be addressed. First, what are the major postulated change processes in child psychotherapy? In order to address this question, three analytically separable, but interrelated, types of change process—interpersonal, emotional, and cognitive—will be considered. Second, what are the core models of pathogenic process that serve as organizing frames for specific case formulations? To this end, a set of prototypical case formulations will be identified. And third, what are the principles for matching therapeutic processes with case formulations? Of particular interest here will be an exploration of the parameters for defining "goodness of fit" between change processes and case formulations.

In summary, it is our proposal that the revitalization of child psychotherapy hinges on restoring the link between specific treatment processes and formulations of pathogenic process. However, the achievement of this goal requires systematic specification of the postulated change mechanisms in child psychotherapy and an elaboration of the basic case formulations that guide clinical practice.

II

~

CHANGE PROCESSES IN CHILD PSYCHOTHERAPY

P ART II CONTAINS three chapters concerned with the explication of basic change processes in child psychotherapy. Typically, discussions of change mechanisms are yoked with treatment brands. One disadvantage of this approach is that therapeutic processes are often disconnected from the basic psychological domain in which they are embedded. In this section, we offer an alternative perspective on change processes by considering them in the context of three interrelated, but analytically separable, psychological domains—interpersonal, emotional, and cognitive. Each chapter is devoted to an analysis of postulated change processes in the context of developmental research on interpersonal, emotional, or cognitive processes. Thus, rather than analyzing therapeutic procedures primarily in relation to their theories of origin, we reexamine change mechanisms in the context of basic psychological processes.

This approach extends the claim of Orlinsky and Howard (1978) that psychotherapy is a form of social interaction that can be understood in terms of processes that apply to all social interactions. We propose that such continuity is not limited to social processes, but includes cognitive, language, and emotional processes as well. In brief, the phenomena relevant to understanding change in therapy are not very different from the phenomena examined by researchers, especially developmentalists, in other systematic areas of psychology.

One of the most significant threats to the vitality of child psychotherapy is that a vast literature on the development of basic psychological processes has not been absorbed by this therapeutic tradition. Thus, a major goal of this section is to resituate models of therapeutic change in the context of research on basic psychological processes. We hope that this approach will lead to increased elaboration and specification of the postulated change processes in traditional child psychotherapy.

Chapter 5 differentiates models of relationship processes in child psychotherapy. Although relationship processes are widely acknowledged as critical change mechanisms in traditional child psychotherapy, multiple perspectives on *how* the relationship affects therapeutic change can be discriminated. In this chapter, three conceptualizations are examined in relation to developmental and clinical research on interpersonal processes—the relationship as support, as alliance, and as technique.

Chapter 6 examines the central role of emotion in child psychopathology and child psychotherapy. It is proposed that many forms of childhood disorders can be understood in terms of problems with the experience, expression, or regulation of emotion. Furthermore, it is argued that adaptive emotional functioning cannot be reduced to the control of negative feelings, but that multiple capacities are involved in the experience, expression, and regulation of emotion. In turn, no one therapeutic procedure can be expected to address the diversity of emotional problems that characterize clinical cases. Thus, multiple models of emotional change processes are examined in relation to developmental research on the experience, expression, and regulation of emotion.

Chapter 7 reexamines cognitive interventions at the level of discourse processes or symbolic interaction. Despite the fact that many cognitive interventions involve the modification of verbal behaviors, symbolic representations, or other language-mediated processes, little attention has been directed to discourse or language processes as change mechanisms. It is proposed that the reorganization of representational and discourse structures through language or symbolic interaction constitutes one of the most fundamental mechanisms of change in child psychotherapy.

5

⁓

Interpersonal
Change Processes

PSYCHOTHERAPY, whether with children or adults, occurs in the context of an interpersonal relationship. For some time, relationship processes have figured prominently in the adult psychotherapy research literature. Based on a review of process predictors of therapy outcome, Orlinsky and Howard (1986) report that the quality of the relationship between patient and therapist is consistently related to treatment progress. Similarly, Luborsky and colleagues (Luborsky, Crits-Christoph, Mintz, & Auerbach, 1988) have maintained that the therapeutic alliance is one of the most robust predictors of treatment outcome.

Perhaps one of the most frequent observations of practicing child psychotherapists is that therapeutic change is closely linked to the development of a positive relationship between child and therapist. At times, a stronger version of this perspective is asserted, namely that with children *the relationship itself is responsible for therapeutic change.* Yet, to date, there is virtually no empirical evidence for this position. Moreover, the global character of this clinical assertion does not easily translate into principles of clinical practice. Such a dictum may suggest to the developing clinician that child psychotherapy is essentially indistinguishable from other close relationships. Thus, one might ask, is child psychotherapy merely a contracted friendship or a form of high quality baby-sitting? If so, is there any need for training in child psychotherapy, and if not, why is the practice of child therapy the province of professionals? In fact, perhaps child clinicians should be selected on the basis of their ability to establish and maintain friendships; and is there any reason to believe that paraprofessionals would be any less skilled in these abilities?

There is little doubt that much of child psychotherapy can be viewed in terms that apply to all social relationships (Shirk, 1988a). In addition, it is likely that individuals with better interpersonal skills and greater interpersonal depth will be more effective child therapists than those with interpersonal problems and preoccupations. Nevertheless, such parallels and probabilities do not reduce the therapeutic relationship to just another social bond. Instead, what distinguishes the therapeutic relationship from other close relationships is the *intentional* use of the relationship to bring about changes in the cognitive, affective, or interpersonal repertoire of the child patient. In contrast to the global assertion that a positive relationship is responsible for therapeutic change, in reality one finds a number of models of *how* the relationship serves this purpose. In this chapter we move beyond global prescriptions to a comparative analysis of models of relationship processes in child psychotherapy.

THE RELATIONSHIP AS A VEHICLE
FOR THERAPEUTIC CHANGE

Although psychotherapists of varied persuasions point to the relationship as a critical component of successful therapy, close examination of this apparent consensus reveals a number of perspectives on the function of the therapeutic relationship. The focal question to be addressed is how is the relationship between child and therapist to be conceptualized as a change process? Stated another way, how might interpersonal processes operate as processes of therapeutic change? To this end, three conceptual models of the therapeutic relationship—relationship as *support*, as *alliance*, and as *technique*—will be examined.

The Relationship as Support

A substantial body of research has shown that social support is linked to mental and physical health outcomes (Cohen & Wills, 1985; Vaux, 1988). One of the most dramatic findings to emerge from this literature is that social support is related not only to well-being, but also to mortality. Such a finding echoes the pioneering work of Spitz and his associates (1945), who demonstrated that survival among institutionalized infants was related to the availability of nurturing relationships and not merely to the fulfillment of physical needs. When viewed from this perspective, supportive relationships constitute one of life's basic provisions.

Social support is typically conceptualized as a form of coping or as a factor that facilitates coping (Compas, 1987). Yet there is considerable controversy about the mechanisms through which social support is related to the prevention or amelioration of psychological problems. In part, this controversy stems from the fact that support comes in a variety of forms and can serve a number of functions (Vaux, 1988). Nevertheless, one of the most prominent models in the literature is the stress-buffering hypothesis (Cohen & Wills, 1985). According to this perspective, the accumulation of stressful events can overwhelm the problem-solving capacities of individuals, thus resulting in symptoms of psychopathology. Support, it is believed, may intervene between stress and symptom formation at several points.

First, support may affect the way children appraise stressful situations or their own coping capacities. Redefinitions of stressful situations, either as less important or more manageable, may have a direct effect on symptom formation by reducing physiologically based stress reactions, or by increasing the probability of problem resolution through increased coping efforts. One possibility is that social support indirectly affects stress by decreasing demoralization which, in turn, leads to renewed problem-solving efforts.

Alternatively, social support could operate through a different path. A growing body of evidence indicates that social support processes are closely linked to the development and maintenance of self-esteem (Harter, 1986). Given the relationship between self-esteem and diverse forms of symptomatology among children and adolescents (Rosenberg, 1979), processes that bolster children's sense of self-worth could protect them from the adverse effects of stress. Consistent with this perspective is evidence that high self-esteem is one of the dispositional characteristics that distinguishes resilient children from those who succumb to adversity (Garmezy, 1985).

Finally, support may intervene between the experience of stress and symptom formation, not through its impact on the individual's psychological state, but by actually resolving the problem, for example, through teaching a needed skill or by providing material resources. In essence, not all support is emotional in character. In fact, it is not uncommon for child clinicians to encounter requests for tangible forms of support (help with transportation, child care, or summer camps) when working with parents who have limited financial resources or who are burdened by other types of social adversity. Similarly, children may view the therapist as a source of instrumental support, that is, as someone who could help with homework or negotiate fewer chores at home.

Research on social support among children and adolescents has produced strong evidence for a direct relationship between support and psychological symptomatology (Compas, 1987). Children and adolescents with greater support evince fewer psychological symptoms than age-mates who lack supportive relationships. However, as Compas has noted, the strength of this relation varies as a function of both child characteristics and type of support investigated. Moreover, despite its theoretical appeal, evidence for the stress-buffering hypothesis with children and adolescents has been rather mixed (Compas, 1987). Not all studies have produced convincing evidence of an interaction between stressful life events and social support in predicting level of symptomatology.

What are the implications of these findings for child psychotherapy? First, the direct relationship between support and children's well-being suggest that social support is essential for children's social–emotional development. Although it is likely that some troubled children alienate potential supporters, it is also likely that some children develop emotional and behavioral difficulties because they lack sustaining relationships. To the degree that the absence of supportive relationships results in psychopathology, evidence of a direct relationship between support and adjustment suggests that the provision of support in therapy could produce beneficial effects. In essence, for children who lack sustaining relationships, who are relationship-deprived, the experience of support in the context of therapy may translate into increased emotional and behavioral adjustment. Alternatively, given the direct relationship between support and symptomatology, supportive therapy might be viewed as a preventive intervention for children who come from high-risk environments.

The mixed evidence for the stress-buffering model suggests a more cautious view of the "sufficiency" of support as an intervention for children who are reacting to stressful life events. A substantial number of children are referred for psychotherapy because of maladaptive reactions to disruptive life events, one common example being disruptions of family functioning due to parental separation or divorce. Such a situation, which often leads to the diagnosis of adjustment disorder in the child, appears to fit the parameters of the stress-buffering model. The supportive relationship offered in child psychotherapy is viewed, often implicitly, as offsetting or moderating the effects of the stressful situation on symptom formation. Yet existing research on the moderating effects of social support suggest that the buffering (i.e., therapeutic) effect of support may not hold in all circumstances. In part, the mixed results in the empirical literature may reflect both the heterogeneity of stressful events *and* the diversity of types of support offered as remedies. The effectiveness of support as a therapeutic process may depend on the goodness of fit between types of problem and types of support. Interestingly, relatively little is known about what types of supportive interactions are perceived by *children* to be most helpful for emotionally distressing situations. Thus, a major question for child therapists involves how to use the therapeutic relationship as a supportive intervention that is responsive to the particular needs of the child. Two

approaches, each reflecting a different conceptualization of child psychopathology, have been prominent in the clinical literature.

Support as Validation

At the heart of the client-centered tradition of child psychotherapy is the
assumption that "the way in which a person thinks and feels about him- or
herself is the most important determinant of behavior" (Wright et al., 1986,
p. 53). Extending self-concept theory into the domain of child psychopathology, these clinicians view emotional and behavioral problems as
markers of underlying disturbances or vulnerabilities in the self. Not
surprisingly then, the client-centered child therapist does not focus on
specific goals or the modification of specific problems (Wright et al., 1986).
Instead, the therapist attempts to provide the interpersonal conditions that
will enable the child to establish positive feelings of self-regard. Viewed
from this perspective, the principal function of the therapeutic relationship is the *validation* of the self.

Implicit in this formulation is the notion that the self is an interpersonal construction. This view has been articulated by Wright and his
colleagues (1986), who maintain: "Every individual is entitled to love and
esteem from significant others. Most of those who find themselves in
therapy are children who were deprived of such a human response or who
somehow misinterpreted it" (p. 56). A similar sentiment can be found in
contemporary psychoanalytic thinking about the developmental origins of
psychopathology. For example, Berger and Kennedy (1975), in describing
the histories of a group of troubled children, observe, "There was only one
factor missing in their lives and this due to their mothers' personality
difficulties; there was no parental pride and pleasure in the child; accordingly, there was a complete lack of the admiring approval from the parents'
side . . . "(p. 280). These clinicians go on to note that "it is a sobering
thought that within the complex mesh of influences that shape the life of
any individual child, the presence or absence as well as the quality of any
single ingredient should have such power to determine the developmental
result" (p. 280). In essence, healthy development is predicated on parental
responsiveness, not just to the child's basic survival needs, but to his or her
emotional needs for admiration, love, and care.

This position has been elaborated by Kohut (1977), who contends that
the developing child's self is structured and sustained by others' empathic
responses. In the absence of admiration and empathic attunement by
others, what Kohut calls "mirroring," vulnerabilities develop in the child's
self. Under these circumstances the child does not develop the capacity to
regulate distressing feelings or the ability to maintain self-esteem. In the
absence of self-regulating capacities, feelings of inner emptiness or depres-

sion are defended against with a variety of attempts to stimulate or soothe the self (e.g., intake of food or drugs, sexual promiscuity, withdrawal, or aggressiveness; Kahn, 1985). Thus, consistent with the client-centered position, self psychologists attribute diverse forms of psychopathology to underlying vulnerabilities in the self that can be traced to deficits in parental responsiveness.

These perspectives on the interplay between the responses of signifi- cant others and the development of the self have a long history that can be traced to the work of Charles Cooley (1902). According to Cooley, the origins of our sense of self are to be found in our impressions of what significant others think of and feel toward us. To use Cooley's phrase, the "looking-glass self" is composed of reflected appraisals of significant others. More recently, this perspective has been extended to infancy by attachment theorists. According to Bowlby (1973), young children develop "working models" of the self and others through ongoing interactions with caregivers. These interactions provide the developing child with comple- mentary information about whether caregivers are caring and responsive, and about whether the self is worthy of care and attention.

Two lines of developmental research have supported the social inter- actional model of self-esteem. Drawing directly upon the work of Cooley, Harter (1986) operationalized the social determinants of self-worth as the degree to which children feel that significant others (parents, teachers, classmates, and close friends) acknowledge their worth through positive regard, approval, and emotional support. Her research indicated that parent and classmate support were highly predictive of self-worth during middle childhood. Extending this line of inquiry, Robinson (1989) found that approval from significant others, in contrast to emotional support and instrumental aid, displayed the strongest relationship with self-worth. In her research, approval is defined as the degree to which others valued, praised, or evinced pride toward the person. These findings suggest that validation by significant others is an important determinant of self-worth. A complementary pattern of findings emerges from the attachment litera- ture. Here retrospective accounts of the quality of early caregiving interac- tions have been shown to be related to adolescents' and adults' self-esteem (Armsden & Greenberg, 1987; Collins & Read, 1990). As expected, caregiver responsiveness and sensitivity were related to positive self-regard.

Given evidence for a relationship between self-esteem and validation by others, how might a therapist operationalize this process in child psychotherapy? That is, how do the actions of a therapist serve to validate the self? Certainly, Robinson's research suggests that basic approval of the child is an essential ingredient. In the context of child therapy, this process often has been discussed in terms of the communication of *unconditional positive regard*. According to Wright et al. (1986), this therapeutic process is less a technique than an attitude or emotional stance of the therapist. It involves the therapist experiencing a warm acceptance of the child, a sense described by some as "prizing" the child as a person, and as "pulling" for the child as he or she struggles with the tasks of emotional development. It is an experience that is probably most simply expressed in "liking" the child, and most directly self-observed in one's affective orientation, that is, whether one "looks forward" to therapy sessions with the child. In essence, validation of the child in therapy is built on the therapist's felt experience.

How, then, does the therapist communicate this felt experience to the child? According to Wright et al. (1986), positive regard is most effectively conveyed through interest, warmth, and empathic understanding. Of these three, empathy has received the greatest attention in the clinical literature. Although numerous studies of adult psychotherapy have shown a link between therapist empathy and patient progress (cf. Orlinsky & Howard, 1986), others have noted that the results of this research are not entirely persuasive (Marks & Tolsma, 1986). Often the relationship between therapist-offered empathy and outcome is rather modest, and the strength of the connection depends on the source of measurement (Orlinsky & Howard, 1986). In part, the absence of consistently strong results may reflect conceptual and operational variations in the definition of the empathy, which remains controversial (Marks & Tolsma, 1986). Some have suggested that empathy is essentially a cognitive process involving the "ability to detect and describe the immediate affective state of another" (Danish & Kagan, 1971, p. 51), whereas others have emphasized the affective and relational components of empathy. For example, Carkhuff and Berenson (1967) maintain that empathy involves "the therapist's ability to allow himself to experience or merge in the experience of the client, reflect on this experience while suspending his own judgments, tolerating his own anxiety, and communicating this understanding to the client" (p. 27). In fact, it is likely that empathy involves both affective and cognitive components. One integrated model has been presented by Kaplan (1983) who emphasizes the dual nature of empathy. She notes, "The affective component comprises feelings of emotional connectedness, a capacity to take in and contain the feelings of the other person. The cognitive component rests essentially on one's integral sense of self and the capacity to act on the basis of that sense of self" (p. 13). In essence, empathy involves an openness to the child's emotional experience without the loss of personal boundaries. Though there is a "coexperiencing" of the child's emotions, the therapist does not lose sight of the origins of the emotion. As Rogers (1961) has observed, empathy involves understanding the client's subjective experience *as if* it were your own, but without losing the "as if" quality.

It should be obvious that the qualities of interest, warmth, and empathy are not unique to the therapeutic relationship, but in fact, characterize sensitive and responsive parent–child relationships. However, parents are faced with a variety of childrearing responsibilities, including the socialization of the child's overt behavior. According to Wright et al. (1986), the therapist's interest, warmth, and empathic understanding attain therapeutic power to the degree to which they are uncontaminated by concerns with behavior management. As Wright et al. (1986) note, "Therapists do not try to condition clients to behave in certain ways under certain conditions; they try to change the child's basic feelings about the self" (p. 57). Free from concerns with behavior management, the therapist can focus on understanding the child's emotional experience. Rather than interpreting or applying consequences to the child's behavior, the therapist attempts to grasp the child's inner experience and to communicate this felt understanding back to the child. It is assumed that the experience of being understood in this affirming manner will facilitate the development of positive self-regard. As Rogers (1977) has noted, "The more this (understanding) exists, the more the individual gains in self-esteem" (p. 139). In the absence of a therapeutic agenda to change the child's behavior, the therapist presumably is in a unique position to validate the child's self. In turn, emotional and behavioral change follow from strengthening the child's sense of self-worth.

This formulation raises a number of important questions. First, it is increasingly the case that children who are referred for therapy present with disruptive behavior disorders. Thus, the therapist is often immediately confronted with serious lapses in self-regulation, not only as a focal referral problem, but in the therapy session itself. For a significant number of children, aggressive and destructive behavior can be a threatening experience for both therapist and child. If, in fact, the process of validation is compromised by concerns with behavior management, it would appear that this form of supportive therapy is suitable only for overcontrolled children, that is, for those who present as inhibited, withdrawn, or depressed. However, as reflected in the clinical and research literatures, this therapeutic process has been applied to a wide array of child patients. The question, then, is how does the therapist attend to problematic behaviors while validating the child's self?

The apparent antagonism between behavioral control and unconditional regard has vexed child therapists for some time. Most client-centered child therapists acknowledge the necessity of setting limits, despite the recommendation for establishing a permissive environment in therapy. However, as Mishne (1983) has noted, recommendations on what constitutes a therapeutic response to a child's refusal to accept a stated limit have been conspicuously missing in this literature. For example, Axline (1947) suggests that therapists maintain their reflective stance and continue to offer comments about the child's felt experience. But few suggestions are offered about what to do if the child fails to respond to such reflections. Others have noted that permissiveness in therapy extends only to *symbolic* behavior, and that direct acting out must be limited (Ginott, 1959). Acknowledging the necessity of limits in therapy, Wright et al. (1986) distinguish between communications directed toward the child's *behavior* and the child's *person*. These clinicians hold out the possibility that one can manage the child's behavior while maintaining unconditional regard for the child as a person. In part, the therapist is faced with differentiating comments about the child's actions from messages about the child's self. Minimally, this means that therapists must not contaminate their efforts at behavior management with judgments about the person who is producing the behaviors. This is a tall order for two reasons. First, it requires significant affect regulation on the part of the therapist. As any seasoned child clinician will observe, "You don't have to practice child therapy for very long before you're faced with provocation or limit testing." Such behaviors are likely to arouse negative feelings in the therapist, and the true test for the child clinician is to manage these feelings without acting on them in subtle, reactive ways. Therapists who have difficulty managing their own negative affect in therapy are at risk for slowing or undermining the progress of their patients (Strupp, 1989). Thus, in the context of negative affect arousal, the therapist is faced with the very challenging task of differentiating behavioral sanctions from ongoing affirmations of the self. To add to the complexity of this situation, it is likely that the child will find it difficult to differentiate these messages as well. Developmental research has indicated that young children, particularly preschoolers, may not distinguish the self as a person from the self as a composite of specific behaviors and preferences. One problem in assessing global self-worth in young children is that they lack the very concept of "personness," a generalization about the self, that is distinct from concrete behaviors (Harter, 1986). Thus, at least in the treatment of young children, therapists' best efforts at making the person–behavior distinction may not be easily grasped by the child.

The apparent antagonism between behavior management and the communication of positive regard may, in fact, be based on a false dichotomy. Children who are "out-of-control," who repeatedly test limits, may lack the internal resources for self-regulation, and in turn, may attempt to elicit containment from the external environment. To ignore the child's need for structure can result in amplifying the child's insecurity and negative view of the self. In essence, the therapist who responds to a "felt" need in the child offers a form of support by enabling the child to regain control. Viewed from this perspective, the provision of behavioral regulation is an example of accurate empathy! It is worth noting that this perspective is based on the premise that self-esteem is a consequence of behavioral competence, and not its antecedent. Thus, in order to facilitate the development of self-esteem, one needs to help the child manage his or her own behavior. Research on links between self-perceptions of conduct and global self-worth have not resolved the issue of causal directionality, though these self-perceptions are clearly related (Harter, 1986). Consequently, although our goal may be the enhancement of self-worth, our interventions may be more effective when directed toward the *determinants* of these self-feelings, such as the child's competencies or interpersonal behaviors (Harter, 1988).

A second line of criticism of the apparent antagonism between behavioral control and positive regard comes from the parenting literature. Research on parenting practices has repeatedly produced two major dimensions of parental behavior, warmth and control (Gerlsma, Emmelkamp, & Arrindell, 1990). Although these dimensions represent two relatively independent factors, control is by no means the antithesis of warmth. Thus, the antagonism between behavior management and the expression of positive regard may be more theoretical than experiential. In fact, this vast literature supports the view that the integration of warmth and control in parenting produces adaptive outcomes for developing children. Of particular relevance here, Maccoby and Martin (1983) have reported that parents who are relatively high on both warmth *and* control tend to have children who evince high self-esteem. In contrast, parents who are "indulgent," who are relatively high on warmth but low on control, tend to have children who are impulsive, aggressive, lack independence, and lack the ability to take responsibility. These maladaptive outcomes raise serious questions about the importance of permissiveness, or at least about the appropriate degree of permissiveness in the therapeutic relationship. If we transpose these findings to the process of child psychotherapy, we might find that high levels of therapist warmth, untempered by a measure of therapist direction or control, do not produce the most adaptive outcomes for troubled children. In fact, such a therapeutic stance may not even be the most effective means for enhancing children's self-esteem.

One important question raised by this challenge is whether there is evidence for the enhancement of children's self-esteem through therapies based on a permissive therapeutic relationship involving relatively high warmth and low control. Outcome research on client-centered child therapy would seem to provide the best opportunity to answer this question. Moreover, unlike other nonbehavioral treatments for children, there have been a reasonable number of evaluations of this approach. Ironically, less than a handful of these studies include a measure of self-esteem among their outcome variables. This is particularly surprising insofar as self-esteem is purported to be the principal target of intervention for client-centered therapists.

Among those studies that have included a measure of self-concept, the results were mixed. One study found no significant change in self-concept among underachieving high school students (Baymur & Patterson, 1960); whereas two studies found some evidence for improved self-concepts among maladjusted school children and delinquent youth, respectively (Dorfman, 1958; Truax, Wargo, & Silber, 1966). Only one study made an effort to ensure that high levels of empathy and warmth were actually offered by therapists, and none evaluated the level of therapist control. Thus, it appears that the permissive posture of high warmth and low control prescribed by client-centered clinicians rests on a weak empirical foundation. When viewed in light of findings from the developmental literature, namely, that high self-esteem is associated with a balance of parental warmth and control, a reevaluation of the therapeutic processes involved in self-esteem enhancement seems warranted.

Unfortunately, the intervention literature provides few leads for such a reformulation. In their meta-analytic review, Casey and Berman (1985) found that the effect of child psychotherapy on self-esteem was extremely small; in fact, the effect did not reliably differ from zero. Of course, these results are based on a limited sample of studies that have included a measure of self-concept as an outcome variable.

One of the major limitations of the prevailing conceptualizations of self-esteem enhancement is the absence of a developmental framework. It may be the case that the assumptions of the client-centered approach are a "good developmental fit" for very young children. But as Pope, McHale, and Craighead (1988) have observed, "The attention and responsiveness of adults may be more important to a three-year-old learning a new skill than the actual quality of her task performance. In contrast, a nine-year-old may be so concerned about getting a job done correctly that positive adult attention may be an ineffective substitute for task failure" (p. 15). In other words, a unitary model of self-esteem enhancement may be misguided. The promotion of positive self-regard may depend on different therapeutic experiences at different developmental levels. To propose that all children with low self-esteem will be equally responsive to a single form of intervention commits what has been called the "developmental uniformity myth" of psychotherapy (Kendall, Lerner, & Craighead, 1984). Moreover, such a proposal ignores the fact that self-esteem is affected by more than one factor. Harter (1986) has shown that self-esteem is a function of children's experience of others' approval *and* their experience of competence. In addition, there may be significant developmental and individual differences in the relative importance of these two broad sources of self-esteem. When viewed from this perspective, therapeutic efforts to enhance self-esteem must be guided by an assessment of the factors that contribute to poor self-regard. One can imagine a number of interventions with somewhat different emphases.

For the child who is relationship-deprived or who experiences others' approval as contingent on achievement, appearance, or success, the provision of a warm, accepting relationship is likely to be pivotal. For the child who lacks specific interpersonal competencies to establish and maintain relationships, the therapeutic power of a warm, accepting relationship is not likely to be sufficient. Instead, the therapist may seek to build interpersonal competencies in order to boost the child's self-esteem. For the child who appears relatively competent, but who evaluates his or her abilities in an unrealistically negative manner, the therapist may attend to the child's self-evaluative processes in the context of a supportive relationship. In essence, the enhancement of self-esteem will depend on a *balance* of competence-building, self-evaluative, and validation processes. The relative therapeutic emphasis, in turn, must follow from an assessment and formulation of the factors that are contributing to low self-esteem.

In summary, the diagnosis of low self-esteem will not, in and of itself, provide the basis for the design and delivery of corrective interventions. Moreover, although warmth and approval may be necessary ingredients for interventions for low self-esteem, given the multiple determinants of self-regard, they may not constitute the complete recipe for successful outcome.

Support as Scaffolding

A second conceptualization of supportive processes in child psychotherapy can be found in the ego analytic tradition. According to Anna Freud (1968), children who present with serious deficits in ego functioning, such as poor impulse control, low tolerance of frustration, limited affect regulation, and weak reality testing, are in need of corrective experiences that will enable them to build basic regulating functions. In this context, support is viewed in "ego-building" terms. The aim of child therapy is to "turn the treatment situation itself into an improved version of the child's initial environment and within this framework aim at the belated fulfillment of the neglected developmental needs" (p. 43). In essence, therapy involves *corrective reparenting* of the child. The therapist attempts to provide the interpersonal conditions, presumably lacking in the child's relationships with other caregivers, that will facilitate the development of basic ego functions.

Consistent with this perspective, Pine (1976) spells out some of the interpersonal conditions for facilitating ego development in his parent–child model of psychotherapy. According to Pine, parents play a number of critical roles in the process of ego development. New capacities are modeled after those of the parent(s); in turn, these capacities may be practiced in relation to the parents, and when used elsewhere, parents may provide support and encouragement for the exercise of these emerging capacities; finally, capacities that first appeared in close relationships, become part of the child's internal psychological repertoire of regulating functions (Pine, 1976). In long-term supportive therapy, according to Pine, all of these processes occur in the relationship with the therapist. Thus, the therapist's supportive function is conceptualized in terms of the facilitative role of the parent in ego development.

These supportive processes often have been discussed in terms of the child's identification with the therapist (Sandler et al., 1980). According to this perspective, the child begins to take on characteristics of the therapist through the development of a positive relationship. However, as Pine (1976) notes, this descriptive account provides little insight into the process by which the therapist's input becomes part of the child's internal psychological functions. Moreover, this account suggests a rather passive role for the therapist. The therapist needs only to establish a positive relationship with the child, and in turn, the child will copy the needed, adaptive attributes of the therapist.

In contrast to this perspective, Pine offers a different vision of supportive interventions. Drawing on research in infant development, Pine notes that the mother typically plays a pivotal role in the regulation of unpleasant affect and impulse. In the absence of fully developed inner resources for controlling affective states, the mother provides an external source of regulation. In essence, the mothering one is an "auxiliary ego" for the child (Pine, 1976). Over the course of development, parents play this role in relation to a variety of emerging functions. For example, the toddler who is inspired to great anger is soothed, in fact restrained, by the parent. The parent may also simultaneously verbalize the child's affective state, thereby providing an alternate expressive outlet for the child's anger. Or later in development, the child who is frustrated by a lengthy task may be helped by the parent who breaks the task into manageable parts and encourages the child in the process. In essence, parents play an *active* role in closing the gap between the child's limited, emerging capacities and the demands of specific situations. For Pine, this is one of the basic supportive functions the therapist can play in child therapy.

Pine offers the example of a young child who had not developed the signal function of anxiety. Again drawing on a developmental formulation, Pine notes that the development of signal anxiety depends on repeated pairings of distress and relief. For the child who has come to anticipate relief when distressed, usually in the form of parental responsiveness, anxiety comes to signal the need for defense, either in the form of active coping or external support. However, for the child who has not experienced relief, initial distress is only a stimulus for greater distress. For such children, there is often extremely low tolerance for unpleasant feelings, in large part, because the arousal of such feelings can be highly disorganizing.

In Pine's treatment of "Emmy," only the most neutral activities could be tolerated. The slightest arousal of negative affect set off screaming or fighting, and months went by in quiet play with little change. Pine conceptualized the therapeutic task as the development of the signal function of anxiety. Three aspects of this process were brought into play. The first was to help Emmy *anticipate* affect arousal by warning her that the therapist was going to raise an emotionally charged topic. Second, the therapist *titrated* the stimulus by introducing emotional material in a graded manner (e.g., by asking only one question). Third, the therapist helped her anticipate *relief* by setting a limit to the potential threat (e.g., only raising one question) and by offering her a method of control (e.g., verbalizing when she needed to stop). Through this interactive process, Emmy gradually was able to tolerate greater affective arousal.

As Pine's case so clearly illustrates, the supportive function of the therapist is an active function. The therapist first must identify areas of functional deficits. Then, based on this assessment, the therapist watches for or actively structures situations in which the child's limited capacity will be evoked. In this interactive context, the therapist offers his or her capacities to supplement the child's own. In essence, the therapist builds a *scaffolding* between the child's functional level and the demands of the situation by offering some of his or her functional capacities in support of the child's efforts. Viewed from this perspective, children develop internal psychological functions, not by passively copying a well-liked therapist, but through active participation with the therapist in situations that were once beyond their functional level.

This conceptualization of support as scaffolding shares a number of assumptions with contextual models of development most prominently found in the work of Vygotsky and his followers. According to Vygotsky (1978), all higher mental functions make their first appearance in a social context. Internal psychological functions are created from patterns of activity that were first performed in social interaction. For example, internal self-regulating language follows a developmental sequence from self-regulating speech issued from others, to overt statements expressed by the self, to internal, subvocal speech. Thus, what was once external becomes internal. However, the process of internalization is not simply a matter of passive transfer from the external to the internal plane (Wertsch, 1985). Instead, psychological functions are created through patterns of shared activity. A basic tenet of Vygotsky's theory is that children's participation in activities with the guidance of more skilled partners allows them to develop more mature approaches to tasks and challenges (Rogoff, 1990). In essence, much of children's development can be viewed as an apprenticeship. According to Rogoff, children develop new skills and functions through "guided participation" with adults who challenge, constrain, and support children in the process of solving problems. Much of this process occurs incidently in the context of everyday tasks, for example, through children helping their parents with chores such as cooking or tending the garden. Other higher level cognitive functions are established through repeated patterns of interaction. For example, parents structure children's developing narration skills by asking questions that organize the child's accounts and enable the child to fill in missing components (Rogoff, 1990). Eventually, the child is able to present complete narratives without the scaffolding of organizing questions. Again, this developmental achievement is not attained through imitation alone, but depends on the active coparticipation of the child with a more skilled partner. As Bruner (1983) has noted, children are not mere spectators to the developmental process, but in fact, are active participants in it.

Transposed to the therapeutic plane, new psychological functions are not built primarily from imitation of the therapist, but are constructed from the child's participation with the therapist in activities that exceed the child's functional capacities. For example, consider the case of a child who is attempting to solve a social problem. The child has found a box containing numerous compact discs. The child, who often views the world from a self-interested perspective, very much wants to keep the discs. However, he has experienced some pressure from parents and peers to find the owner. During a session, he asks the therapist what he (the therapist) would do. The therapist has a number of choices. After hearing the child's dilemma, he could verbalize his own internal deliberations if faced with the same problem and hope that the youngster would incorporate significant parts into his own thinking. Such a strategy would be highly consistent with an imitation-based approach to therapeutic change. Or in keeping with the principle of shared participation, the therapist could engage the child in joint problem solving. In this case, the therapist might ask the child about how he would feel if he kept the discs or if he returned them. During this particular session the child evidenced little concern for the other person's feelings. Instead the situation was construed as either getting a desired object or giving it up in response to external pressure. In an effort to engage the child in more mature problem solving, the therapist involved the child in a role play. Now it was the therapist who had found the child patient's discs. The therapist verbalized the desire to keep the discs, and the child played out the complementary role of the person who had lost them. In essence, the therapist did not provide the child with a solution to the problem but structured an activity that provided the child with an opportunity to address the problem in a new way. In this case, the therapist was less concerned with the specific solution of the dilemma than with engaging the child in social perspective taking.

The social-contextual approach to development offers a number of basic principles that are relevant to the practice of child therapy. Given the view that internal psychological functions are built from repeated patterns of interaction, attention is directed toward joint activities between child and therapist. Rather than simply following the child's lead, the therapist watches for or devises situations that will engage the child's developing functional capacities. This may involve helping the child tolerate increasing levels of frustration, or manage anxiety-provoking situations, or reevaluate perceptions of social reality, to mention only a few possibilities. In this context, the therapist offers his or her functional capacities (e.g., coping strategies) to the child as an auxiliary backup to the child's own. For example, in assisting a child with frustration tolerance, the therapist may help the child verbalize his or her feelings, or may offer encouragement to the child to remain on task. In brief, the therapist provides a scaffolding for the child's developing capacities.

As a therapeutic approach, supportive scaffolding rests on two other principles. The first is that development, including development in the context of therapy, involves the construction of children's functional *competencies*. It is assumed that deficits in these competencies undermine adaptive functioning. Thus, one of the first tasks for the child clinician is to identify the functional deficits that are implicated in the child's present-ing problems. For example, are the child's difficulties in school activities related to problems with affect regulation, anxiety tolerance, or social problem solving? The identification of underdeveloped competencies will then provide a focus for therapy. Needless to say, this can be a very challenging task. In fact, the question of which type of functional deficit is most commonly associated with which type of childhood disorder is one of the most pressing, and currently unresolved, issues for developmental psychopathology. Although the research literature can provide some useful leads, it is advisable for the child clinician to cast a broad net when considering possible sources of difficulty.

One attempt to bring order to this complex task has been offered by Strayhorn (1988), who has identified nine groups of competencies that are critical for child mental health. Each cluster of functional competencies was further analyzed into specific subskills. For example, for the skill of relationship building, Strayhorn identified 10 subskills, including the accurate assessment of the trustworthiness of others and the ability to engage in social conversation. As this example illustrates, some of the capacities seem to translate into skill parameters more readily than others. Nevertheless, Strayhorn's approach underscores two critical points for child therapists. First, one must move beyond the child's presenting problems. Identification of the deficits, and not simply diagnosis of covarying symptoms, will provide the therapist with an action plan for therapy. Second, effective therapeutic intervention will depend on adequate specification of the child's functional deficits. It will not be enough to diagnose the child as having trouble with impulse control or frustration tolerance. These molar concepts represent a starting point in the assessment process and must give way to an analysis of the mechanisms involved in each competency. For example, poor frustration tolerance might stem from problems with verbalizing negative feelings or from highly critical self-evaluations in difficult situations. The challenge for the child therapist is to identify such gaps in the child's functioning and then to devise situations in which new competencies can be built.

The therapist's approach to scaffolding competencies should be informed by a second principle, what Vygotsky (1978) has referred to as the "zone of proximal development" (p. 86). Vygotsky defined this concept as the *distance* between the child's actual developmental level, operationalized in terms of the child's independent problem solving, and the child's potential developmental level, operationalized as the child's level of problem solving in collaboration with a more capable partner. According to Vygotsky, instruction or learning opportunities that occur in the zone of proximal development yield the most beneficial effects. In essence, development moves forward through children's participation in activities that are slightly beyond their level of competence. Thus, the second therapeutic principle is that exposure to activities that slightly exceed the child's independent capacity should produce beneficial effects when the child is supported by a more skilled partner.

For the child therapist this principle implies a careful assessment of the child's functional capacities, and the deliberate attempt to provide therapeutic learning opportunities at their outer edge. This might mean, for example, that in working with an impulsive child, the therapist seeks opportunities, perhaps in contexts of low emotional intensity where the child shows some capacity for self-control, to introduce planning and anticipation of consequences. As the child evinces greater capacity to independently carry out these functions, the therapist seeks opportunities for their exercise in more challenging situations.

A basic assumption of this approach, and one that stands in sharp contrast to the client-centered perspective, is that adaptive functions require active input from social partners in order for them to mature. It is not assumed that the provision of an emotionally supportive environment is sufficient for the maturation of psychological functions. Although emotional support is essential for therapeutic learning, the construction of psychological functions is built out of coparticipation in activities that are slightly beyond the child's level of competence. This joint activity constitutes the *work* of child therapy.

In summary, two models of supportive processes have been prominent in the child clinical literature. The first emphasizes the enhancement of self-esteem through therapist validation and emotional support. The second views the therapist's supportive actions in terms of scaffolding the child's emerging psychological functions. Although the type of deficit differs in these two approaches—self-esteem versus ego functions—both assume that interactive processes serve a compensatory function.

The Relationship as Alliance

Anna Freud (1946) has observed that an "affectionate attachment" between child and therapist is a "prerequisite for all later work" in child therapy (p. 31). In this clinical assertion we find a reformulation of the function of the therapeutic relationship. Unlike the client-centered perspective, the development of a therapeutic relationship is not conceptualized as *an end in itself,* but rather is viewed as a *means to other ends.* Here the relationship, conceptualized as an alliance, refers to the emotional connection between child and therapist that enables the child to *work* purposefully on resolving emotional and interpersonal problems. The relationship itself is not the curative factor, as the client-centered formulation implies, but is a necessary condition for the conduct of therapeutic work. In this conceptualization, a distinction is made between the affective quality of the relational bond and participation in therapeutic tasks. A positive or affectionate relationship between child and therapist facilitates the child's involvement in the work of therapy.

This conceptualization of the therapeutic relationship has reappeared in recent cognitive models of child therapy. For example, Stark, Rouse, and Livingston (1991) have observed that depressed children can be difficult to engage in cognitive-behavioral treatment; consequently, "the establishment of a solid therapeutic relationship, as held by clinical wisdom, can help motivate the youngster and promote compliance" (p. 174). It is interesting to note how far this perspective departs from traditional behavioral wisdom on treatment collaboration. Here one finds an emphasis on extrinsic rewards or consequences for the maintenance of treatment involvement. In contrast, cognitively oriented child therapists have begun to acknowledge the importance of relational factors in promoting treatment collaboration. It is possible that different motives for treatment participation could have a differential impact on treatment progress and the maintenance of treatment gains.

The basic assumption shared by dynamically and cognitively oriented child therapists is that the quality of the relationship between child and therapist can have an important bearing on the child's level of engagement in the tasks of therapy. In essence, the alliance between child and therapist is conceptualized as a *working* alliance. The relationship is a catalyst for change insofar as it enables the child to work on specifiable therapy tasks.

What separates these two approaches is not their respective conceptualizations of the therapeutic relationship, but their divergent formulations of
the tasks of therapy. Construed broadly, one finds an emphasis on the
expression of feelings, the verbalization of experience, and the promotion
of self-awareness in the psychodynamic tradition. In contrast, cognitively
oriented child therapists frequently focus on the development of cognitive
strategies or the correction of maladaptive cognitive beliefs. Nevertheless,
both assume that a bond between child and therapist is essential for task
collaboration.

The question, then, is what constitutes the therapeutic bond? When
child clinicians refer to the existence of a positive therapeutic relationship,
do they simply mean that the child "likes" the therapist? According to Anna
Freud, the alliance involves more than affectionate feelings for the therapist (Sandler et al., 1980), although such feelings are an important ingredient of a positive bond. Instead, a working alliance is based on the child's
experience of the therapist as a *helper.*

As Sandler and colleagues observe, a therapeutic alliance has been
formed when it appears that the child is operating from the belief that "I
really need to change, and you are the person to help me to change" (p.
55). Thus, in addition to positive feelings for the therapist, a working
alliance is predicated on the child's acknowledgement of problems and
recognition of the therapist as an aid in problem solution. From this
perspective, the denial of problems or the rejection of the therapist as an
agent of change constitutes evidence for a weak working alliance, even in
the context of affectionate feelings for the therapist.

Although relationship processes largely have been ignored by child
therapy researchers, there is some evidence that problem acknowledgement is predictive of alliance formation with children. In a study of
51 seriously disordered child inpatients, Shirk and his colleagues (Shirk,
Saiz, & Sarlin, 1993) found that children's acknowledgment of a need for
personal change at the time of admission was related to the quality of the
therapeutic bond, from both the child's and the therapist's perspectives, 3
weeks into treatment. These initial results suggest that children's perceptions of their own difficulties will have an important bearing on their
willingness to engage in therapy. Conversely, children who do not acknowledge emotional or interpersonal problems are unlikely to participate in a
process whose aim is to produce change.

How are we to reconcile this view of the alliance as a "working
relationship" with the fact that children rarely refer themselves for treatment, and often do not acknowledge the existence of problems? Typically,
the prompt for seeking child therapy comes from an adult, often a parent
or teacher, who is more distressed about the child's problem than is the
child. In other words, children rarely enter therapy with the "mature"

motive of seeking relief from distress by working with a designated helper. Instead, problems often are minimized, particularly early in treatment, and at times, the therapist is viewed suspiciously as another adult who is attempting to control the child's behavior. These problems were not lost on Anna Freud. Rather than assuming that children enter treatment eager to engage in therapeutic work, she proposed that therapists consider the initial phase of treatment as a "preparatory" period for therapy proper (A. Freud, 1946).

This perspective has filtered into the contemporary practice of child psychotherapy, but all too often it seems that the preparatory, "relationship-building" period centers exclusively on the development of positive feelings between child and therapist. Practically, "preparation" is translated to mean that the therapist joins the child as a friendly playmate who does nothing to upset the emerging relationship, for example, by introducing disturbing issues. In turn, the process of therapy often appears to bog down in endless sessions of board games and other activities that seem peripheral to the child's difficulties. In fact, the therapy has not "bogged down" but has been shaped by a definition of treatment that omits any reference to therapeutic work. Although one cannot assume that children will orient immediately to the therapist as a helper, equally one cannot expect children to spontaneously discuss their problems and difficulties if the therapist makes no effort to define the relationship as a helping relationship. In other words, the preparatory period of child therapy involves more than the development of a positive, generic relationship; it involves the development of a positive, *helping* relationship. The therapist's goal is not simply to be viewed with a positive emotional valence, although this goal can be challenging with some children and is essential for all else in therapy, but instead is to be regarded as person who can be helpful with emotional and interpersonal difficulties.

How, then, does the therapist attain this role in relation to the child? In discussing the treatment of an uncooperative 10-year-old boy with mixed emotional problems, Anna Freud (1946) describes the gradual development of a working alliance. In this case, the boy lacked "the sense of suffering, confidence in analysis and decision in favor of it" that are necessary for engagement in treatment (p. 8). Consequently, in early sessions, her principle aim was to follow the child's lead in conversation and activity and to match his affect as closely as possible, in order to do "nothing else but to make myself interesting to the boy" (p. 10). As sessions progressed, she attempted to prove herself useful by first writing letters for him on her typewriter, then by serving as a scribe for his stories, and still later by mediating conflicts with his parents. In the treatment of a little girl, she actually crocheted clothes for the child's dolls during early sessions. As Anna Freud succinctly notes, "I developed in this way a second agreeable quality—I was not only interesting, I had become useful" (p. 10). By responding to the child's interests and by serving some of the child's needs, the therapist assumes the qualities of an understanding, helpful person. The challenge, then, is to transform this general positive orientation to the therapist into a collaborative relationship whose main goal is to address emotional and interpersonal problems. It is at this point that therapy often appears to get stuck.

Perhaps the greatest obstacle to the establishment of a working alliance is the fact that children often do not experience their presenting problems as distressing. The absence of emotional distress undermines one of the most compelling motives for collaboration in psychotherapy. Although the therapist and other adults in the child's life may reach consensus about the child's problems, the child's perspective on the situation may diverge widely from those around him or her. Thus, the child therapist is faced with the daunting task of engaging the child in a set of problem-solving activities without a shared definition of the problem. An essential ingredient, then, in the establishment of a working alliance with a child is the development of shared goals for treatment.

This task may be one of the most difficult, yet least discussed, problems in child psychotherapy. First, there is the problem that the child's aims may be quite different from the parents'. Whereas the parents may be seeking greater compliance and fewer challenges to their authority, for example, the child may be interested in relief from parental demands. Second, the parents may locate the problem in the child, for example, as reflecting willful hostility, whereas the child views the problem in terms of unrealistic parental expectations. Obviously, both accounts must be considered by the child therapist, since truth in such situations rarely resides in one perspective. However, as a starting point in building a working alliance, it can be useful for the therapist to focus on helping the child differentiate his or her own goals for treatment from the goals of referring adults. By offering the child one's best efforts to meet these goals, the therapist is positioned as an ally of the child. This does not mean, however, that the therapist has to accept the child's goals without qualification, particularly if this means joining the child in the denial of obvious problems. Instead, the negotiation of a mutually shared definition of a problem is the central task of this phase of therapy. And for the purposes of establishing a working alliance, the initial consensual goals may not be the most important goals for treatment. Instead, the aim, at this point in treatment, is to define the therapy relationship as a working relationship, and this can be facilitated by initially addressing goals that may be somewhat peripheral to the central problems presented by the child. Nevertheless, by forging an alliance around such goals, the therapist's role as a helper with emotional or interpersonal problems becomes more clearly defined.

Arriving at mutually agreed-upon goals for therapy is no small feat with children. It may entail reframing the child's understanding of the problem situation. For example, when faced with a child who views conflict with his or her parents in terms of the parents' basic unreasonableness, the therapist need not accept the child's causal analysis in order to establish an alliance. Instead the therapist attempts to identify the child's desire for change by acknowledging and sympathizing with the child's wish for fewer family hassles. The goal for therapy, then, can be redefined in terms of reducing the number of hassles that arise in the family. In essence, the therapist holds out the possibility of relief from a negative situation. This, in turn, sets the stage for eliciting the child's help in understanding all the potential contributing factors, including both the child's and the parent's, to these problematic interactions. Therapist and child can then begin to work together toward a mutual goal.

For many referred children, the problems that led their parents to seek therapy are congruent with the child's own self-image. The task, then, for the therapist, is to help the child view the presenting problems as a source of distress (Sandler et al., 1980). According to Anna Freud (1946), children who are "one with their symptoms" are extremely difficult to engage in treatment; consequently, the therapist must induce "a split in the child's inner being" (p. 12). Essentially this means creating distance between the child and his or her symptoms. In one case Anna Freud describes the personification of a child's problems by giving them a name. Implicit in this intervention is the differentiation of the child's self-image. Problematic parts of the child's self are encapsulated and separated from other aspects of the child's personality. For example, with a child who engages in periodic antisocial acts, it can be useful to distinguish the "reckless" or "angry" part from other parts of the self. Such a maneuver can have the effect of making the symptoms foreign to the child. However, in order for the child to attain some distance from the symptoms, it is important to identify and contrast the problematic aspects of self with other, positive parts of the child's presentation.

At times, differentiation of symptomatic aspects of self is not sufficient to promote treatment engagement. Instead, the therapist must find a way to alter the meaning of the child's symptoms so the child will view them as a target for change. In one case, Anna Freud (1946) compares a boy's temper outbursts to the uncontrollable rages of a madman. The child, who viewed his symptoms with some pride, was taken aback. The symptom was now perceived as a challenge to the child's capacity for self-control. Given the developmental press toward mastery and competence in preschool and school-age children, and toward autonomy among adolescents, framing symptoms as challenges to self-determination can decrease children's comfort with their problems. For example, it can be useful to present child patients with evidence that they are not in charge of their symptoms, or that the symptoms lead to constraints on their autonomy. A variation on this theme is to help children examine the impact of their problems on other goals. Although it is often difficult to help children consider their problems in light of future consequences, a focus on the immediate impact of their difficulties can be useful. Pragmatically, this may mean showing children that change in a presenting problem will enable them to gain something for themselves (e.g., fewer restrictions or more supportive interactions). Conversely, change could entail loss for the child. Consequently, it is important for the therapist to consider the functional aspects of the child's symptoms, and to explore possible negative consequences of change.

More recently, an alternative approach to preparing children for psychotherapy was devised. Rather than focusing on children's perceptions of their problems, these investigators (Bonner & Everett, 1982; Weinstein, 1988; Coleman & Kaplan, 1990) emphasized the importance of prognostic and role expectations for children's engagement in therapy. In an early study, Day and Reznikoff (1980) found that inappropriate expectations about treatment were related to premature therapy dropout. Based on this finding and Frank's (1974) work on the centrality of expectations for treatment success, several attempts have been made to prepare children and their parents for therapy through audio- or videotape preparation. Although the content of these tapes vary, they tend to focus on providing information about the structure of therapy and the role expectations of participants. Overall, tape preparation appeared to have positive effects; children's knowledge of the structure and process of therapy was increased (Weinstein, 1988; Coleman & Kaplan, 1990), children's attraction/receptivity to the therapist was enhanced (Bonner & Everett, 1982), and children's expectations about treatment outcome were elevated (Bonner & Everett, 1982). Unfortunately, there is virtually no evidence that these positive cognitive changes translate into increased engagement in child therapy. In the only study that examined the impact of preparation on therapy process, Weinstein (1988) did not find a relationship between preparation and adaptation to the client role. Consequently, the usefulness of videotape preparation for promoting alliance formation remains an open question.

Alliance formation is not simply a function of the child therapist's skillful application of treatment strategies. The alliance is a dyadic construct, and its formation cannot be reduced to the actions of one participant. Children vary enormously in their willingness to participate in treatment and thus exert their own influence on the formation of a working alliance. One important source of variation in children's orientation to therapy is to be found in their attachment histories. Viewed from an attachment perspective, children's capacity to enter into a helping relationship should be related to their early experiences with affectionate and caring others (Frieswyk et al., 1986). One would expect continuity between the quality of early care and a child's subsequent willingness to engage in a helping relationship. Children who have experienced unreliable, unresponsive, or punitive interactions with early caregivers are likely to bring expectations based on these interactions to other caregiving encounters. The inability of some children to experience the therapist as a benevolent helper, and their difficulties with forming a positive working alliance, can be viewed as a remnant of these early experiences. The formation of an alliance, then, hinges on reworking expectations derived from early caregiving interactions. In essence, a corrective relationship experience is a precondition for some children to utilize the therapist as an ally in problem solving. From another perspective, the reworking of such basic interpersonal expectations through a corrective relationship is not the prelude to therapy proper but, in fact, is the essence of child psychotherapy. This distinction brings us to our final conceptualization of interpersonal processes as change processes.

The Relationship as Technique

It has been common practice for psychotherapy researchers to divide sources of therapeutic influence into two factors. The first, usually referred to as technical or specific factors, includes specifiable interventions or actions delivered by the therapist; the second typically includes interpersonal processes that are thought to be common to virtually all forms of psychotherapy. Given this breakdown, it should not be surprising that comparative outcome studies have focused on variations in therapeutic technique. However, as Strupp (1986) notes, the partitioning of sources of influence into technical and interpersonal processes is based on a false dichotomy. He goes on to contend that "such interpersonal variables as empathy, warmth, and caring should be regarded as specific as traditional techniques" (p. 515), particularly given the substantial variation in therapist delivery of these qualities. Consistent with this position, Strupp defines psychotherapy as "the systematic use of a human relationship" (p. 513) for the purposes of promoting change. As implied in this definition, relationship processes can be utilized in a technical manner. In contrast to the perspective that interpersonal processes constitute the facilitating context for technical interventions, or more coarsely, the grease for the mechanisms of change, this view posits the technical use of the therapeutic relationship as the principal change process.

The conceptual foundation for this perspective is grounded in an interpersonal formulation of psychopathology. This view has been succinctly summarized by Strupp (1986), who proposes that patients suffer "from the ill effects of past interpersonal experiences which have been internalized and now guide (their) behavior like computer programs or subroutines" (p. 518). Similarly, in his comments on therapeutic process, Bowlby (1988) has pointed to the patient's working models of self and others, derived from early relationships, as the source of interpersonal problems and distress, and as the main target for intervention.

These observations reveal a number of the basic tenets of an interpersonal perspective. First, psychopathology reflects the cumulative effects of problematic interpersonal experiences (Strupp, 1989). From this perspective, current interpersonal functioning must be viewed in the context of past relationships. Second, the link between past and present interpersonal experiences is through *representations* in the form of internalized working models, schemas, or core beliefs about self and others (Safran, 1990). Third, psychiatric symptoms, such as depression or anxiety, are associated with maladaptive internal representations that influence both emotional experience and interpersonal behavior (Bowlby, 1988; Guidano & Liotti, 1983; Safran, 1990).

Supportive evidence for an interpersonal model of child psychopathology is beginning to emerge. First, there is growing evidence of connections between children's early relationship experiences and the development of social and emotional problems. One promising line of research has begun to uncover links between the quality of early parent–child attachment and the development of psychopathology in childhood. For example, Lewis, Feiring, McGuffog, and Jaskir (1984) found strong negative associations for boys between security of attachment measured at 1 year of age and both internalizing and externalizing symptoms assessed at age 6. Similarly, Lyons-Ruth, Alpern, and Repacholi (1993) found that the strongest single predictor of hostile behavior toward peers in the preschool classroom was the child's disorganized/disoriented attachment status at 18 months of age. There also is growing evidence that children develop representations related to past interpersonal experiences. Main, Kaplan, & Cassidy (1985) have shown that children's early attachment security is related to their "working models" of their parent's accessibility at age 6. Similarly, research with abused children has revealed relationships between the experience of maltreatment and representations of interpersonal relatedness (Lynch & Cicchetti, 1991). Evidence for relationships between interpersonal representations and child psychopathology is beginning to appear. For example, Kobak, Sudler, and Gamble (1991) have found a relationship between representations of attachment figures and depressive symptoms among adolescents. Research by Dodge (1980) has revealed links between interpersonal expectancies in the form of judgments of hostile intent and children's aggressive behavior. Finally, Shirk and Eason (1993) demonstrated associations between self–other schemas and variations in the expression of emotional distress among young adolescents. Overall, the pattern of evidence is consistent with an interpersonal model of child psychopathology. Nevertheless, given the limited number of studies, additional research is needed to provide a solid empirical foundation for this perspective.

Perhaps the most important construct in the interpersonal model is interpersonal representations. These representations are viewed as the link between current interpersonal problems and past interpersonal experiences, and constitute the principal target for therapeutic change. Interpersonal representations have been conceptualized in a number of ways. For example, Safran (1990) defines the *interpersonal schema* as "a generic cognitive representation of interpersonal events" (p. 89). Similarly, Baldwin (1992) proposes that *relational schemas* refer to "cognitive structures representing regularities in patterns of interpersonal relatedness" (p. 461). Bowlby (1973) maintains that children develop *internal working models* that contain beliefs about the availability and responsiveness of caregivers and complementary beliefs about the value of the self in relation to caregivers. Common to all three conceptualizations is the focus on *relationships* as opposed to representations of self or other persons in isolation (Baldwin, 1992). In attempting to differentiate the elements of interpersonal representations, Baldwin hypothesizes that individuals develop both interpersonal scripts, that is, generalizations about interactional patterns, and self–other schemas that reflect generalizations about self and others in relational contexts. In other words, individuals construct representations of interactional sequences and role expectations for the persons, including the self, who are participating in these sequences (Baldwin, 1992). Such representations are based on repeated experiences with similar patterns of interaction. Thus, children who are repeatedly dismissed by their parents when they express anxiety or sadness can be expected to develop generalizations about what can be anticipated from others when they express distress, and associated beliefs about the affective consequences for the self. It is possible that such schemas are represented in conditional form, such as, "When I show my feelings, others will put me down and I will feel unloved." The strength and generality of these beliefs are likely to be related to the pervasiveness and recurrence of such interactions.

Interpersonal representations are not viewed as static mental categories (Baldwin, 1992; Safran, 1990). Instead, they are hypothesized to exert significant influence on emotional experience, interpersonal perception, and the regulation of behavior (Baldwin, 1992; Bowlby, 1973; Main et al., 1985). Recent research has shown that interpersonal representations have an impact on memory processes, the interpretation of ambiguous social situations, and the activation of emotions (see Baldwin, 1992, for a review). Moreover, these effects are attained without the conscious awareness of participants; that is, interpersonal representations function as *implicit* rules for the organization of experience and the regulation of emotion and behavior.

How, then, can the therapeutic relationship be used to produce change in maladaptive interpersonal representations? It is assumed that children's social interactions, including interactions in therapy, will be influenced by interpersonal representations such as relational schemas or internal working models. Children can be expected to bring, albeit without conscious awareness, sets of interpersonal representations to their interactions with their therapist. Maladaptive representations will give shape to the interaction between child and therapist. Consider, for example, the child who has experienced unreliable care and has developed expectations about the unresponsiveness of others. It would not be surprising to find this child approaching therapy with caution and relating to the therapist in a guarded manner. Similarly, for the child who has experienced high levels of control, the therapist's efforts to interview the child might be construed as highly invasive, and it is likely that struggles around limits would be a common form of therapy interaction. In brief, both the child's perceptions of the therapist's intentions and behavior *and* the child's pattern of relating to the therapist will be influenced by internal representations derived from past relationships.

Interventions into repetitive interpersonal patterns have been discussed by the analytically oriented in terms of *transference analysis,* where "transference" refers to the "transferring of thoughts, feelings, and fantasies about some childhood figure onto the therapist" (Westen, 1988). In essence, the child relates to the therapist *as if* he or she were relating to another significant figure. The main thrust of analytic interventions, then, is to help the child gain insight into the distorting effect of this "as if" form of relating through interpretations that link current (transferred) behavior with past relationships (Sandler et al., 1980). Some within the analytic community have challenged the importance of such interpretations in child treatment (Kennedy, 1971), whereas others outside of it (e.g., Shirk, 1988a) have raised questions about children's ability to comprehend the complex connections in these interpretations.

The principal alternative to the traditional interpretive approach is the "corrective relationship" model. This approach is guided by the assumption that maladaptive representations will be replaced or repaired through *interactions* that do not replicate the relational patterns upon which they were based. In order to provide a "corrective relationship" experience, the therapist must offer a pattern of interactions that will *disconfirm* the child's dysfunctional interpersonal representations. In essence, the therapist uses the relationship in a technical or strategic manner.

This approach has been elaborated by the Mt. Zion Psychotherapy Research Group (Weiss et al., 1986) and extended to the treatment of children (Gibbons & Foreman, 1990). Weiss and colleagues (1986) propose that interpersonal and emotional problems arise from pathogenic beliefs derived from interactions with significant others. For example, in a child who has grown up with a mother who is debilitated by chronic illness, one might find the unconscious belief: "My needs are a burden to others and will cause them pain." In turn, such beliefs guide behavior; in this case, the child might routinely assume a self-sacrificing role by attempting to be the caregiver in close relationships. Weiss et al. (1986) further propose that individuals bring pathogenic beliefs to therapy and unconsciously "test" them in relation to their therapist. In testing these beliefs, patients carry out trial actions that elicit responses from their therapist that either confirm or disconfirm their underlying belief. For example, in the case of the self-sacrificing child, he or she may attempt to become the therapist's helper by organizing the toys or by being concerned about the other children who visit the therapist. If the therapist allows him or her to occupy such a role, no corrective information will be provided by the new relationship. Although therapist and child may develop what appears to be a warm, collaborative relationship, the pathogenic relational pattern is replicated and progress is obstructed. In this case, the therapist should refrain from allowing the child to occupy the "little helper" role by redirecting attention to the child's own needs. As Safran (1990b) notes, the therapist "unhooks" himself or herself from the client's interpersonal pull by intentionally refraining from engaging in behavior that is complementary to the client's.

As this example illustrates, there is not a "prototypically correct" therapeutic relationship. This view runs contrary to generic prescriptions for therapist neutrality, activity, or even unconditionality. Instead, the therapist must organize his or her manner of relating to the child within the framework of the child's pathogenic beliefs. From this perspective, Rogers's (1957) well-known, interpersonal conditions might not be the right conditions for promoting change with certain patients. For example, imagine an adolescent who has experienced chronic parental underinvolvement. Based on this experience, the adolescent develops a pathogenic belief: "Others will be indifferent to my efforts and behavior." Not surprisingly, the adolescent often acts in ways that appear to show little concern for the feelings of others. In therapy, the teen is often late for sessions, and on occasion fails to keep an appointment. In fact, these behaviors represent a test of the adolescent's pathogenic belief that others will be disengaged. Unconditional acceptance by the therapist, in this context, would parallel the teen's prior experience and would confirm the associated belief. Therapeutic progress, on the other hand, would follow from therapist actions that disconfirm the underlying belief, in this case, by the therapist vigorously addressing the pattern of late appointments. In so doing, the therapist provides a relationship experience that is discrepant from the relational patterns predicted by the child's pathogenic beliefs. In this respect, the relationship *is* the therapeutic technique.

A major question for this approach is whether a discrepant relationship experience will be sufficient to promote therapeutic change. Although this is ultimately an empirical question, confidence in the efficacy of this approach hinges on several issues. The first concerns the openness of patients to new, discrepant information. Weiss et al. (1986) appear optimistic on this issue, in part, because of their assumption that patients enter therapy with an unconscious "plan" to master their interpersonal conflicts. Accordingly, tests of the therapist are viewed as opportunities for disconfirmation of pathogenic beliefs. In contrast, there is substantial evidence that rigidly held schemas bias the processing of new information in ways that are congruent with schematic beliefs (Baldwin, 1992; Safran, 1990). This research suggests that patients will enter therapy with a bias toward confirming their beliefs rather than disconfirming them. Moreover, there is growing evidence for the stability of interpersonal schema (Main et al., 1985; Safran, 1990). Beliefs that have been built from recurrent maladaptive interactions or traumatic events are not likely to change easily. Instead, it would seem that efforts to correct such representations would involve equally strong disconfirming experiences. Taken together, these factors mitigate against the effectiveness of time-limited, relationship therapy, particularly with children whose ongoing interactions with parental figures potentially reinforce the representations that led them into treatment.

A related issue concerns the degree to which change can occur without the awareness of underlying, problematic beliefs or schemas. As an alternative to the insight model, the corrective relationship approach emphasizes experiential learning. The modification of maladaptive representations occurs through repeated interactions that are inconsistent with pathogenic beliefs. Change occurs, not by the patient being told about problematic beliefs, but by his or her experiencing their lack of validity in interaction. The question then is whether the therapist needs to communicate to the child his or her hypotheses about the beliefs that influence the child's behavior, or might the therapist conduct treatment as a kind of interpersonal choreography whose steps are determined by the hypotheses but not explicitly communicated to the child? In the adult literature, it appears that the interpersonal actions of the therapist are augmented by metacommunications about interactional patterns and the beliefs underlying them (Kiesler, 1988; Weiss et al., 1986). Given the emergent nature of children's self-understanding, as well as their disinterest in examining motives and expectations (A. Freud, 1965), many child therapists deemphasize the importance of the child's insight into pathogenic beliefs. As Anna Freud has observed, it is not uncommon to find children who remember little about the content of therapy despite having been changed by the process. Although children may attain some cognitive under-standing of the links between their behaviors and the interpersonal representations underlying them, such insights are viewed as the by-prod-uct of other processes that are responsible for change. For the interperson-ally oriented child therapist, the critical change process is the technical use of the therapeutic relationship.

CONCLUSION

The therapeutic relationship is viewed as one of the most important vehicles for change by child therapists. Over time, a number of conceptu-alizations of the function of the therapy relationship have evolved. When viewed as a form of social support, the therapeutic relationship often serves a compensatory function. Children are provided with supports either for the maintenance or enhancement of self-esteem or for the development of self-regulating structures. When conceptualized as an alliance, the thera-peutic relationship is treated as a means to other ends. A positive bond between child and therapist serves the function of promoting collabora-tion on specifiable therapy tasks. Finally, when conceived as a treatment technique, the relationship is utilized strategically. The therapist provides the child with opportunities to engage in relational patterns that discon-firm problematic beliefs and assumptions. Despite important differences in these perspectives, there is substantial agreement that relationship processes are critical change processes.

Nevertheless, a marked discrepancy exists between the clinical signifi-cance of the therapeutic relationship and the number of studies on relationship processes in child psychotherapy. The absence of research on relationship processes in child therapy is strikingly inconsistent with cur-rent interest in interpersonal processes by developmental psychopatholo-gists. Here a major line of research is concerned with the interpersonal origins of child psychopathology. In this context, one might expect sub-stantial interest in relationship processes in child therapy. Instead, what one finds is a conceptually rich clinical literature largely unsupported by empirical evidence. As shown in this chapter, the therapeutic relationship is not a unitary construct; instead one finds multiple conceptualizations of its function in child psychotherapy. Research aimed at evaluating the contribution of relationship processes to treatment outcome should be sensitive to these important differences. Such empirical efforts should enable us to move beyond the global assertion found in clinical wisdom—that a positive relationship is essential for change—to a more precise understanding of the change processes embedded in therapeutic relation-ships.

6

Emotional Change Processes

CHILDREN ARE frequently referred for psychotherapy because of problems with emotion, and many childhood disorders can be viewed as involving difficulties with the experience, expression, or regulation of emotion. Moreover, it is not uncommon for the process of child therapy to be cast in terms of helping children deal with their feelings. For many years this clinical prescription meant facilitating the release of emotion through play or talk with an accepting therapist. However, the role of emotion in child therapy has evolved as our understanding of emotion processes has been advanced by new conceptual models supported by empirical research. No longer is the child therapist limited to catharsis as a means for promoting emotional change. As the domain of emotional functioning is differentiated, and the course of its development mapped, new avenues for intervention are opened. In this chapter, we examine research on children's emotional development in order to provide a framework for conceptualizing emotional change processes in child psychotherapy.

EMOTION IN CHILD PSYCHOTHERAPY

Despite the importance of emotion in child psychotherapy, emotion processes have been treated rather unsystematically in the child psychotherapy literature. One noteworthy trend, discernible in child therapy texts from the last 40 years, involves a shift in the conceptualization of emotion in child maladjustment. Emotional *overcontrol*, prominent in early formulations of child psychopathology, has been supplanted by an emphasis on emotional *undercontrol.* For example, early models of play therapy emphasized the importance of pent-up feelings in the development of a broad spectrum of childhood disorders (Axline, 1947). Similarly, psychoanalytic accounts of child maladjustment often focused on maladaptive defenses that block the appropriate expression of affect and, in turn, result in symptom formation (A. Freud, 1966). Thus, what one finds in the early child-therapy literature is an emphasis on the denial, distortion, or displacement of emotion. Clinical problems encountered by child therapists were understood to involve the overcontrol of affective experiences. Not surprisingly, then, discussions of therapeutic technique emphasized methods for facilitating the experience and expression of emotion.

In recent years, child therapy's preoccupation with unexpressed feelings has given way to heightened concerns with the undercontrol of disruptive emotions. Problems as different as depression and conduct disorder have been conceptualized by contemporary child therapists in terms of ineffective regulating structures or strategies. And though it is common to array childhood disorders along an internalizing to externalizing dimension (Achenbach & Edelbrock, 1983), what appears to distinguish many of these problems is the relative prominence of either *emotional* or *behavioral* undercontrol. Some have taken this perspective a step further and have proposed that a fundamental component of disruptive behavior disorders is the dysregulation of emotion, especially the undercontrol of anger (Cole & Zahn-Waxler, 1992). In turn, when emotional undercontrol is a central construct for understanding child psychopathology, methods for managing and containing emotional arousal are prominent in discussions of child-therapy technique.

Although there is increasing emphasis on emotional undercontrol in diverse forms of child psychopathology, it is unlikely that the full spectrum of childhood disorders can be reduced to a unitary emotion-processing problem. A recurrent problem in the history of child therapy has been the overextension of unitary treatment models and methods to disorders that do not share the same pathogenic processes. For example, the application of nondirective play therapy to learning disabled or conduct-disordered patients has not yielded a pattern of significant results (Weisz et al., 1987), in large part, because these disorders do not share the same pathogenic processes as disorders involving inhibition and constriction. Similarly, standardized treatment packages involving social problem-solving and social skills training have been widely applied to patient groups (e.g., depressed children), even when there is evidence that not all children in these groups show such deficits (Stark et al., 1991). One risk of the increasing emphasis on emotional undercontrol as the organizing framework for understanding child psychopathology is that it, too, could become overextended to disorders that involve significantly different emotion processing problems. To assume that all disorders involve the same general type of emotional problem (e.g., either over-control or undercontrol) would extend the uniformity myth to the emotional domain. Instead, it is likely that different types of disorders involve different types of emotion-processing problems. In fact, even *within* a specific disorder, it is possible that there will be variation in the types of emotion-processing problems encountered.

For example, children who have experienced serious maltreatment often present in therapy with very constricted affect. Such restriction makes sense in light of their traumatic experiences; indeed, their emotional survival may depend on their ability to seal off disturbing experiences and the related feelings. In fact, this type of emotion-processing problem is one of the cardinal features of posttraumatic stress disorder. Included among the diagnostic criteria for this disorder are the restriction of affect and the numbing of responsiveness. However, not all maltreated children show this pattern of emotional expressivity. Rather than emotional restriction, some maltreated children display heightened emotional arousal, as reflected in poorly modulated outbursts or exaggerated anxiety responses. Thus, within the same disorder, in this case, posttraumatic stress disorder, emotion problems involving both overcontrol and undercontrol are in-cluded among its defining features. As is evident, the diagnosis alone will not provide a sufficient basis for selecting an emotion-focused strategy that emphasizes either increased expressivity or increased control. To make such a decision, we must discern the type of processing problems that underlie the child's difficulties. As Greenberg and Safran (1989) have maintained, our basic question should be, "What type of emotional pro-cessing problem in therapy can be corrected by what type of intervention?" (p. 22). A major task for child psychotherapists, then, is to determine what type of emotional processing difficulties are involved in the child's present-ing problems, and to assess the degree to which they depart from develop-mental expectations.

Interventions for Children's Emotional Problems

Interventions into children's emotional processes have been guided, to a large degree, by two rival theoretical traditions (Cole, Michel, & O'Donnell, 1994; Dodge & Garber, 1991). The first dates to the early Greek philoso-phers but attains contemporary status in psychoanalytic theory (Cole et al., 1994). In this tradition, emotions are an "irrational, animistic, visceral phenomena" (p. 73); in brief, they are disturbers of organismic peace. Skillful, adaptive functioning is threatened by uncontrolled emotion, and the absence of regulation results in psychopathology (Dodge & Garber,

1991). In contrast, the second tradition, originating in the work of Darwin, posits emotion as an essential contributor to adaptive functioning. Emotions organize human experience and function to coordinate organismic needs with environmental demands (Cole et al., 1994). For example, emotions orient us to what we want or to what we need to avoid. Viewed from this perspective, emotions are critical sources of information. Emotion, itself, is "a type of control system that provides feedback to the organism about its responses to situations and helps it to adapt to the environment" (Greenberg & Safran, 1987). Thus, to be cut off from one's emotions is a serious threat to adaptive functioning.

As framed by these two traditions, emotion is both regulating and in need of regulation (Cole et al., 1994). Clinical approaches based on the former assumption tend to emphasize expressive interventions, whereas approaches based on the latter tend to focus on methods of emotional control. Recently, however, developmental psychopathologists have suggested that such a dichotomous view might not capture the complexity of children's problems with emotion (Cole et al., 1994; Dodge & Garber, 1991). According to Cole and her colleagues (1994), there has been a tendency among child clinicians to equate emotion dysregulation with inadequate control of negative affects. This view, however, captures only one dimension of emotion dysregulation. As Cole et al. point out, adaptive emotion processing is not limited to the reduction of the intensity or frequency of negative states, although this capacity is essential for psychological well-being. Instead, emotion regulation includes "the capacity to generate and sustain emotions in order to carry out activities and to communicate and influence others" (p. 83). For example, accessibility to anger can be essential for appropriate self-assertion. As Cole et al. note, to focus only on emotional restraint "overlooks the fact that deficiencies in the capacity for spontaneity and immediacy can be as dysfunctional as deficiencies in the capacity to attenuate strong emotions" (p. 83). For example, children who are distanced from their affective experiences are likely to have difficulty attuning to the emotions of others or communicating their own needs and wishes to others, and such deficiencies are likely to interfere with adaptive social interactions.

Emotion dysregulation, then, cannot be equated with either emotional overcontrol or emotional undercontrol. Instead, adaptive emotion regulation involves multiple capacities including, at minimum, the ability to access and sustain emotions that are congruent with contextual demands, and the ability to modulate the intensity and duration of emotions (Cole et al., 1994). Children's problems with emotion, then, can take many forms. These include, but are not limited to, problems with affect modulation, emotional constriction, limitations in the capacity to understand contextual cues for emotion expression or control, and emotional lability.

However, interventions for children's emotional problems have focused on two broad classes of processing difficulties: limitations in the capacity to experience emotions and problems in the management of emotional expressions.

EMOTIONAL EXPERIENCE

Treatment plans for child cases often include references to "helping the child put feelings into words," "talking about upsetting experiences," "identifying feelings," and "promoting insight into emotional reactions." The shared goal of such interventions, it seems, is to increase the child's capacity to process emotional experiences. The capacity to attend to, understand, and talk about emotion has received considerable attention in the adult psychotherapy literature under the rubric of "emotional experiencing" (Greenberg & Safran, 1987). Although there is some disagreement about the precise meaning of this construct, emotional experiencing appears to involve the patient's capacity to focus inwardly on immediate feelings and to integrate this affective experience with personal meaning. One of the most consistent findings to emerge from the adult literature is that "successful therapy clients started, continued, and ended therapy at higher levels of experiencing than did less successful clients" (Greenberg & Safran, 1987, p. 76). Thus, successful psychotherapy, at least for moderately distressed adults, appears to be related to the capacity to focus on and to understand emotional experience. When viewed from a developmental perspective, the link between emotional experiencing and treatment outcome represents a significant challenge for therapists who are working with clients whose capacity for such emotion processes is only emerging.

What does emotional experiencing entail? First, it involves the recognition or identification of feelings, and accurate identification of feelings implies the capacity to differentiate variations in feeling states. Closely connected with this aspect of emotional experiencing is the capacity to verbalize or describe variations in internal states. The child must acquire a network of emotion-denoting words that can be applied to felt experiences. Finally, experiencing, as it has been defined, involves more than labeling affective experiences. Instead, experiencing entails an ability to grasp the meaning of emotional experiences. One important aspect of emotional understanding involves insight into the source or causes of feeling states. For example, the child who attributes his or her irritability to the lack of sleep imbues this felt experience with a very different meaning than the child who frames similar feelings in terms of loss or thwarted ambitions. It is important to note that although these aspects of emotional experience are frequent targets of intervention for child therapists, children at different developmental levels enter therapy with widely varied capacities for addressing their feelings.

Emotion Recognition

Consider, first, the child's developing capacity to recognize different feeling states. In a provocative experiment, Kreutzer and Charlesworth (1973) exposed infants between the ages of 4 to 10 months to an experimenter who simulated different facial expressions accompanied by affective verbalizations. By 6 months of age, infants paid more attention to sad than angry, neutral, or happy expressions. These infants also reacted with more frowning and crying to negative emotional displays than neutral or positive expressions suggesting something about what the infant might be experiencing in reaction to these discrimination. However, evidence for early differentiation of emotions has not resolved the issue of what these emotions mean to the infant (Zahn-Waxler, Cummings, & Cooperman, 1984). During the second and third year of life, children show increasing complexity in their discrimination of emotion experiences. One critical development in this area is the relatively rapid acquisition of emotion-denoting words to describe the internal states of self and others (Bretherton, Fritz, Zahn-Waxler, & Ridgeway, 1986). Evidence from maternal diaries indicates that between 18 and 36 months of age, children begin to label their own and other's feelings, talk about past emotional experiences, and begin to talk about the antecedents and consequences of emotions in a rudimentary manner (Bretherton et al., 1986).

During the preschool and elementary-school years, children increasingly show the ability to identify the appropriate emotion that would be elicited in emotionally evocative situations, for example, losing a pet (Shantz, 1983). In the preschool period, happy and sad situations are distinguished more consistently than situations involving anger or fear. During the elementary-school years, identification of another's emotion improves with age, provided the emotion is congruent with the situation (Shantz, 1983). However, when situational cues and affective displays are incongruent, older children appear to impose their own affective reaction onto the situation (Kurdek & Rogdon, 1975). Such a finding highlights the salience of situational cues for inferring affective states, perhaps even the child's own, during the elementary-school years.

A critical question for child therapists is whether the referents of children's emotion language are the same as those of the therapist's, that is, whether emotion words refer to different emotional experiences at different developmental levels. Although therapist and child may use the same emotion label, the emotional experience that the label captures may be quite different. Two lines of developmental research suggest different answers to this question.

Support for developmental continuity in emotion concepts comes from two sources. First, congruence between child and adult assignment of emotion terms to specific evocative situations suggests comparability in referents for emotion labels. For example, Barden, Zelko, Duncan, and Masters (1980) examined the experiential determinants of emotions in kindergarten and third- and sixth-grade children. There was consensus among children at all ages that experiences such as success and nurturance elicit happiness. However, evidence for congruence between adult and child assignment of emotion words varied across types of emotional experiences, and in general, congruence increased as a function of child age. Also, most research on the experiential referents of emotion has focused on the identification of relatively simple emotions such as happy, sad, and mad. A second, and perhaps stronger, source of evidence for developmental continuity is found in studies of children's classification of emotions (Russell & Ridgeway, 1983). Research on adult's classification of emotions has revealed that emotion concepts are systematically related and that these relationships can be represented in a two-dimensional space where the axes refer to dimensions of hedonic valence (pleasure–displeasure) and arousal (aroused–sleepy). In a series of studies, Russell and Ridgeway found that children as young as third graders organized emotion words in much the same way as adults. The interrelationships among emotion words fell in a circular order corresponding to variations on the dimensions of valence and arousal. Moreover, the pattern of relationships among emotions (e.g., sad is more similar to afraid than to tired) closely approximated the adult pattern. These results suggest that elementary school children describe their emotional states along the same basic dimensions as do adults.

In contrast to this perspective, research by Harter and her colleagues suggests that the meaning of various emotion labels, particularly labels for more complex emotional blends, differs over the course of development. For example, in research utilizing open-ended interviews, children were asked to provide a description of pride and shame. Although many 4- and 5-year-old children used these emotion words in everyday interaction, most youngsters of this age could not describe these feelings (Harter & Whitesell, 1989). More importantly, the meaning of pride and shame appeared to change with development. For younger children, descriptions of pride and shame involved an experience of how others would react to the self's behavior. For older children, pride and shame concerned their own reactions to their behaviors. In essence, for younger children the experience of pride and shame entails the reaction of an audience, but for older children these feelings are independent of others' reactions. Although the difference is subtle, it has interesting clinical implications. One could imagine a child who discloses feelings of shame about a certain experience, such as failing to make a team. For the younger child, the experience is likely to involve a sense of disappointing others, and the therapist might reasonably encourage the child to check the reality of others' reactions. In contrast, checking the reality of others' reactions would not follow from the older child's disclosure of shame. Instead, the experience captured by the same emotion label is likely to refer to the child's own reaction to failure. In this case, the therapist might reasonably explore the child's own standards and the tendency to evaluate the self harshly. Similar differences are suggested with other emotions. For example, Renouf and Harter (1990) found that the vast majority of preteens describe depression as a blend of anger and sadness. However, it is not clear that younger children's experience or report of depression involves the same emotional elements. First, young children tend to focus on one dimension of an emotional experience rather than on the interplay of feelings (Harter & Whitesell, 1989). Second, even for relatively simple emotions like sadness, there appear to be important differences in what emotion terms connote. For example, Glasberg and Aboud (1982) found that older children were far more likely than younger children to link sadness with feeling *bad* about the self.

How, then, do we reconcile these sets of findings? On the one hand, it appears that there is evidence for continuity in the denotative structure of emotion concepts between middle childhood and adulthood. However, findings showing important developmental differences in the attributes associated with various emotion labels support the existence of discontinuity in the connotative organization of emotion concepts. Because child therapists are not merely concerned with the accuracy of children's descriptions of their emotional experiences, but are highly interested in the *meaning* of such experiences, an awareness of possible connotative differences in emotion concepts is essential for understanding children's accounts of their feelings. For the child therapist, then, understanding and facilitating emotional experience in therapy cannot be equated with eliciting affect labels.

Much of the existing developmental research has focused on children's recognition of relatively simple emotions, for example, happy versus sad. However, many of the experiences presented by children in therapy involve a complex combination of emotions. For example, it is not uncommon to encounter an abused child who oscillates between strong feelings of fear, anger, and love for the maltreating parent. And as this example suggests, children in therapy are often confronted with the problem of conflicting emotions. Harter (1977) found that young children in play therapy often showed substantial difficulty with acknowledging the co-occurrence of positive and negative emotions. These children typically denied the simultaneous experience of two emotions, particularly when they occurred in relation to significant others. For example, when disappointed by a friend, the child might report intense anger but be unable to acknowledge the existence of any feelings of enduring affection. From a clinical perspective, such difficulties might be construed in terms of unstable relational capacities that characterize more serious forms of psychopathology. However, research has revealed that children's ability to recognize and acknowledge the existence of conflicting feelings follows an expected developmental sequence that is linked to advances in cognitive functioning (Carroll & Steward, 1984; Donaldson & Westerman, 1986; Harter & Buddin, 1987).

Harter and her colleagues (Harter & Buddin, 1987; Harter & Whitesell, 1989) have conducted a series of studies on children's understanding of simultaneous emotions. This work has revealed a consistent sequence for the emergence of understanding co-occurring emotions. Two dimensions appear to be critical in this developmental sequence: the valence of the two emotions, that is, whether they are both positive or negative or are of opposite valence; and the number of targets toward which the emotions are directed, that is, whether each feeling is directed toward a separate target or the same target. Five levels of understanding have emerged from research that varies these two dimensions. At Level 0, the child does not understand that one can simultaneously feel two emotions, regardless of valence. The mean age for children in this group was about 5 years. Children at Level 1 (mean age = 7.3) begin to show some awareness of simultaneous emotions, but their understanding is limited to emotions with the same valence directed toward a single target. At the next level (mean age = 8.7) children understand that emotions with the same valence can be directed toward different targets simultaneously, but deny the experience of simultaneous opposite-valenced emotions. This limited understanding gives way to an appreciation of simultaneous emotions with opposite valences at Level 3 (mean age = 10.1). However, at this level the emotions are directed at different aspects of an event, for example, "I was happy that summer vacation was here, but sad that I wouldn't see my teacher." Finally, at Level 4 (mean age = 11.3) children understand that opposite-valenced emotions can be directed toward the same target, for example, "I was upset by what the coach said, but glad he was honest with me." According to Harter and Whitesell (1989), this developmental sequence can be understood in terms of Fischer's neo-Piagetian skill theory (1980); that is, understanding simultaneous emotions involves the coordination of multiple representations. As Harter and Whitesell (1989) note, "Each of the levels in this analysis involves developmental change with regard to the number and type of representations that the child can simultaneously control, coordinate, and integrate" (p. 86). Each level reflects an increasing cognitive demand on the child which, in turn, translates into an age-related developmental sequence.

These developmental findings carry important implications for the child's recognition of emotional experiences in psychotherapy. It is frequently the case that complex clinical situations (e.g., divorce, maltreatment, or peer rejection) elicit multiple rather than single feelings. However, school-age children's developing cognitive capacities may limit their ability to attend to the complex interplay of feelings. Instead, the therapist might be confronted with a child who focuses exclusively on one affect, for example, anger in the context of peer rejection, and denies the presence of other emotions such as sadness. In this situation, the process of denial must be examined carefully. Although it is tempting to attribute the child's difficulty with acknowledging multiple feelings to defensive processes, the inability to acknowledge multiple emotions, particularly conflicting feelings, could reflect representational limitations.

Donaldson and Westerman (1986) have found that even when children recognize the co-occurrence of conflicting feelings, school-age children (under age 10) have problems understanding that contradictory feelings interact and modify each other. From their perspective, the recognition of ambivalence, an experience that has been viewed by psychodynamic theorists as integral to the child's capacity for sustaining stable relationships, is a complex developmental achievement. According to Donaldson and Westerman, the child's understanding of ambivalence involves the recognition of the coexistence of conflicting feelings directed toward the same object at the same time, an awareness that these feelings interact (e.g., dampen or heighten each other), and an understanding that feelings evoked by the immediate situation interact with enduring emotions. In other words, the capacity to recognize and understand ambivalence involves more than the recognition of simultaneous conflicting feelings. Given the complexity of this concept, it is not surprising that young elementary-school children fail to demonstrate an understanding of ambivalence. Consistent with the findings of Harter and her colleagues, these results suggest that the child's ability to identify emotional experiences in therapy will be constrained by developmental processes.

Two caveats should be considered at this point. First, the preceding developmental research has been concerned with the child's recognition of complex emotion experiences, and not with children's felt experience per se. It is likely that children experience multiple and conflicting emotions early in development; in fact, it is likely that some disordered child behavior reflects the interplay of conflicting affective states. However, children's capacity to apprehend and talk about such experiences, as is often requested in child psychotherapy, is limited by their level of cognitive maturity. Second, it is important to remember that the recognition of emotional experience in therapy is not simply a function of the child's developing cognitive abilities; that is, the *capacity* to recognize feelings should not be equated with the *willingness* to acknowledge and talk about emotional experiences. Children vary in their tendency to avoid emotionally charged material, and a number of investigators have shown that this tendency changes with development (Brody & Carter, 1982; Smith & Rossman, 1986).

Glasberg and Aboud (1982) investigated young children's acknowledgement of sadness. The youngest children in their sample, kindergartners, distanced themselves from sadness and reported that they had not experienced the emotion. Older children, age 7, were far more likely to acknowledge sadness as a part of their past experience. The older children were also willing to acknowledge both sadness and happiness as aspects of their personalities. In contrast, the younger children presented uniformly happy portraits of themselves. Glasberg and Aboud suggest that younger children's unwillingness to acknowledge negative emotions is consistent with findings of global, positive self-evaluations among children of this age. Indeed, Harter (1988) has found that preschool and early elementary-school children's reports of their own competencies are often highly inflated. Alternatively, it also may be the case that young children's tendency to keep their distance from negative emotion is a function of their rudimentary cognitive and emotion regulation processes. As Harter (1977) had noted, the dichotomous nature of young children's thinking makes them vulnerable to perceiving themselves as "all bad" if they acknowledge some negative personal characteristic or emotion. Moreover, young children may be less able than older children to differentiate *representations* of negative feelings (e.g., describing past experiences that made them sad) from reexperiencing the sadness. Consequently, the recollection of a sad experience might rearouse the distressing feelings more readily in younger than older children. In essence, young children may be highly vulnerable to mood induction; thus in order to avoid the rearousal of sadness, they maintain their distance from self-perceptions and memories that could evoke such feelings.

Brody and Carter (1982) also have shown that children tend to censure negative and intense feelings when attributing affect to themselves. In this study, Brody and Carter examined the quality and intensity of emotion attributed to either the self or to an ambiguous protagonist in a series of emotionally evocative stories. Their results revealed that children at all ages, in this case, ages 7 to 11, attributed more sad and scared feelings to the ambiguous protagonists than to themselves in the same stories. In addition, more intense feelings were ascribed to the other than to the self. This pattern of results was viewed by Brody and Carter as reflecting the prominent role of defenses in children's management of negative emotions. The findings also suggest that children will find it difficult to acknowledge and *directly* talk about intense, negative emotions in the context of child psychotherapy. In this regard, these developmental findings are consistent with clinical accounts of seasoned child therapists, who have maintained that an *indirect* path, for example, through play or fantasy, is the least obstructed route to facilitating children's understanding of their emotional experiences.

Emotional Understanding

In addition to focusing on and recognizing emotions, emotional experiencing involves integrating affective states with personal meaning. One important aspect of integrating meaning with emotions is the child's causal understanding of emotional experiences (Thompson, 1989). In fact, several approaches to child psychotherapy emphasize the importance of the child's causal understanding of emotion. In the psychodynamic tradition, interpretations often make links between feelings and antecedent events and experiences (Shirk, 1988a). Similarly, cognitively-oriented therapists focus on the child's causal attributions as a potential source of maladaptive emotional response (Stark et al., 1991). Though the aims and techniques of these two approaches differ significantly, children's causal understanding of their emotional experiences is pivotal in both.

Conducting causal analyses of emotional experiences is not likely to be a novel activity for children in therapy. Bretherton and Beeghly (1982) showed that causal utterances about emotion can be found in the everyday language of toddlers. In fact, among very young children, causal statements about internal states primarily referred to emotion. This, of course, does not mean that children at different developmental levels are relatively equivalent in their ability to understand the causes of emotion. Instead, recent research has revealed a number of important developmental trends in this type of emotional understanding.

One of the most important transitions involves a shift from viewing feelings in situational terms to conceptualizing them in mediational terms (Harris, Olthof, & Meerum Terwogt, 1981; Nannis, 1988); that is, as children mature, there is increasing recognition that feelings are not simply evoked by situations, but also are mediated by internal processes. Harris et al. (1981) found that children age 6 and younger believe that events directly elicit emotions, whereas by age 11, children recognize that internal processes such as memories and preexisting feelings influence their reactions to events. Increasing recognition of internal processes entails several important changes in children's reasoning about emotion. First, there is increasing complexity in children's inferences about emotions in themselves and others. Thompson (1989) found that young elementary-school children (second graders) tend to focus on situational outcomes (e.g., success vs. failure) to infer emotions. Given the implicit assumption that feelings directly follow from events, it makes sense that young children principally examine situational characteristics to infer emotions. By fifth grade, however, children rely to a far greater degree on "attribution-dependent" inferences; that is, they go beyond outcome information to an analysis of the causal antecedents for particular outcomes, for example, whether the outcome is the result of luck, effort, or ability. Consequently, older children's emotional inferences become more differentiated; they move away from global concepts, such as happy or sad, to more specific emotions, such as proud, ashamed, grateful, or relieved. Accurate inferences of more differentiated emotions depend on a consideration of internal processes and not just overt outcomes. Interestingly, young children did infer, at times, more specific emotions such as pride and guilt, but they did not consistently link these feelings with the appropriate causal cues. These findings suggest that young children may draw very different inferences about the emotional significance of situations than their therapists as a result of less mature information processing capacities. In fact, if children utilize causal cues differently than adults, and there is reason to believe that this tendency is exacerbated in some clinical populations (Dodge & Frame, 1982), then child patients could be quite perplexed by their therapists' labels for their emotional experience. Of equal importance, if therapists are confused by what appear to be idiosyncratic emotional reactions by their child patients, clarification might be attained by exploring the child's causal understanding of the situation.

A second important change associated with the developmental shift to viewing emotion in mediational terms is the increasing recognition of the enduring nature of feelings. Although Harris (1983) has shown that children as young as age 7 recognize that distress can persist after a precipitating event has ended, Donaldson and Westerman (1986) have found that younger children have difficulty coordinating feelings evoked by immediate situations with feelings related to prior experiences. In fact, Harris' younger subjects were inclined to discount the emotional impact of an earlier event on current feelings. Similarly, younger children's lack of differentiation between feelings and emotion expressions. (e.g., "If you're not crying, you're not sad") suggests a rather transitory view of emotion. Yet child therapists often are concerned with the emotional *residue* of past experiences; that is, child therapists frequently work from the assumption that disordered child behavior is instigated by a reservoir of unexpressed emotion carried over from earlier experiences. In other words, the therapist assumes that emotion can be "conserved" despite lapses in time and changes in outer expression. This assumption about feelings is not likely to be shared by a child who views emotions as tightly linked with situations and expressive behavior. Given this discrepancy between child and therapist assumptions, we should not be surprised by the disinterest many child patients show in our efforts to uncover difficult feelings we assume they are harboring. For the child who understands emotion in situational terms, this therapeutic task would make little sense. To be sure, this is not to say that children are not affected by enduring feelings. Clinical experience shows that children often transpose difficult feelings aroused in one situation onto another. Rather, the importance of these developmental differences for therapy is that we cannot expect children to actively engage in a therapeutic task they cannot understand. Instead, as child therapists, we must provide children with the "scaffolding" to enable them to address emotional issues. In this case, the therapist may need to provide the child with a metaphor (e.g., a passenger who is weighed down by luggage that holds old feelings) or a visual representation, such as a "feelings bin," in order to engage the child in this therapeutic process. Minimally, it is important to remember that younger children understand feelings in close connection with the situations that evoked them and in terms of the reactions that followed. Thus, the difficulties encountered when we attempt to address feelings that are not currently evoked or displayed should not be attributed to defensive processes until it is clear that the child shares our assumptions about the "conservation" of emotion.

These developmental constraints on children's ability or willingness to focus on emotional experiences suggest that "emotional experiencing" in child therapy might be best conducted "on-line," that is, as the feelings are aroused in the therapeutic situation. This perspective is consistent with the therapeutic emphasis of nondirective play therapy (Axline, 1947). Rather than focusing on the child's emotional responses to past events, the therapist responds to the child's expressed emotion in the present (Wright et al., 1986). Similarly, one of the advantages of dyadic or group forms of therapy, such as Selman's (1980) pair therapy, is that peers often evoke emotional reactions that children would not disclose in traditional therapy. Rather than depending on the child's representation of prior events and their associated feelings, the pair therapist can respond to emotional experiences as they occur in ongoing social interaction. Of course, dynamically oriented child therapists have long emphasized the relative importance of feelings that are elicited in relation to the therapist. It is assumed that such feelings are linked to core affective patterns that organize the child's interpersonal experience and behavior, and thus constitute the "royal road" to emotional change (Chethik, 1989).

It is possible, however, that what is gained in emotional accessibility is lost in emotional understanding. Children who are experiencing strong emotion may be less able to grasp its meaning than children who are reflecting on past emotional experiences. Harris and Lipian (1989) found precisely this pattern with medically ill children. They compared the emotional understanding of children, ages 6 and 10, who were facing an emotionally charged situation, hospitalization for illness, with children who had been sick but were now recovered. Although both groups were queried about emotions related to an illness experience, it was assumed that the latter group would no longer be experiencing the relevant emotions to the same degree as the hospitalized group; that is, they would be reflecting on past experiences with illness. Harris and Lipian computed a "maturity score" reflecting the overall sophistication of responses to questions about mixed emotions, masked feelings, and strategies for changing feelings, and found that the mature replies of healthy 10-year-olds were far less prevalent among hospitalized children, despite comparability in overall intelligence and social class. In fact, the replies of the hospitalized 10-year-olds were quite similar to the responses of the healthy 6-year-olds. Although part of this pattern might be attributed to differences in the severity of the illness each group considered, a similar pattern held for responses to hypothetical situations. Harris and Lipian concluded that the hospitalized children evinced a consistent pattern of slippage or regression in their understanding of emotion. In the context of negative affect arousal, the hospitalized children showed less maturity in their emotional understanding than children who were no longer experiencing the negative feelings, but instead were reflecting on a prior negative experience. Although this study focused on a limited range of negative emotion, the results suggest that children's understanding of emotion is affected by their current experience of emotion.

Taken together, these developmental patterns pose an interesting challenge for the therapist who wishes to help children deal with strong feelings. On the one hand, the typical middle childhood patient is likely to maintain his or her distance from strong, negative feelings. Attempts to get the child to focus on emotionally-difficult past experiences are likely to be met with some resistance. Consequently, many child therapists attend to emotion as it is expressed in the present. On the other hand, if the aroused emotion is strong, it is likely to undercut the child's ability to understand the experience in a mature manner. It takes relatively little clinical experience to recognize the constraints on emotion processing when a child is overwhelmed with rage or sadness.

One solution to this dilemma, it seems, is to break the process of "emotional experiencing" into a sequence of processing steps. At least three components can be identified. The first involves *elicitation* of emotions. Clinical experience suggests that direct questioning of clinic-referred children often produces superficial responses. Instead, the therapist may be well advised to attend to the spontaneous expression of emotion in the treatment relationship, or to indirect expressions of emotion in the context of symbolic play. When the emotion is aroused, the therapist's principal task is to bring it to the child's attention. The second component, then, involves the *registry* of emotion; that is, when strong emotion is aroused, the therapist's main task is not to analyze its source and meaning with the child, but to register its occurrence by providing a verbal label. The third component, *reflection* on the meaning of the experience, should occur after intense arousal has been managed. Again, clinical experience suggests that reflection on the meaning of emotional experiences is facilitated when the therapist draws the child's attention to a pattern of emotional episodes that have been registered across sessions. As this model implies, "emotional experiencing" with children is a process that occurs over time. From this perspective, one marker of therapeutic progress is the child's increasing ability to process emotional episodes as they occur.

Clinical Approaches to Emotional Experience

Many developing child clinicians become frustrated by their lack of success in addressing emotion in therapy. In clinical supervision it is not uncommon to hear reports of thwarted efforts to help the child deal with feelings. One of the most common experiences can be summed up as follows: "I asked him how he felt and all he did was shrug his shoulders; when I asked again, he just said 'fine' and nothing else." The question, then, is: Are there approaches to children's emotional experience that might yield a more productive response? The developmental literature suggests a number of guidelines for therapists who attempt to facilitate children's experience of emotion in psychotherapy.

First, inquiries about emotion should be *contextualized.* Developmental research indicates that children, particularly elementary-school children, rely on situational cues for the identification of emotion. Questions such as, "How did it make you feel?," although useful as a follow-up to a child's account of an important event, rarely elicit as much emotion as the account itself. Thus, rather than approaching emotion from the more abstract (i.e., removed) perspective of emotion labels, it can be useful to ask the child about the concrete details of an important event. In this way, the emotional experience is embedded in a situational context. For example, in a recent session, an 8-year-old boy from a very disadvantaged background reported that his cousin was going to live with the family for several months. The family's resources were already stretched to the limit, and one of the child's major concerns involved deprivation and the availability of emotional and material provisions. Consequently, it was not hard to imagine that the arrival of the cousin would arouse considerable emotion. However, when asked, "How do you feel about her coming?," the boy simply said, "It's okay."

Was this a defensive response, or had the therapist failed to provide the facilitating context for the child's emotional experience? In this situation, the latter appeared to be the case. When the therapist focused, instead, on the concrete implications of the cousins arrival—for example, "Where will she sit at dinner? Will there be enough for seconds? Who will get to choose the TV shows?"—the child's responses betrayed strong feelings. The felt experience was elicited by the situational (concrete) context, and then the therapist was able to help the child identify and label the emotional experience.

A second guideline derived from the developmental literature involves the usefulness of providing *scaffolding* for children's emotional experiences. Children's performances on emotion tasks in developmental research are highly sensitive to task demands (Fischer, 1980), such that simply asking children to talk about their emotional experiences may mask the complexity of their emotional understanding. One of the best examples of scaffolding children's understanding of emotion is reported by Harter (1977) in a case study of play therapy. In this case, a 6-year-old child, who was referred because of poor school performance, presented with great difficulty in dealing with conflicting feelings. Her spontaneous play was characterized by the repetitive theme of a punitive teacher who chastised her student for incompetence and misbehavior. The child's play revealed both an intense emotional experience and an undifferentiated representation of the self. In essence, the child cast the student as all dumb, with no redeeming qualities that could conflict with this uniform portrayal. In an effort to introduce greater complexity into this representation, her therapist depicted parts of herself, including different emotions, graphically. These graphic depictions of mixed feelings eventually were absorbed into the thematic play. (The child instructed the class on the meaning of the depictions!) Over the course of therapy these depictions were applied to new emotional experiences and enabled the child to represent conflicting emotions. As Harter noted, the concrete, visualizable depictions provided the child with structure for organizing her emotional experiences. Similar beneficial effects of concrete scaffolding have been reported in the child clinical literature, for example, using a "feelings thermometer" to help the child differentiate levels of emotional intensity (Stark et al., 1991).

A third guideline involves the use of *indirect* methods for facilitating emotional experience. Developmental research indicates that children are more likely to acknowledge negative emotions in an ambiguous, but similar, protagonist than in themselves (Brody & Carter, 1982). This finding supports one of the basic assumptions of play therapy, namely, that thematic play is a better medium for facilitating emotional experiences with children than is verbal interaction (Axline, 1947). According to this perspective, child therapists should be prepared to operate within the *child's* favored medium when it comes to addressing strong emotions. This does not mean that the therapist should abandon attempts to engage the child in talk about feelings, but rather that emotional accessibility will often be increased by providing the child with multiple methods for representing his or her emotional experiences.

Finally, the developmental literature suggests that children, especially preschoolers and young elementary school children, will find it difficult to represent and focus on past emotional experiences. The therapist's implicit assumption of "emotion conservation" is not likely to be shared by young child patients who yoke emotions with eliciting situations and affective displays. Consequently, if the goal is to enhance emotional experiencing, child therapists will find it more fruitful to focus on "presented" emotion than on discussions of past experiences. A critical task for child therapists, then, is to provide the medium through which past emotional experiences can be presented in therapy. Traditionally, child therapists have focused on the spontaneous presentation of emotion in thematic play or in inter-action with the child. However, it also is important to consider other, less spontaneous methods for eliciting emotional experiences. Assorted possi-bilities include structured thematic play (Buchsbaum, Toth, Clyman, Cic-chetti, & Emde, 1992), role plays, and the production of "docudramas" that capture significant life events.

With these developmental considerations in mind, let us now turn to two prominent therapeutic approaches to children's emotional experi-ence. One important dimension that distinguishes therapeutic approaches to children's emotion involves the degree of structure provided by the therapist. Anchoring the structured end of the continuum are those approaches, often grouped under the label of "affective education," that utilize a well-defined, emotion-focused curriculum. A basic assumption of this type of approach is that troubled children lack the *skills* to recognize and verbalize their emotional experiences (Stark et al., 1991). Therapy, then, is framed in terms of teaching children the requisite skills for processing emotional experiences by guiding them through a sequence of emotion-focused activities.

One of the best examples of this approach is offered by Stark and his colleagues (1991) in their comprehensive treatment package for childhood depression. Affective education is the first therapeutic procedure utilized in this approach, and children are presented with a series of five games (usually in group format) that focus on emotion recognition, labeling, and display. For example, links between feelings and behaviors are emphasized in the game, "emotional charades." In this game, a player draws an emotion card from a deck and portrays the emotion to either the therapist or other children. Special attention is directed toward the behavioral cues that signal the felt emotions. Other games emphasize links between thoughts and feelings. And as Stark et al. note, the content of these games can be tailored to the specific needs of the child.

In contrast to this approach, and at the other end of the structured–unstructured continuum, is traditional child play therapy. Children's difficulties with emotional experience are not conceptualized in terms of skill deficits, but rather are viewed in terms of the *conditions* that have separated the child from fully experiencing his or her feelings. A basic assumption of this approach is that troubled children have learned that it is unacceptable to acknowledge and express specific emotions, and that these "accumulated" feelings undermine adaptive functioning (Axline, 1947, p. 16). Therapy, then, is framed as an opportunity for the child to experience the full range of emotions without fear of sanction. Rather than providing the child with a set of emotion-focused activities, the therapist offers the interpersonal conditions of permissiveness and nonjudgmental acceptance. No attempt is made to actively elicit feelings from the child. Instead, the therapist's activity centers on responding to the child's emotional expressions. As Axline (1947) maintains, the principal task for the therapist is to attend to feelings expressed both directly and indirectly by the child, and then to reflect these feelings back to the child in a supportive manner. Although this therapeutic approach is often labeled "nondirective," the therapist consistently directs attention to the affective tone of the child's play or verbal statements, rather than to its thematic content (Wright et al., 1986). For many children, content is figural against an affective background; however, the goal of the play therapist is to reverse this relationship by focusing on feelings.

Although these two approaches share the therapeutic aim of promoting children's experience of emotion, their treatment methods diverge widely and reflect markedly different conceptualizations of pathogenic process. Affective education, with its emphasis on teaching processing skills, typifies treatments based on a skill deficit model. However, when defensive processes are framed as the pathogenic culprit, the focus of treatment shifts from teaching skills to eliciting felt emotion. Not surprisingly, then, these two approaches entail substantially different treatment processes and, thus, offer the child therapist alternatives for overcoming some of the developmental obstacles to working with emotion in therapy.

First, the developmental literature suggests that it will be important to provide adequate scaffolding in order for children to address their emotional experiences. Here the two approaches differ significantly. Play therapy relies on the spontaneous presentation of feelings through play, games, or verbal interaction, whereas affective education provides a hierarchy of structured activities for identifying and labeling emotional experiences. For the child who avoids affective material in therapy, structured activities may provide a method for gradually introducing emotion into sessions. For the child who readily engages in thematic play, such activities may be unnecessary, and in fact, could obstruct the child's processing of personally relevant emotions. Thus, the provision of structure is not always the appropriate intervention; instead, it depends on the needs of the specific child. In this respect, it is important to note that what might be gained by increased scaffolding (structure) could be lost in emotional immediacy; that is, play therapists tend to focus on feelings as they are expressed; in contrast, therapists who rely on an affective education approach tend to emphasize "hypothetical" or role-played emotional experiences. On the one hand, role-played activities could provide the child with an *indirect* method of dealing with troublesome feelings, and thereby overcome another developmental obstacle in therapy, namely, the child's inclination to maintain distance from negative emotions. However, such indirect activities might not provide the child with the opportunity to integrate his or her processing skills with actual "felt" emotion. In this respect, one of the advantages of play therapy is that it provides the child with an opportunity to reflect on emotional experiences as they occur. Of course, play therapists also rely on indirect methods for eliciting feelings (e.g., through symbolic play), and a recurrent issue for those practicing this approach involves the degree to which indirectly experienced and expressed emotions must be directly acknowledged by the child (Shirk, 1988b).

How, then, does the child therapist choose between these two approaches to facilitating the experience of emotion? First, the decision to utilize either an affective education or play-therapy approach should be based on an assessment of the degree to which the child's difficulties with the recognition, labeling, and understanding of emotional experiences are a function of skill deficits or defensive processes. Second, the therapist should consider the degree to which the treatment procedures are aligned with the child's specific problems with emotional experience. For example, if the child has difficulty integrating emotional understanding with the actual experience of feelings, then reliance on role plays and structured activities is not likely to be sufficient. Instead, the therapist will need to provide the child with the opportunity to process emotional experiences "on-line," that is, as they are felt by the child. Finally, the therapist must consider the degree to which the treatment procedures attend to developmental obstacles often encountered when addressing emotion in child therapy. For example, if the child is highly avoidant of emotional material (e.g., he or she engages in endless sessions of board games), then providing the child with a graded series of emotionally evocative activities could provide the structure and support needed to address difficult feelings. Although the developmental literature suggests a number of guidelines for facilitating children's emotional experience, it is important to remember that such developmental considerations must be aligned with the specific needs of the individual child.

Given the importance assigned to the recognition, labeling, and understanding of emotional experiences in models of child therapy, it is surprising how little research has been conducted on these processes among troubled children. To date, the clinical hypothesis that troubled children are less able to process their emotional experiences, either by virtue of skill deficits or distorting defenses, lacks a firm empirical foundation. Most of the existing, albeit limited, literature has focused on the identification of others' emotions. For example, Zabel (1979) found that emotionally disturbed children were more inaccurate in their recognition of emotion depicted in facial expressions than were their nondisturbed peers. These results parallel findings by Camras, Grow, and Ribordy (1983) that abused children were less accurate than nonabused children in their ability to identify emotion from affective displays. Although this research suggests that maladjusted children are vulnerable to one type of emotion-processing problem, little is known about the mechanisms that contribute to the inaccurate identification of emotion. Of equal importance, it is not clear whether such inaccuracies are common to all forms of maladjustment or are specific to certain disorders. Furthermore, evidence for one type of emotion processing problem in maladjusted children should not be generalized to other aspects of their emotional experience. For example, Taylor and Harris (1983) found no differences between disturbed and nondisturbed boys' understanding of the interplay between emotion and memory. Taken together, these results suggest that maladjusted children may not evince problems in all areas of emotion processing. Given the narrow scope of existing research, however, expected patterns of processing difficulties have not been identified. For example, it is not clear whether children who have difficulties with the recognition of others' emotions will show similar problems with their own feelings. Thus, the identification of patterns of emotion processing problems remains a challenging task for child therapists who hope to promote children's recognition, labeling, and understanding of emotion.

EMOTION REGULATION

Intake interviews with parents of clinic-referred children often are replete with references to emotion dysregulation. "He's a time bomb just waiting to explode"; "She's wound so tight I don't know what she's feeling"; "Talk about a short fuse, I don't think he has a fuse"; "Every little thing makes her so upset, we should buy stock in Kleenex." Given the ubiquitous nature of emotion regulation problems among clinic-referred children, some have argued that such problems are at the core of child psychopathology (Cole et al., 1994). Consistent with this perspective, others have proposed that stable regulatory styles constitute one of the most important defining features of different types of disorders (Malatesta & Wilson, 1988). It has become increasingly common to conceptualize "internalizing" disorders such as dysthymia or generalized anxiety disorder in terms of emotion dysregulation. For example, the depressed child appears to have problems with the control of sad feelings or the maintenance of positive affect, or perhaps both. Recently, however, greater attention has been directed to the role of emotion dysregulation in the disruptive behavior disorders as well (Cole & Zahn-Waxler, 1992). Of central concern has been the disruptive child's difficulties with the control of anger. Thus, to ignore emotion processes in the treatment of disruptive children would be a significant oversight. Instead, both internalizing and externalizing disorders appear to involve emotion-regulation problems. This view is buttressed by the recurrent finding of a significant overlap between emotional distress and disruptive behavior in parent ratings of child behavior problems (Achenbach & Edelbrock, 1983).

Although it is common to equate emotion regulation with the control of negative feelings, adaptive emotional functioning involves both the ability to access and maintain emotions that are congruent with contextual demands, and the ability to modulate the intensity and duration of emotions that could disrupt cognitive and interpersonal processes. In the child psychotherapy tradition, there is a long history of theory and application of treatment methods for helping children attain adaptive emotional functioning. A brief review uncovers many attempts to utilize children's play as a medium for releasing (Levy, 1939), limiting (Bixler, 1949), structuring (King & Ekstein, 1967), or transforming (Erikson, 1963) problematic emotions. Currently, however, much of child psychotherapy appears to be guided by one of two alternative perspectives on emotion regulation—psychodynamic or information-processing models.

Psychodynamic Perspective on Emotion Regulation

Conflict is a cornerstone of psychodynamic theory, and according to Vaillant (1986), Freud emphasized the role of disruptive emotions in his model of psychological conflict. In the face of dysregulating impulses and emotions, humans develop methods for maintaining psychological equilibrium. This fragile balance is achieved through the evolution of regulatory processes known as "mechanisms of defense" (A. Freud, 1966). According to Vaillant (1986), defenses represent the individual's primary means of managing impulse and affect; they operate outside of awareness; they are distinguishable from one another; and although they serve an adaptive function, when overused, they are a salient feature of major psychiatric disorders. Chandler and his colleagues (Chandler, Paget, & Koch, 1978) have defined defenses as alternative systems for "distorting or transforming the appearance of more candid but less acceptable thoughts and feelings" (p. 197). For example, the child who experiences intense anger toward a parent might redirect such strong feelings toward a parent substitute, such as a teacher, through the defensive process of displacement. In addition to the *redirection* of emotion, as in displacement or turning against the self, defensive operations can involve the *negation* (denial), *submersion* (repression), *reversal* (reaction formation), *neutralization* (sublimation), *detachment* (isolation and intellectualization), or *reorigination* (projection) of emotional experience. As these processes imply, defenses regulate emotions by transforming them, and the failure to activate defensive processes results in the direct translation of emotion into behavior (acting out).

How, then, does the child develop this system for transforming disruptive emotion? According to Freud (1946), the origins of the defenses are linked to the development of the ego. In psychoanalytic theory, the young child's behavior is energized by unmodulated affects and impulses. However, behavior based on blind response to such impulses invariably leads to conflict and dangers in relation to the social world. The ego, as a system of regulation, develops through interaction with representatives of the external world, namely caregivers. As a means of both avoiding potential dangers (sanctions from caregivers) and maintaining relatedness, the ego "interpolates between desire and action" (Freud, 1946, p. 106), and the principal method at its disposal are the mechanisms of defense. Thus, defenses are the offspring of the primordial conflict between impulse and constraint, between egocentric wish and social limitation.

The question of defense "choice," that is, what leads a child to utilize one set of defenses rather than another, has perplexed dynamic theorists since the issue was first raised by Anna Freud (1966). She suggested that the activation of particular defenses might be tied to specific affects and impulses, for example, repression against sexual feelings versus reaction formation against aggressive impulses. Others such as Winnicott (1965) have drawn attention to variations in mother–infant interaction as the matrix from which the child's affect-regulating processes emerge. And beginning with Anna Freud, a number of theorists have proposed that defenses evolve through a developmental sequence propelled by maturational processes (Cramer, 1983; Stolorow & Lachman, 1978; Vaillant, 1971). For example, Vaillant (1971) identified four levels of defense—narcissistic, immature, neurotic, and mature—involving maturation on two dimensions: movement from distorting reality to altering internal affect, and from distorting affect to redirecting emotion into socially acceptable channels. In his 20-year follow-up study of college-aged men, Vaillant (1977) found an increasing use of mature defenses over time. Thus, primitive and immature defenses, that is, those that distort reality or affective experience, are commonly found among very young children. However, their appearance later in life signals developmental arrest or regression.

There has been relatively little research on the development of children's defenses. Cramer (1979, 1983, 1987) has proposed that defense mechanisms can be ordered along a developmental continuum based on the cognitive complexity of the defensive (transformative) process. Relatively immature defenses involve simple negation or reversal. For example, in using denial, the child withdraws attention from distressing stimuli, or with the use of language, negates a frightening aspect of a situation (e.g., upon seeing a boy about to receive an injection, the child proclaims, "It's just a little needle"). Denial may also involve simple reversal. For example, in fantasy, the frightened child might transform fear into heroic courage, or failure into glorious achievement. At a somewhat higher level are defensive processes that involve reciprocal transformations (Chandler et al., 1978). Here the object of the affective reaction is transformed, for example, by redirecting anger toward another (displacement) or toward the self. Among the most complex defense is projection. Here multiple transformations are involved. The child's affect, typically anger, is not only denied but also it is translocated to another person who directs it toward the self. Cramer (1983) includes principalization (e.g., rationalization and intellectualization) and identification at the highest level of defense. However, it is not clear that these defenses entail greater cognitive complexity, that is, involve more transformations, or simply are associated with the development of language skills.

One of the most consistent findings to emerge from this literature is that the use of denial decreases with age (Brody, Rozek, & Muten, 1985; Cramer, 1987). For example, Cramer (1987) found that denial was most frequently used by preschoolers and declined thereafter. However, Smith and Rossman (1986) noted that knowledge of a child's tendency to utilize denial *in general* may not be particularly predictive of the use of this defense under stress or in specific problematic situations. For example, in their study, older children were more open than younger children to acknowledging negative affects in response to more abstract questionnaire items; however, this greater openness did not preclude their use of denial in specific stressful situations.

There is less consistent evidence for the development of other defenses. Cramer (1983, 1987) has uncovered patterns of defense utilization that are inconsistent with her proposed model. For example, in one study, projection was used more by early adolescents than late adolescents; and in another, older school-aged children used "turning against the self" less frequently than younger children. These results are at odds with a developmental model based on variations in defense complexity. It should be noted, however, that Cramer relied on chronological age as the sole indicator of developmental level. It is possible that some of these inconsistent findings are attributable to variations in cognitive development that are not accounted for by age alone. More importantly, there is evidence that utilization of a particular defense may not be fully explained by its level of complexity. One of the most robust findings to emerge from these studies is the association between defense utilization and gender. Among young children, males are more likely to direct affect externally (turn against the object), whereas females are more likely to use reversal (Cramer, 1983). Among adolescents, these sex differences are even more prominent. Males tend to externalize conflict through projection and turning against the object, whereas females are more likely to redirect affect toward the self (Cramer, 1979). It is likely that socialization practices associated with gender account for these differences.

A second limitation of the existing literature is the overemphasis on individual maturational factors to account for defense development and utilization. One of the few attempts to examine the contribution of relational processes has been research on sexual identification and defense utilization (Cramer & Carter, 1978). Although defense utilization was not found to be related to sex-role attitudes, there was evidence that gender identity was associated with defensive processes. For example, males who utilized projection to a greater degree than others evinced stronger masculine gender identification. Similarly, females who showed strong feminine gender identification were more inclined to utilize defenses that minimized external conflict than less feminine-identified females. These findings, albeit preliminary, suggest that defense utilization may be associated with variations in identity formation.

Recent developmental theory and research on emotion regulation (ER) have emphasized both the evolution of "within-child mechanisms that underlie activation of ER, and factors external to the child that facilitate ER" (Kopp, 1989, p. 344). For example, Kopp (1989) notes that aspects of emotion regulation are biologically preadapted for the management of distress such as gaze aversion, nonnutritive sucking, and body rubbing in infants. These basic "prewired" mechanisms evolve into elemental cognitive mechanisms through associative learning; for example, the infant discriminates and remembers events that evoked distress and utilizes the basic cognitive strategies to modify the experience, for example, distracting oneself by playing with a toy. With increasing representational and cognitive development, toddlers utilize planful cognitive activities to regulate distress, for example, by anticipating outcomes and attending to predictive cues for impending distress. The evolution of these "within-child" mechanisms emerge slowly because of their close links with cognitive development (Kopp, 1989).

However, as Kopp (1989, p. 345) emphasizes, "Infants and young children must have external support for regulating their emotions." In the early months of development, only the caregiver can relieve distress resulting from hunger, wet clothes, or gas pains. Initially, caregivers are reactive; they rely on tactile and kinesthetic calming methods, such as stroking or rocking; but this approach typically gives way to the use of expressive vocalizations, during which messages about managing distress are conveyed (Demos, 1986; Kopp, 1989). As infants increase in their communicative competence, caregivers begin to differentiate signals of distress (boredom vs. hunger), and infants begin to associate the expression of distress with the caregiver's potential to change their emotional state (Kopp, 1989). Recurrent patterns of responsiveness, or lack of responsiveness, to infants' signals of distress are gradually incorporated into sets of expectations about caregiver availability and reliability (Ainsworth et al., 1978). In addition, caregivers vary in the strategies they employ in response to infant distress (Demos, 1986). For example, some caregivers vary their techniques in response to different forms of distress (e.g., pain, illness, boredom, or fear), whereas others tend to rely on a narrow repertoire of calming strategies. In one study, Demos described a mother who only used physical contact and food in response to all forms of distress. In more extreme cases, the infant's distress is a catalyst for parental distress, which results in reactions (e.g., anger) that actually escalate the infant's distressed state (Cicchetti, Ganiban, & Barnett, 1991). As these examples suggest, the context of early emotion *coregulation* is fertile ground for the development of individual differences in emotion regulation processes.

Recently, this view has been elaborated by attachment theorists, who provide a relational perspective on the development of defenses (Cassidy & Kobak, 1988; Kobak & Sceery, 1988; Kobak, Cole, Ferenz-Gillies, Fleming, & Gamble, 1993). Although attachment theory is often presented as a framework for understanding continuity in interpersonal relations, emotion regulation is an inherent component of attachment behavior. First, the goal of the attachment system is the affective state of "felt security" (Sroufe & Waters, 1977). Second, individual differences in the means by which this affective state is achieved stem from variations in parental sensitivity and responsiveness to the infant's affective signals. Infants who experience distress *and* the availability of comforting caregivers learn that emotions can be regulated by seeking support from others (Kobak & Sceery, 1988). However, in less fortunate circumstances, in which the distressed child recurrently experiences inconsistency, unavailability, or rebuff, alternative strategies for regulating distress may emerge (Ainsworth et al., 1978). According to Kobak (Kobak & Sceery, 1988; Kobak et al.,

1993), insecure infants and children, who are unable to reliably attain felt security through access to the attachment figure, develop characteristic strategies for reducing distress. For children who have experienced parental inconsistency, responsiveness might be elicited by *hyperactivating* the attachment system. Such children might be expected to exaggerate signals of distress in order to attain parental responsiveness. As a generalized pattern of emotion regulation, such children might be prone to excessive emotional displays (Kobak et al., 1993). In contrast, children who have experienced rejection or rebuff when distressed might employ a *deactivating* strategy that serves to minimize conflict with the caregiver (Kobak et al., 1993). Such children could be expected to attenuate signals of distress and ultimately to avoid others as potential sources of comfort or support.

Cassidy and Kobak (1988) have proposed that a number of defensive processes have their origins in the avoidant or deactivating attachment strategy. According to Bowlby (1980), attachment behavior that does not elicit comfort or support arouses anger and anxiety. However, the expression of these feelings to a rejecting parent risks further rebuffs, or in the case of maltreated children, possible retaliation. In this psychologically (and possibly physically) dangerous context, avoidance and the masking of negative affect may serve to maintain the fragile relationship with the caregiver (Cassidy & Kobak, 1988); that is, the infant uses an avoidant strategy as a defense in order to minimize conflict with the caregiver. As Cassidy and Kobak note, in order to avoid anticipated conflict, the child learns "to cut-off, repress, or falsify the expression of negative affect" (p. 304). It is possible that avoidant strategies evolve with cognitive development such that more primitive mechanisms (denial and repression) give way to other affect-restricting processes, such as isolation and intellectualization. However, the origins of different defensive organizations are to be found in variations in the coregulation of distress emerging from recurrent infant–caregiver interactions. In essence, attachment theory redirects attention to the relational context of emotion regulation.

Interventions for Transforming Defenses

Although many psychodynamic case studies underscore the importance of transforming or building defenses as an important component of child psychotherapy (cf. Chethik, 1989), there have been very few empirical studies linking defensive processes and child psychopathology. In one study with psychiatrically hospitalized adolescents, Noam and Recklitis (1990) found relationships between externalizing symptoms and defenses that locate conflict outside the self (turning against the other, projection), and between internalizing symptoms and defenses that locate conflict within the self. Similarly, Winfrey (1993) found that clinic-referred aggressive children tend to externalize their conflicts. Although these limited findings suggest that defensive processes may affect symptom expression (i.e., the *type* of symptoms expressed), developmental psychopathologists have yet to demonstrate a relationship between defensive style and severity of child psychopathology. In contrast, clinical practice has been guided by an intervention model that emphasizes both defense flexibility (ego resiliency) and defense maturity. The former has as its aim the facilitation of adaptive emotional control that is congruent with situational demands; the target of the latter is to reduce the distorting influence of defensive processes on reality testing and social judgment. The maladaptive nature of defensive rigidity is best exemplified by extreme cases. Children with overly brittle, restrictive defenses are unable to engage in normative tasks of develop-ment, such as competition or exploration, whereas children who consis-tently fail to mobilize defenses, and subsequently "act out," tend to be distracted and overwhelmed, and if the unchecked emotional content is hostile, tend to be rejected by peers and adults alike. Similarly, children who rely on defenses that distort their affective experiences typically find it difficult to sustain friendships, for example, they misconstrue others' intents, or because these distortions engender unusual preoccupations, they are isolated by peers or find it difficult to focus on age-appropriate tasks (e.g., schoolwork).

Transforming Maladaptive Defenses

What methods are available to child clinicians for transforming children's maladaptive defenses? A review of the child treatment literature reveals a number of therapeutic strategies. Perhaps the most well-known approach is found in the writings of psychoanalytically oriented child therapists who have emphasized the *unconscious* nature of defensive processes. Here the implicit assumption is that processes that operate outside of awareness cannot be rationally controlled. Thus, modification of defenses is contin-gent upon bringing them into awareness and promoting the child's under-standing of their operation. In a rather strong version of this perspective, Cramer (1983) maintains that "the effectiveness of a defense mechanism depends on its disguise function not being understood; once an individual understands how a defense is disguising an unacceptable thought or feeling, it is no longer a successful defense" (p. 79). In essence, the therapist's task is to help children recognize what they are doing with their emotional experiences. Traditionally, this has meant clarifying and inter-preting the defensive process to the child (Kernberg & Chazan, 1991; Sandler et al., 1980). Typically, such interpretations highlight linkages between thoughts, emotions, and behaviors (Shirk, 1988a).

For example, in a recent case with a 10-year-old boy caught in the middle of visitation conflicts between his divorced parents, it became necessary to modify one of his overused defenses. The child, angered by his father's high expectations (especially around sports), was resistant to weekend visitation. However, he was also frightened to express his anger directly toward his father. As a result, he developed a passive–aggressive stance toward his father (e.g., waking late on ski mornings) and displaced his anger onto his mother, who needed to comply with the court-imposed visitation plan. In addition to working with the father around his high expectations and short temper, individual therapy with the child focused on his expression of angry feelings. In session we identified the "buildup" of anger and frustration, and his fears about expressing these feelings to his father. With some "detective" work, he was able to acknowledge that at times he got very angry at his mother over "little things." After connecting the felt anger toward his father with the expressed anger toward his mother, we dubbed this process "dumping," which provided a salient marker for self-monitoring of this defensive process.

It is worth noting that children at different developmental levels will not be equally capable of understanding interpretations of psychological defense mechanisms (Shirk, 1988a). According to Chandler et al. (1978), defenses vary in their level of structural complexity; that is, some involve more transformations than others; thus children at different stages of cognitive development will vary in their ability to decode defensive trans-formations. In fact, their research provided strong support for the hypothesis that children's understanding of defense mechanisms is a joint function of their level of cognitive development and the structural complexity of the psychological defense (Chandler et al., 1978).

Although the traditional analytic approach emphasizes insight into defensive processes as the primary means of transforming them, others have argued that insight alone is not sufficient (Chethik, 1989; A. Freud, 1966). According to this perspective, the neutralization of a defense must be complemented by the development of a more adaptive defense. In other cases, typically characterized by more severe psychopathology (e.g., borderline disorder), the latter process is the critical therapeutic task; that is, the goal of treatment essentially involves *building* defenses where none exist.

A number of approaches to defense construction have been presented in the child clinical literature. All appear to share the common goal of promoting ego development, that is, facilitating the development of internal controls that redirect emotions into socially acceptable channels. For example, Kernberg and Chazan (1991), in their work with conduct-disordered children, emphasized the development of symbolic functions such as play and language. As they note, therapy enables the child "to expand his capacity for play and to channel acting-out behaviors into the realm of

symbols and words" (p. 18). This perspective draws heavily on the traditional analytic assumption that verbalization is indispensable for adequate
control of affect and impulse (A. Freud, 1965). Thus, rather than relying
on primitive defensive processes such as denial or repression to manage
strong emotions, the child is encouraged to discharge such feelings through
words, fantasies, or play (Kernberg & Chazan, 1991). Through this process,
sublimation is cultivated as an adaptive defense.

Others have emphasized the supportive function of the therapist in
the process of defense building (Chethik, 1989; Pine, 1976). As an emotional support, the therapist "lends" his or her adaptive skills to the child
during therapeutic interactions. For example, the therapist might attempt
to help the child anticipate conditions of high arousal, distinguish between
real and fantasized dangers, contain the direct expression of emotion, and
to soothe the child when disruptive emotions are evoked.

In one case involving a 7-year-old child who had been exposed to
dramatic episodes of interparental violence, initial efforts by the therapist
to help the child address these disturbing events through symbolic play
resulted in marked emotional regression during therapy. The child literally
fell over backwards, covered her eyes, and refused to continue to talk. It
was evident that she lacked the regulatory processes needed to manage
such distressing memories. The aim of therapy, then, shifted to the
facilitation of adaptive regulatory strategies. The therapist made an agreement with the child that she would not probe such painful memories until
the child felt comfortable enough to address them. However, she did inform
the child that an important part of therapy would be learning how to deal
with strong feelings. Together they agreed that the therapist could ask one
question about feelings in each session. The child, in turn, opted to respond
to the therapist by writing brief responses on a note pad. As the child gained
greater confidence in her ability to tolerate these questions and control
her level of arousal, she permitted, in fact, she encouraged, the therapist
to ask more than one "feelings" question each session. Over time, the
therapist increased the potential emotionality of her questions and permitted the child to respond by drawing pictures. As this process progressed,
the child reported to the therapist that she often thought of her (the
therapist) when she was in emotionally upsetting situations, and that such
thoughts helped her deal with her feelings. As this brief vignette shows,
the therapist provided the child with a supportive experience in which she
helped the child anticipate arousal, modulated the intensity of arousal, and
facilitated the development of methods for processing emotion (writing
words or drawing pictures). As a consequence, the child's brittle defenses
were softened, and denial and avoidance were replaced by a more realistic
appraisal of emotional events. In essence, the therapist functioned as a
"coregulator" of the child's affective experience, much in the same way

parents provide this type of external support to very young children. Over time, it is assumed that the child internalizes the regulatory contribution of the therapist through repeated encounters with emotionally evocative material. And as this case so nicely demonstrates, the child carried the image of the therapist and their work together into emotional situations outside the clinic.

In contrast to this more global approach to facilitating emotion regulation, Santostephano (1989) has proposed that adaptive emotional functioning is predicated on the development of a specific set of "cognitive controls" (p. 77). Essentially, cognitive controls function to integrate information from the external environment and the internal environment of thoughts, fantasies, and feelings. Drawing on the work of G. Klein (1954), Santostephano emphasizes that children develop characteristic patterns "to avoid, select, compare, and cluster information in order to adapt to and use the requirements of a situation" (p. 37). Cognitive controls include such processes as *focal attention,* the manner by which the child scans a field of information; *field articulation,* the manner in which relevant and nonrelevant information is processed; and *leveling–sharpening,* the degree to which past and present information is fused or distinguished. The developmental task is to balance the flow of information from internal and external environments in order to regulate action. Development is characterized by an initial orientation toward the internal environment, with external information experienced through the filter of fantasy and private symbols. During middle childhood controls are reoriented outward in order to provide insulation against the disruptive world of fantasy and feeling (Santostephano, 1989). With entry into early adolescence, controls become more flexible and coordinate information from both the internal and external environment. According to Santostephano, much of child psychopathology can be understood in terms of failures to integrate information from these two environments because of inadequate cognitive controls. For example, the child who is oriented to the inner world of fantasy is unable to coordinate thoughts, feelings, and actions with the realistic demands of specific situations. The treatment of such a child would not focus on *what* the child is experiencing, but rather on *how* the child organizes experience (Santostephano, 1985). Therapy, then, involves a program of graded tasks whose aim is to restructure each cognitive control. For example, in order to build the child's capacity for focal attention, and thus enable the child to attend to information from both internal and external environments, the child may be asked to track moving targets of varied complexity, first while seated and later while walking. In essence, the target of cognitive control interventions is the form of the cognitive processes rather than their contents. Thus, in contrast to traditional dynamic therapies, cognitive control therapy attempts to transform maladaptive patterns of emotion regulation by directly building cognitive processes that are assumed to control affective experience.

In contrast to models of defense transformation that focus exclusively on restructuring internal processes, others have emphasized interventions that modify the *conditions* for defense mobilization. Clinicians who draw on an attachment framework suggest that one method for transforming maladaptive defenses, specifically, defensive avoidance, is to alter the interpersonal conditions that maintain this affective orientation. Thus, instead of focusing on building cognitive controls or other internal regulating structures, these clinicians emphasize the important role of ongoing "threats," perceived or real, to affect expression (Cassidy & Kobak, 1988). From an attachment perspective, avoidance develops as a method for minimizing conflict between child and caregiver. The expression of negative feelings threatens the continuity of the caregiving relationship; consequently, such feelings are cut off. In turn, the anger engendered by the lack of parental responsiveness is displaced or expressed in a passive–aggressive manner. As Kobak and Cassidy note, "A primary therapeutic goal is to increase the individual's ability to acknowledge and communicate emotions" (p. 317), and this is accomplished through the therapist's tolerance of the expression of negative affect. In part, therapy aims to restructure the child's working model or maladaptive assumptions about the expression of emotions. The therapist's sensitivity and responsiveness to the child's emotional processes provide a corrective experience, and presumably disconfirming information, about the necessity of avoiding negative feelings. However, in addition to individual therapy with the child, collateral family interventions are geared toward the acknowledgment and expression of negative emotion within the "safe" confines of supportive family therapy (Kobak & Waters, 1984). Thus, the child has the opportunity to experience new responses to emotional expression, and to participate in the restructuring of emotional interactions with family members that presumably maintain the avoidant pattern. In essence, this two pronged approach attempts to alter both internal and external sources of threat to adaptive emotional expression by modifying internal working models and ongoing family interactions.

In summary, then, defense mechanisms are viewed by psychodynamic theorists as the core system for regulating impulse and emotion. It has been hypothesized that variations in child psychopathology can be understood in terms of the unique organization, or lack thereof, of defense mechanisms (A. Freud, 1966). Consequently, the transformation of defenses is a common goal of psychodynamic child therapy (Chethik, 1989). A number of clinical approaches have developed to alter, build, or relax children's defenses. For some children the goal may be the promotion of more mature defenses, whereas for others, the aim may be far more basic, namely, to build a system of inner controls where few or none exist. Not surprisingly, a number of therapeutic strategies have developed to meet these different goals, including defense interpretation, coregulation of emotion by the therapist, cognitive control training, and the reworking of sources of threat that signal defense mobilization. Given the centrality of defense mechanisms in psychodynamic formulations of child psychopathology, it is surprising that psychodynamic child outcome studies have not included measures of defense among their outcome variables. Consequently, the utility of the foregoing interventions for defense transformation awaits confirmation by future research.

Information-Processing Perspective on Emotion Regulation

The most prominent alternative to the psychodynamic approach to emotion regulation is the information-processing perspective (Dodge, 1991; Garber, Braafladt, & Zeman, 1991). In contrast to the hydraulic metaphors of the psychodynamic tradition (flooded with emotion, leaky defenses), the core metaphor for this framework is the computer. Undoubtedly, some may question the goodness of fit of computer metaphors for emotional processes. Typically computers do not conjure emotional imagery (except perhaps frustration). Instead they tend to be viewed as unfeeling, calculating pieces of hardware. Consequently, it may seem ironic that the information-processing perspective represents the major alternative for understanding emotion regulation. In fact, some have suggested that one of the most neglected components of this framework is emotion itself (Gottman, 1986). Recently, however, Crick and Dodge (1994) have maintained that "emotions are an integral part of each information-processing step" (p. 81), and that the framework is applicable to understanding cognitive, behavioral, and emotional phenomena.

The social information-processing perspective emerged as an alternative to global models of children's social maladjustment (Dodge & Frame, 1982). For example, rather than viewing children's problems with peer relations in terms of deficits in broad capacities such as role-taking ability, information-processing theorists proposed that adaptive social functioning hinges on an interrelated set of information-processing skills (Dodge & Frame, 1982; Crick & Dodge, 1994). Inherent in this formulation are two basic assumptions: (1) Complex social processes can be analyzed into simpler, component elements; and (2) these elements can be understood as discrete *skills*. Consistent with the model, these basic assumptions have been applied to emotion regulation. In contrast to models that focus on the development of global constructs, such as ego controls, the information-processing perspective differentiates the process of emotional regulation into multiple components. Furthermore, these components are conceptualized as regulatory skills.

One of the clearest explications of this approach can be found in Garber's (Garber et al., 1991) application of this model to the regulation of sad affect. As mentioned, emotion regulation is conceptualized as an interrelated set of component skills. According to Garber and colleagues, adaptive emotional regulation involves a sequence of information-processing steps including the following:

> (1) perception, or the recognition that affect is aroused and needs to be regulated; (2) interpretation, or the cognitive interpretation of what is causing the emotional arousal and what or who is responsible for altering the negative affect; (3) goal setting, or the decision as to what if anything, needs to be done to alter one's affect; (4) response generation, or the generation of concrete responses to achieve the goal, which can be affected by one's knowledge of appropriate responses and one ability to access this knowledge; (5) response evaluation, or the evaluation of the response generated with regard to their expected outcome . . . ; (6) enactment, or the actual skill one has to implement the chosen response. (pp. 210–211)

For example, consider a child who has just received a poor grade on a term paper she was invested in; and to top it off, she discovered at lunch that she had not been invited to a big party over the weekend. Having been challenged on two important fronts, competence and acceptance, it is likely that the child would be distressed. Competent emotional regulation, then, involves the activation of a sequence of regulatory skills. First, the child must *recognize* and identify her emotional distress. In this case, she might experience a blend of sadness and anger as a function of perceived failure and rejection. In fact, the *interpretation* of the experience as failure or rejection will be an important contributor to the specific type of affect experienced. At this point, in order to regulate the distress, the child must engage in *goal setting*. Among a range of possible goals, the child could opt to resolve the problem, for example, by approaching her peers to find out why she had not been invited or by talking to the teacher about the term paper (problem focused); or she could attempt to alter her mood directly, for example, by expressing it or by engaging in a distracting activity (emotion focused); or she could reach out to others for support (social focused). Depending on the chosen goal, the child would then need to *generate a response*. For example, if the goal were an immediate improvement in her mood, she might opt to buy a desired compact disc or indulge in eating a favorite food. However, as the child prepares to generate a response, additional information-processing takes place. *Response evalu-*

ation involves an assessment of the probability that the response will alleviate the distress, and a judgment about her ability to execute the selected response. In our case, if the child had few friends and a conflictual relationship with parents, it is likely that the goal of obtaining support would be evaluated unfavorably. The child would be confronted with the probability that such a strategy would be doomed to failure, and other alternatives would need to be considered. Finally, *enactment* of an regulating strategy will depend on the child's assessment of her ability to carry out the selected response option. For example, the child might believe that she lacks sufficient appeal to elicit support from others. Such efficacy beliefs, in turn, are likely to affect the execution of the regulatory strategy (Bandura, 1977).

Although the example may suggest that the distressed child engages in a series of deliberate information-processing tasks, it is quite likely that these processes occur quite rapidly, and for the most part, remain outside of awareness. Repeated experiences with specific affects, particularly intense affects, or affect-eliciting situations may routinize certain information-processing patterns, such that the entire sequence is carried out with great automaticity. In this respect, the cognitive operations inherent in emotion regulation may be analogous to Beck's (1976) automatic thoughts; that is, they occur rapidly and without substantial focal attention. However, by slowing the process, and by breaking it into elemental components, this approach highlights the different points at which emotion regulation could go awry.

According to the information-processing model, emotional maladjustment could stem from *deficits* in any of the component skills in the emotion regulation sequence (Garber et al., 1991). At this point, it is too early to know if some deficits are uniquely associated with certain forms of child psychopathology, or if the number of deficits is predictive of severity of psychopathology; however, research is beginning to illuminate the contribution of some of these processes to adaptive emotional functioning. One area that has received considerable attention is the generation of response strategies for emotion regulation (Band & Weisz, 1988; Rossman, 1992).

Drawing on the work of Kopp (1989), who identified five types of emotion-regulation strategies among toddlers, Rossman (1992) interviewed 6- to 12-year-old children in order to establish an inventory of emotion-regulation strategies. Responses from these open-ended interviews were evaluated and transformed into an emotion coping questionnaire. The questionnaire was then administered to a large sample of school-age children. Factor analyses of the children's responses revealed six distinctive emotion regulation strategies. As Rossman (1992) noted, the six strategies could be grouped into three categories: (1) social support from either caregivers or peers; (2) affect communication (express distress or anger); and (3) autonomous regulation (distraction/avoidance or self-calming). For example, the distraction/avoidance factor reflected the child's attempt to withdraw attention from the reality of the stressor through the use of games or fantasy. Self-calming strategies included more self-directed activities, such as verbal self-reassurance, to enhance mood. In contrast, social strategies, such as the caregiver strategy, involved interactions with parents (e.g., talking with Mom or Dad about feeling bad) as a means of relieving distress. Finally, expressive strategies included such behaviors as screaming, yelling, or crying.

Not all emotion-regulation strategies were equally adaptive in the face of stress; that is, some of the strategies moderated the negative relationship between stress and self-esteem—the higher one's life stress, the lower one's self-esteem—whereas other strategies left children more vulnerable when stressed (Rossman, 1992). For example, self-calming and caregiver strategies compensated for the negative impact of stress on self-worth. In essence, this strategy protected the child's feelings of self-worth under conditions of high stress. In contrast, the distraction/avoidance strategy actually left children more vulnerable at higher levels of stress. Finally, the communicative strategies of expressing distress or anger were associated with lower self-esteem. As Rossman noted, showing your feelings may not elicit the kind of help that contributes to arousal reduction and a positive sense of self. These results suggest that certain forms of childhood distress may be associated with maladaptive emotion-regulation strategies, and thus may represent a critical target for clinical intervention.

Along these lines, Garber and her colleagues (1991) compared the emotion-regulation strategies of depressed and nondepressed children. In brief, children were asked to generate strategies for dealing with both positive and negative affects. Overall, depressed children were more likely than nondepressed children to generate avoidance strategies for sadness and fear. In response to anger, these children also tended to generate more avoidance strategies and negative behavioral expression than nondepressed children. In contrast, nondepressed children were more likely to generate active problem-solving and active distraction strategies than depressed children. Interestingly, depressed and nondepressed children did not differ in the strategies they generated for maintaining positive emotions. When viewed in the context of Rossman's findings, it would appear that depressed children's strategies are less adaptive than the strategies of their nondepressed counterparts. Certainly, these results suggest that an important component of childhood depression involves the generation of emotion-regulation strategies. As Garber et al. noted, it is not clear from these results whether depressed children lacked adaptive strategies or whether their distress undermined the utilization of more adaptive strategies; that is, the degree to which maladaptive regulatory strategies contribute to the onset of depression was unclear. However, given the higher rates of maladaptive regulatory strategies among depressed children, these findings suggest that depressed children will have difficulty recovering from a negative emotional experience once it has occurred.

Although research on the information processing model of emotion regulation remains in progress, new interventions that draw on the assumptions of this framework are currently evolving. Moreover, consistent with the basic tenet that emotional regulation involves a set of interrelated skills, these interventions tend to involve multicomponent treatment packages. As an illustration of this approach, a treatment program for childhood anxiety disorders will be reviewed.

Clinical Interventions for Emotion-Regulation Skills

According to the information-processing model, dysregulation of emotion could result from deficits or utilization problems in component, affect regulatory skills, including identification of arousal, cognitive interpretation of arousal, generation of regulatory strategies, strategy evaluation, and strategy enactment. Anxiety disorders represent one form of emotional dysregulation that can be understood from an information-processing perspective. For example, anxious children might misinterpret various forms of arousal as anxiety, could overgeneralize expectations about anxiety-evocative situations, could utilize ineffective regulatory strategies, and might hold negative beliefs about the efficacy of their coping strategies. Interestingly, research on affect regulation among anxious children is just beginning to emerge. For example, Rabian, Petersen, Richters, and Jensen (1993) found that children with anxiety disorders show greater *anxiety sensitivity* compared to nonclinical controls. Anxiety sensitivity refers to the belief that the experience of anxiety signals further catastrophic consequences such as illness, embarrassment, or additional uncontrollable anxiety. Such "fear of fear" could lead to maladaptive regulatory strategies, such as avoidance, and could exacerbate the intensity of an anxiety episode. Consequently, an important component of treatment might involve helping anxious children monitor their cognitions subsequent to anxiety arousal. Here the self-monitoring and causal analysis would not focus on attributions for affect arousal, as in the treatment of depression, but rather on the catastrophic cognitions that follow negative arousal. In fact, despite considerable evidence for the co-occurrence of anxiety and depressive symptoms among children (Wolfe et al., 1987), there is emerging evidence to suggest that these two disorders may not share the same problematic cognitive processes. For example, Kaslow, Stark, Printz, Livingston, and Tsai (1992) found that the "negative cognitive triad" (negative view of self, world, and future) that characterizes depressed children's thinking is far less prominent among anxious children. Similarly, Stark, Humphrey, Laurent, Livingston, and Christopher (1993) found that depressed and anxious children differ in their schemas and automatic thoughts. As these authors have noted, such differences support Beck's (1967) content specificity hypothesis; that is, each disorder is characterized by unique problems in information processing. These results, although obviously in need of replication and specification, lend further credence to the view that treatments for different disorders must be based on models of underlying pathogenic process.

Kendall and his colleagues (Kane & Kendall, 1989; Kendall et al., 1991) have developed a cognitive-behavioral treatment program that emphasizes the information-processing factors associated with children's anxiety. In this program, children receive training in the recognition of anxiety and its associated cognitions that, in turn, serve as cues for utilizing effective anxiety management strategies. The program emphasizes four major components:

> a) recognizing anxious feelings and somatic reactions to anxiety, b) clarifying cognitions in anxiety-provoking situations (i.e., unrealistic or negative attributions or expectations), c) developing a plan to help cope with the situation (i.e. modifying anxious self-talk into coping self-talk as well as determining what coping actions might be effective), d) evaluating the success of the coping strategies and self-reinforcement as appropriate. (Kane & Kendall, 1989, pp. 501–502)

In essence, the program embraces most of the cognitive components of the information-processing framework.

Therapy involves active participation by child and therapist in role plays, skills training, and practice. For example, in order to help the child differentiate anxious feelings from other feelings, the therapist discusses the idea that facial expressions and body postures are clues to people's feelings. The therapist then presents the child with pictures of people showing different emotions, including anxiety, and together they attempt to identify the expressed emotion. The child is then encouraged to engage in role plays in which he or she expresses different feelings, including anxious or worried feelings. Finally, therapist and child begin to create a "feelings dictionary" by cutting out pictures that display emotions from magazines (Kendall, Kane, Howard, & Siqueland, 1989). Such emotion differentiation may be critical for anxious children, who could misinterpret various forms of arousal as anxiety. In later sessions, the therapist works with the child around the development of alternative regulatory strategies. Among the most important is training the child in self-relaxation skills. As part of this intervention, the therapist attempts to attain the collaboration of the parents in helping the child practice relaxation skills at home. However, the therapist also supports the development of a "problem-solving set"; that is, the therapist explores alternative actions that might be taken to change the anxiety eliciting situation. In general, the goal of this treatment component is to engage the child in active problem solving. Consequently, the therapist first works with the child around problem solving in nonstressful situations, for example, "You've lost your shoes somewhere in the house. How would you go about finding them?" (Kendall et al., 1989, p. 33). The establishment of an active problem-solving orientation to anxiety-eliciting situations may be a critical component of the program in light of Garber's findings (Garber et al., 1991) that distressed children were less likely than nondistressed children to engage in active problem-solving strategies to alleviate depression. The same tendency may be found among anxious children as well. In fact, much of this program can be viewed as graded experiences in self-efficacy. At the core of the program is the STIC (show-that-I-can) task. Each session involves assignments that provide the child with the opportunity to be effective. In the first session, the child is given a notebook and is simply asked to bring it to the next session, with a brief example of when he or she really felt great; later the child is asked to keep a journal of anxious experiences, and still later, the child is asked to practice the coping skills in an anxious situation. Thus, not only does the program build regulatory skills through graded, manageable task assignments, but also it provides the child with the opportunity to be active and increase self-efficacy beliefs.

The foregoing description of therapy sessions represents only a small sampling of the treatment protocol; however, it illustrates the active, skill-building nature of this type of treatment. It is worth noting that therapies that require high levels of involvement in therapy tasks can be severely undermined by low levels of child investment. Consequently, it is likely that the success of such programs will hinge on the development of a positive working relationship (alliance) between child and therapist. Although skill-oriented clinicians typically have focused on specific treatment activities to remediate child problems and have emphasized the use of reinforcers to maintain collaboration, there is growing recognition of the importance of the treatment alliance for the success of structured interventions (Stark et al., 1991). In fact, there is evidence in the adult therapy literature that even in highly technical interventions such as cognitive therapy, the quality of the therapeutic relationship has a major impact on clinical improvement (Burns & Nolen-Hoeksema, 1992). Thus, whereas it is possible to differentiate change processes analytically—in this case, emotional and interpersonal change processes—in the actual conduct of child therapy these processes are closely intertwined.

CONCLUSION

It is not uncommon for children to be referred for psychotherapy because of difficulties with the experience, expression, or regulation of emotion. Even children whose focal problems are most readily conceptualized behaviorally, for example, children with disruptive behavior disorders, often evince serious deficits in emotion regulation. For these children, and children whose problems involve other difficulties with affect such as the avoidance, restriction, or lability of feelings, a central goal of psychotherapy should be the development of adaptive emotional processes. It is clear that adaptive emotional functioning cannot be equated with the capacity to modulate negative feelings, although this capacity is essential to the maintenance of relationships and to one's sense of psychological well-being. Instead, adaptive emotional functioning involves multiple capacities including, at minimum, the ability to access and sustain emotions that are congruent with contextual demands, the ability to recognize one's feelings and to understand their meaning, and the ability to modulate the intensity and duration of emotions. Although some clinic- referred children present with problems in each of these areas, many show specific patterns of deficits. Consequently, as child therapists, we must determine which type of emotional-processing problem is to be the target of our intervention, and then select a therapeutic strategy that is congruent with our conceptualization of the pathogenic process.

As reviewed in this chapter, child therapy is no longer limited to cathartic techniques to promote emotional change, although such techniques may be appropriate for certain cases. Instead, as child therapists, we can choose among a range of approaches, including expressive play therapy, affect education, cognitive control therapy, interpretive methods, and regulatory skill building, to name only a few. To restate the position of Greenberg and Safran (1989), our basic question should be: What type of emotional change process will most directly address the emotional-processing problem presented by the child? By no means is this a simple question, and unfortunately as child therapists, we are currently challenged on two fronts to answer it. First, despite the importance of emotional processes in child psychopathology, research is only beginning to address the types of processing problems associated with various childhood disorders. Second, there have been very few advances in assessment methods for children's emotional functioning. Although there has been a proliferation of methods for the assessment of child symptoms—structured interviews, self-report scales, teacher-rating scales—child practitioners tend to rely on parent reports, observations, and responses to traditional projective tests to assess emotional processes. Although these approaches are useful in the assessment of children's emotional functioning, a more systematic battery of emotional processing tasks, perhaps analogous to batteries for attentional processes, would increase our capacity to identify specific emotional-processing problems. In turn, these assessment procedures could be used as measures of treatment progress. Not surprisingly, few studies of child psychotherapy have included measures of emotion processes as outcome variables. To the degree that children's maladjustment can be understood as involving problems with the experience, expression, or regulation of emotion, and to the degree that these processes constitute a target for intervention, researchers *and* practitioners should administer measures of emotion processes in order to ensure that the putative change processes they have implemented are producing their intended effect.

7

⎯

Cognitive Change Processes

With the cognitive revolution in general psychology, the rise of cognitive and cognitive-behavioral treatments was virtually assured. Cognition, from learning to memorial to attentional and constructional processes, attained an elevated status in theories of the genesis and remediation of child psychopathology. Deficits or distortions in cognitive *structures* (e.g., schemas for encoding new experiences or the capacity of working memory for the attainment of reading competence and conversational regulation), cognitive *processes* (e.g., social problem-solving procedures or disambiguation of conversational implications), and cognitive *products* (e.g., biased attributions or the conferral of inappropriate deference in requests), have been implicated in a wide variety of childhood disorders (e.g., Kendall, 1991). For example, depressed children appear to filter their own performances through a negative cognitive schema that results in misperceptions of their own competencies (Kendall, Stark, & Adam, 1990). Children with attention-deficit/hyperactivity disorder evince verbal mediational and problem-solving skill deficits that appear to contribute to their impulsivity (Tant & Douglas, 1982) and which contribute to their poor conversational regulation. And aggressive children tend to show a cognitive bias involving the misattribution of hostile intent (Dodge, 1985) and a tendency to misread nonverbal facial and other more molar "gestalts" of ongoing interaction (Russell, Stokes, Czogalik, Jones, & Rohleder, 1993).

As the previous examples suggest, cognitive deficits or distortions appear to underlie many of the typical forms of childhood maladjustment that clinicians regularly diagnose and treat. Cognitive deficits also play a role in specific pragmatic, reading and spelling, expressive and receptive language disorders that child clinical psychologists unfortunately often overlook or are ill-equipped to diagnose and treat.

In order to address these cognitive problems, "cognitive-behavioral interventions seek to provide experiences that attend to cognitive content, process, and product so that the child/adolescent builds a structure that will have a positive influence on future experiences" (Kendall, 1991, p. 9). Although a variety of treatment procedures are utilized by cognitive-behaviorists, including direct and symbolic modeling, role plays, practice and rehearsal, most cognitive-behavioral interventions can be characterized as remedial or compensatory instruction. Perhaps reflecting its origins in learning theory, cognitive-behavioral interventions are primarily psychoeducational. Although the focus is on cognition rather than overt behavior, the central change process involves *teaching* new or alternative cognitive skills or processes. In fact, the cognitive-behavioral therapist has been described as a "consultant, diagnostician, and *educator*" (Kendall & Panichelli-Mindel, 1995, p. 107, emphasis added).

Clearly, the focus on teaching new skills or processes through "exposure to multiple behavioral events with concurrent cognitive processing" is a critical cognitive change process, and has been well documented elsewhere (Kendall, 1991, p. 19). However, the intensive focus on teaching or training cognitive skills has tended to engulf the field of cognitive interventions and has drawn attention away from other cognitive change processes that may be as, or more, central in most forms of child psychotherapy. As linguists are apt to point out, the greatest feat of learning, the attainment of language competence, is regularly achieved with little "programmed instruction," but proceeds with what we might term "good enough conversational exposure." Good enough conversational exposure, as we will try to suggest, enables infants and children to build necessary internal structures and interpersonal competencies that enable them to participate adaptively in the paramount activity of human beings—conversational interaction.

Remarkably, despite the fact that many cognitive interventions involve the verbal modification of verbal behaviors *within the context of conversational exchange,* relatively little attention has been directed to discourse or language processes as potential change mechanisms. We might term this the "double blindedness" of most child therapies, for not only cognitive, but dynamic and client-centered technical interventions are typically "administered" verbally (at least symbolically as in symbolic play), *and* they all occur, not only in the context of an interpersonal relationship, but also within the encompassing context of relatively nontechnical language or conversational interaction. In the next section, we will attempt to explicate how language processes and patterns of symbolic interaction in child treatment constitute important cognitive change processes.

LANGUAGE INTERACTION AS A CHANGE PROCESS

We might ask why is it important or even necessary to try to formulate cognitive change processes at the level of discourse or symbolic competencies? First, as we have noted, cognitive interventions are delivered through a symbolic medium, typically either discourse or play. Moreover, many of the goals of such verbal interventions involve either changing verbal behaviors of the child clients, whether they be covert self-statements or interactional verbal social skills, or in transforming nonverbal behavior into more developmentally advanced verbal behaviors, as in the treatment of physically aggressive children. Second, and of equal importance, is the fact that language and discourse processes are deeply implicated in the etiology and maintenance of child psychopathology. Third, normal developmental processes, tasks, and achievements are characterized in terms of, and result in, specific forms of symbolic, often conversational, interactions. Language processes thus importantly constitute child psychotherapy, promote normal development, and are responsible for or correlated with childhood dysfunction.

Language Problems and Childhood Psychopathology

Perhaps surprisingly to some readers, there is a remarkably close relationship between behavioral and emotional disturbance and language problems. As many as half of the children who have language disorders also have psychiatric disorders (Cantwell & Baker, 1987). Moreover, as many as half of the children who are diagnosed with psychiatric disorders also have language disorders, which are often unsuspected or overlooked by psychiatrists or psychologists. Note, even these estimates may be conservative, since many assessments of language do not include meticulous evaluations of children's pragmatic language abilities, that is, their ability to use language appropriately across the many social contexts in which conversation and discourse are required.

There are many studies that document the importance of language and discourse in child problems. For example, in a study that attempted to distinguish hyperactive, hyperactive plus conduct-disordered, anxiety-disordered, and comparative subjects on a host of measures of cognition, attention, motor coordination, inpulsivity, and reading recognition, few group differences remained when a measure of verbal ability was used as a covariate (Werry, Elkind, & Reeves, 1987). In other words, as Hinshaw (1992) suggests, one of the major deficits of youngsters with externalizing problems may be in the area of verbal abilities.

For example, Davis, Singer, and Morris-Friehe (1991) compared 24 delinquent adolescent males to a matched control group on measures of discourse and language proficiency. They reported that "the delinquent youth performed significantly below their nondelinquent peers on both the informal language sample, which evaluated language in a more functional, descriptive context, and the comprehensive standardized measure . . ." (p. 260). In a more recent study, Piel (1990) found that the best predictor of physically aggressive behavior among a sample of second and third graders was language delay, and that verbal aggression, as opposed to physical aggression, was predicted by language maturity. Conversational skill and language proficiency seem to be able to transform physicality into symbolization as a predominant means of conflict resolution. Even among physically abused children, the most aggressive showed significantly more reading and expressive language delays than the less aggressive (Burke, Crenshaw, Green, Schlosser, & Strocchia-Rivera, 1989). These findings of the association of language problems with externalizing disorders are not specific, for there seems to be even stronger evidence that internalizing disorders and language problems are also associated (e.g., Stevenson, Richman, & Graham, 1985). For example, Evans (1987) compared the discourse of reticent children and their normal peers with their teacher during the school year. She found that the reticent children not only speak less than the normal controls, but also speak more often about topics in the "here and now" and failed to elaborate or continue topics when given a speaking turn. Like others (e.g., Friedman, 1975), Evans suggested that reticence might be the product of subtle language or discourse delays/deviations rather than the other way around.

Similarly, Kemple, Speranza, and Hazen (1992) investigated the concurrent and predictive relationship between discourse competence and peer acceptance in preschool. The authors reported finding strong concurrent relationships between peer nominations and specific discourse strategies. For example, the correlation between liked scores and children's noncontingent responses was in the range of $-.5$ across the 2 years, but the correlation between disliked scores and children's noncontingent responses was in the range of .35 across both years. Moreover, the predictive relationships on some discourse measures approached levels nearing those we would expect for reliability coefficients, not lagged predictors! Children's liked scores in the second year were predicted by their acceptance scores (i.e., acceptance of the topic initiated by others) the year before ($r = .72$). The authors aptly summarized their findings:

> Social acceptance was related to communication behaviors which contribute to coherent discourse: clarity of direction of an initiation to an intended recipient and the tendencies to (a) make responses which are contingent to a peer's preceding initiation, (b) accept rather than reject a peer's initiation, and (c) keep the interaction moving by reinitiating when rejecting a peer's initiation. (p. 373)

Children with medical conditions and those who suffer from posttraumatic stress disorder subsequent to abuse also talk differently than their normal peers. In investigating the narratives of children and adolescents with and without early-onset hydrocephalus, Dennis, Jacennik, and Barnes (1994) reported finding significant differences in the narratives' cohesiveness and coherence. "In relation to their age-matched peers, then, children with hydrocephalus produce narratives that are difficult to process, unclear, uneconomic, and less fully elaborated for meaning" (p. 129). Similarly, Densmore and McCabe (1994) found that the narratives of children with posttraumatic stress disorder were less likely to resolve ordinary experiences and more likely to end abruptly at a narrative evaluation high point. Listeners, as in the case with hydrocephalus, would consequently experience a break in ordinary discourse expectancies, and increase the child's risk for social isolation or other interpersonal problems.

The case for the close association of language problems with childhood psychopathology extends beyond the broadband characterizations (e.g., internalizing–externalizing) of child problems or sequelae from trauma. For example, we have not yet considered the most conspicuous childhood disorder in regard to pervasive language and expressive problems, problems that could only result from what have been termed "structural deficits." Childhood autism is, in fact, defined in terms of problems in language communication. Here, not only are there severe deficits in language acquisition and communicative functioning, but also a corresponding deficit in terms of orientation to the rhythms or exchange structure of the interpersonal world. In fact, frame-by-frame videotapes of autistic children and their mothers have confirmed that the normal interactive dance, the ability to fit into the exchange scaffolding that the parents provide, is seriously lacking.

Moreover, in study after study, results have been presented that indicate that autistic children also have a specific deficit in terms of the acquisition of a theory of mind, that is, the theory that self and others act with intention, attain perspectival knowledge, and distinguish between the matter-of-fact world and one of dreams and fantasy. For example, Baron-Cohen, Leslie, and Frith (1986) compared nonclinical children and low ability children with Down's syndrome with high-ability autistic children on a set of picture-sequencing tasks. One of these could be understood and solved on the basis of mechanical information only, one could be understood and solved on the basis of descriptive or behavioral information only, and one could be understood and solved on the basis of psychological–intentional information only. On the two former tasks, the autistic children did as well as or better than the controls but far worse than either group on the sequencing task involving the psychological and intentional information. "This same pattern was also seen in the language used by the children in narrating the stories afterwards. In contrast to the controls, the autistic children used causal and behavioral language, but hardly ever mental state language" (p. 113). Without the exchange structure and the experience of being scaffolded into the culture's theories of mind, the autistic child literally does not fit into the pulse of communicative social life.

This finding can be further dramatized. Roth and Leslie (1991) compared normal 3- and 5-year-olds to autistic adolescents in their level of understanding of brief conversations. They reported that normal 5-year-olds

> display a sophisticated understanding of the beliefs of the protagonists. Three year olds showed a much more limited comprehension but were able to attribute propositional attitudes [such as conveyed by the sentence "He believed it would rain"]. Our autistic adolescents did not display even this limited understanding of the conversational situation. (p. 315)

To understand interaction, to sequence it correctly, it seems that children need to develop theories of mind, and to do so very early in the course of normal development, within dyadic exchange structures with caregivers. Autistic children, with their deficits in language development, their difficulties in engaging in the exchange structure, and their deficient theories of minds, could only have severe handicaps in adjusting to the social world.

But problems in theories of mind, in reasoning about one's own and others' beliefs, desires, intentions, and so on, are not exclusively the province of autistic children, with their serious structural deficits. It is well known that conduct-disordered children have distorted social information processing that has to do with the interpretation of intention (e.g., Dodge, 1985). Furthermore, they have problems in perspective taking, moral reasoning, and in empathy relative to their normal peers (e.g., Campagna & Harter, 1975; Ellis, 1982; Jurkovic & Prentice, 1977; Selman, 1980). These capacities are all part and parcel of, result from, or are constituted by, theories of mind and the language of internal states upon which they are based. Not only deep structural flaws in ego functioning such as are evident in autism, but also the more common psychopathologies of childhood involve language and theory-of-mind deficits and distortions.

Language Processes and the Promotion of Development

If we return to the very earliest interaction between caregiver and infant and focus on the remarkably attuned character it has, we can see that this primary exchange structure is the fundamental building block upon which social representations and language interaction are based. The obvious processes involved in baby talk to children have long been articulated:

These processes involve simplification, clarification, and expressivity (Ferguson, 1977). Interestingly, if we ask where does knowledge of such baby talk come from; that is, where parents and older siblings learn to use it with babies, at least one renowned author suggests that it comes from parents imitating their infants (Brown, 1977)! In a sense, the sensitive parent or older sibling is reflecting back to the infant in words what the infant has expressed in motor or vocal expressions—much like the client-centered therapist. This, of course, makes good sense more generally, as the structure of the caregiver's life comes to look as if it follows rather than simply regulates that of the infant. In point of fact, there seems to be a mutuality of imitation and microadjustments to each other from the very start. As Stern (1985) and attachment theorists have pointed out, satisfactory attunement in these early exchanges can have profound impact on later interpersonal and cognitive adjustment.

For example, there is an extensive literature detailing the impact of parental restrictiveness and mother–infant patterns of communicative exchange on early cognitive abilities in toddlerhood (e.g., Ruddy & Bornstein, 1982, see the following as well). However, as Olson, Bates, and Kaskie (1992) demonstrated, the influence of early patterns of communicative exchange between caregivers and infants on cognitive abilities extends further into the school-aged years. Importantly, as they reported, "These relations were not artifacts of variations in family SES [socioeconomic status], children's early temperament, or developmental status" (p. 309). Consequently, normal development of cognitive abilities is at least partially based on good enough conversational exposure.

But from a discourse point of view, these early exchanges are establishing some of the rudimentary ground rules for participation in the conversational life of the culture, ground rules that make the development of self and social relatedness possible. These ground rules pertain not just to turn taking and the roles and rights associated with speakers and hearers, but also for core presuppositions that we all assume to be operative in literal conversations, and that allow us to interpret them correctly, or to identify them as systematically distorted. Several sets of core conversational maxims have been proposed. Grice (1975), for example, has enumerated nine maxims that are grouped into four categories. Maxims of quantity state that contributions to conversations should be as informative as is required and should not be more informative than required. Maxims of quality state that what one states should not be known to be false or to lack sufficient evidence. The maxim of relation states that one's contribution should be relevant. Last, the maxims of manner state that one's contribution should avoid obscurity and ambiguity in expression, and should be brief and orderly.

These early infant–caregiver exchanges, even those that precede language, can be seen to be doing the work of imparting, establishing, and enforcing these maxims. Such work is normatively accomplished before entering school. For example, as Conti and Camras (1984) have shown, 19% of preschoolers already understand many maxims of conversational interaction. In first grade, over 80% of their children understood many conversational maxims; and by third grade, all of the participants understood the maxims. One can surmise that systematic lack of adherence to maxims at these ages would be tantamount to creating conversational nonsense and the conditions giving rise to social disconnection and maladjustment.

Thus, the mastery of language per se and theories of mind in particular must also be accompanied by a mastery of conversational exchange structures. Like language and theories of mind, mastery of the exchange structure occurs naturally, given a "good enough" discourse context. Can "good enough" discourse contexts and early interactions with a caregiver still result in benefits if other social or economic risk factors are present? That is, does discourse and conversational interaction have a buffering or therapeutic value that we can observe even in everyday life? In a study on the environmental influences on early language development, Morisset, Barnard, Greenberg, Booth, and Spieker (1990) examined high-risk families longitudinally during the period of raising a very young child. The typical single mother was in a low socioeconomic category, had not completed high school, and was supported by public assistance. "They tended to live chaotic and disorganized lives, to live in crowded conditions, move frequently, experience many crises, accidents, illnesses, and high levels of marital (or partner) discord" (pp. 130–131). Interestingly, they assessed several communication variables, including the mother's conversational skills and the quality of the mother–child interaction. They reported finding that the mother's conversation skills and the mother–child interaction were the best predictors of the children's overall language ability at 36 months. These were better predictors than even attachment status. In fact, this too makes good sense, when we remember that the quality of early mother–infant interaction predicts attachment status and not the other way around (Stern, 1985).

Particular forms of language, such as narratives, are also crucial in development and rely on scaffolding procedures. One must learn to recount and project stories about events that are not occurring in the present situation. In other words, we must all learn how to be historians and forecasters early in life if we are to free ourselves from the confines of immediacy, and if we are to obtain a coherent sense of self that persists through time and circumstance. Moreover, if we are to share our experience with others who have not "been there," we must learn how to talk about events so that others can make sense of them. Studies have shown that mothers who elaborate early child narratives, that is, attempt to prolong or extend the narrative topic under discussion, have young children who produce more narrative information than those children of mothers who simply repeat the narratives (Fivush, 1991; Fivush & Fromhoff, 1988; Hudson, 1991). Similarly, when a mother expands the child's topic, repeating what the child has said but now adding new syntactic and semantic information, the child seems to imitate what the mother has modeled and, more importantly, to spontaneously produce new, more complicated topics later on (Scherer & Olswang, 1984). Interestingly, central cognitive skills are affected as well: A child who is asked more questions about past events ends up having better memory skills than those asked fewer questions (Ratner, 1984); and the more a child expresses about an event, the better the event will be remembered (Bauer & Wewerka, 1995).

Discourse interaction thus sets the stage for the internalization of a range of individual competencies. The transformation proceeds from the social plane of interaction to the internal plane of representation. Thus, Vygotsky (1962) has noted that even egocentric speech and play should be seen as "a phenomenon of the transition from interpsychic to intrapsychic functioning, i.e., from the social, collective activity of the child to his more individualized activity—a pattern of development common to all the higher psychological functions" (p. 133). Play also is implicated in specific areas of cognitive development, such as vocabulary expansion and development of object permanence in forming and mastering event schemas, and in problem solving (see Russ, 1995).

As Mead (1934) pointed out long ago, these higher functions include the development of a concept of the self: It is necessary to first internalize others' attitudes communicated toward oneself before and as a condition of the development of a sense of self. Here, for Mead, participation in play and especially in games provided the developing child the opportunity to symbolize the attitudes of others toward him- or herself and thus to do the work of internalization necessary for building a sense of self.

In addition to play and games, recent researchers and theorists have pointed out that the early coconstructed narratives between toddler–preschoolers and caregivers provide the context in which the self is developed. Consistent with Mead and Vygotsky's theories, these early coconstructed narratives are mainly about interpersonal events and the relations in the events between self and other. Not insignificantly, these events are situated in the past, and their conarration is said to help develop the continuity of experience necessary for the development of a sense of self (Miller, Mintz, Hoogstra, Fung, & Potts, 1992).

Consequently, there seems to be powerful evidence from developmental psychology that exchange structures, narratives, theories of mind, and play and games are central to the progressive development of children's sociocognitive functioning. If these structures of everyday normal social experience are so crucial in development, then they would seem to have the potential of being therapeutic in the context of child treatment. They would seem to form the foundation or context in which more specialized skills might develop through explicit instruction. In this sense, these structures and the functions they serve seem to be one of the most powerful sources for promoting development. In fact, from an evolutionary and cross-cultural perspective, it is clear that these structures and functions have been selected and have endured century after century—and not more specific, secondary, change strategies such as thought-stopping, explicit problem-solving instruction, and instructional challenges of errant attributions or invalid logical derivations.

Language-Based Intervention Strategies

Unfortunately, since there is so little research on the process of child psychotherapy, we cannot base recommendations for language-based intervention strategies on well-established or definitive programs of empirical evidence. However, in a suggestive meta-analysis (Russell, Greenwald, & Shirk, 1991), results indicated that treatments significantly affected the language proficiencies of the children, and that the effect sizes associated with treatments that conformed to normal conversational form were larger than those associated with treatments that used specialized conversational "instructional" frames. As we review each of the strategies of intervention having to do with exchange structures—theories of mind, narrative, and play—we will amass further rationales, as well as developmental and clinical evidence, to suggest that these strategies can promote cognitive–linguistic development and facilitate adjustment. It is to that task that we now turn.

Communicative Exchange Structures

In a series of recent process studies of adult and child therapy, Czogalik and Russell (1994a, 1994b, 1995) and Russell, Bryant, and Estrada (in press) reported that the P-technique factor that accounted for most of the variance in the therapists' discourse had to do with information exchange, and not traditional therapeutic techniques such as interpretation or reflection or instruction. The structure of therapist participation was organized first around the microprocesses that constitute basic communicative exchanges. In the study of therapists treating children, this was interpreted to indicate that sessions were organized around a basic underlying structure that resembles question–answer, request–reply or topic–comment sequences. This was said to make good sense from a discourse-analytic perspective: Question–answer, request–reply, or topic–comment sequences are thought to be the underlying prototype of all linguistic exchange.

Could there be therapeutic value in accentuating this basic structure of exchange? First, we should note that child therapy sessions that were judged to be most effective accentuated this underlying exchange structure more so than in sessions judged to be least effective. In the good sessions, therapists worked harder to continue commenting on topics of discussion in a neutral, descriptive way, and to highlight their responsiveness and attentiveness as active listeners than in poor sessions. Moreover, when shifting topics from something nonspecific to a focus on the child client, they tended to have specific rather than nonspecific informational goals. Can the greater emphasis on continuity and responsiveness, in conjunction with specific request about new information about the client, serve some therapeutic function?

Developmental psychology would seem to indicate that such exchange is crucial to the acquisition of a number of basic functions and capacities. For example, the importance of caregiver and infant attunement in verbal and nonverbal exchanges has been amply documented empirically and elaborated theoretically (e.g., Stern, 1985). In summarizing a microanalytic study of mother–infant interaction, Bateson (1979) established that

> the mother and infant were collaborating in a pattern of more or less alternating, nonoverlapping vocalization, the mother speaking brief sentences and the infant responding with coos and murmurs, together producing a brief joint performance similar to conversation, which I called proto-conversation. The study of timing and sequencing showed that certainly the mother and probably the infant, in addition to conforming in general to a regular pattern, were acting to sustain it or to restore it when it faltered, waiting for the expected vocalization from the other and then, after a pause, resuming vocalization, as if to elicit a response that had not been forthcoming. (p. 65)

Even prior to language acquisition, such repeated exchanges have been argued to facilitate the development of a core sense of subjective self. The constraints on the cognitive capacities of infants at this early age should not be overestimated. Infants as young as 6 months of age have been shown to have cued recall memory for affective experiences involved in peekaboo games (Nachman & Stern, 1983).

More surprising is the fact that infants as young as 6 weeks old imitate facial expressions of their caregivers, and even after a 24-hour delay, imitate from memory (Meltzoff & Moore, 1994). Memory constraints on imitation may not be as substantial in early infancy as once thought. What gets developed may be social-cognitive processes and the developing understanding of schemas or working models of persons.

What could the imitative exchanges between caregivers and infants be accomplishing? Meltzoff and Moore (1994) suggest that imitation serves an identity function. As they note, "Infants use imitation as a way of reidentifying and communicating with persons they see before them. . . . Imitation is to understanding people as physical manipulation is to understanding things" (p. 96). Two further elaborations can be made here. First, infants actively attempt to make sense of their interpersonal world, and use imitation to solve a question concerning the continuity of their interpersonal experience. Second, following such theorists as Mead and Vygotsky, we can assume that such attempts at establishing continuities serve a dual identity function, namely, to identify their interactional partner as the selfsame person as in previous exchanges and to establish the foundations of their own personal identity and coherence of self over different occasions of exchange. This can be dramatized by recalling that "the organization of the infant's body motion is sustained in parallel with the duration of a speech sound [emitted by the caretaker] and changes to a new organization when that sound changes" (Condon, 1979, p. 139).

In other words, how the infant organizes and experiences itself in the sensorimotor realm is at least partially a function of the vocal and imitative exchanges it engages in with its caretaker. The interactive exchange and the fine attunements between infant and caretaker that characterize it when it is working well serve as the catalyst for the development of cognitive structures pertaining to self and other and their relatedness in the social world.

In fact, according to Stern (1985), "The communicative power of selective attunement reaches almost all forms of experience. It determines which overt behaviors fall inside or outside the pale [of intersubjectively validated objective and subjective states]" (p. 208). For example, infants as young as 3 months old do not immediately cry or fall apart when overstimulated, but engage in defensive or coping responses, such as turning their heads away from an overzealous communicative partner. However, if the partner persists, becoming a "disregulating other," the infant's adaptive attempts at coping will be frustrated and will not be integrated into his or her evolving interpersonal repertoire. Here both expectancies about others and confidence in one's coping strategies can become problematic (pp. 194–196).

More generally, these early interactive exchanges can be seen as the behavioral and symbolic vehicles by which the root organization of adaptive or maladaptive cultural practices are first encountered and slowly acquired by the infant. Note here that attunement in interactive exchanges entails the division of public communication into roles, speaker and hearer, and implicitly assigns rights and obligations to those fulfilling them. Although it is true that in these early exchanges the work of caregivers often serves a regulatory function, as is fitting for their parental and adult status, it is also true that infant behaviors are communicative, vary in accord with parental input, and exact measurable influence on the caretaker's behavior. Even so, it is very early in development, with the acquisition of communicative gestures, such as the social smile, mutual gaze, pointing behavior and rudimentary language that the preponderance of regulation is tempered by the ascendance of mutuality in sharing subjective states and in purposefully influencing each other's subjective experience. For example, social referencing has been observed to occur before the end of the first year, when infants seem to deliberately seek emotional information from their caregivers on how they themselves should respond to a joint topic or to ambiguous stimuli (Campos, 1983). In a sense, these early exchanges, in setting out the parameters of the *fundamental exchange structure* of everyday life, also serve from the very beginning to scaffold infants and their world of sensorimotor experience into the symbolic world of adults and the contigency of the interpersonal world.

What is important to grasp here is that there is nothing "metacognitive" or truly reflexive or explicitly teleological here. The child and caretaker are engaged in, and not reflecting upon or theorizing about, the sphere of communicative praxis. Their activity is prereflective. The exchange practices, the sphere of communicative praxis, embody and organize skills, habits, and styles of interaction that include cognitive schemas (of self and other) and scripts of repeated activities. Long before infants can reflect cognitively, their activity has been patterned and organized in practices or strategies of communicative exchange, adaptive or maladaptive as they may be. These recurrent exchanges provide the basic foundation for social relatedness.

The heavy emphasis on communicative exchange in traditional child therapy can consequently be seen as an attempt to "repair" or help the child relearn the fundamental, but implicit, structures embedded in these early interactions. In this sense, we view the goal of such work to be structural change in the child's internal representation of the fundamental exchange structures that underlie, and provide the basis for, social participation in everyday life.

Are there relevant contents in this exchange structure that serve a therapeutically corrective function? If we look closely at some of the work of Carl Rogers and an expert child clinician, we may get a clue as to another key cognitive change mechanism in child treatment. We choose Rogers's work because it most explicitly uses the exchange in ways that seem to parallel that of caregivers, in that it redescribes (i.e., reflects) the previous verbal and nonverbal activity of the client at the same time as it affirms or accepts it in a nonrestrictive way. In several microanalytic studies of his well-known, videotaped session with Gloria, we (Essig & Russell, 1990; Collins, Day, & Russell, 1992) focused on particular aspects of the language Rogers used. These aspects, in the Essig and Russell study, pertain to the linguistic ways in which speakers elaborate the subjective meaning of events that serve as topics of their discourse. Two classes were investigated, what were called "specifications" and "predications," that are roughly equivalent to elaborations within simple and complex sentences, respectively. For example, the simple sentence "He went to school" might be subjectively elaborated, as in "He wanted to go to school," or "He anxiously went to school," or "He might go to school." This sentence might also be subjectively elaborated by adding another verb phrase to it, making it a complex sentence. For example, the following types of sentences were coded for the addition of markers of subjectivity: "He thought that he would go to school," "He learned that he would go to school," "He was upset that he had to go to school." They would also be coded if they took the following forms: "I think that you might go to school," "I expect that you will have to go to school," or "You seem angry that you have to go to school." Note that in all of these sentences the basic event of going to school is placed in an elaborated psychological perspective that has to do with necessity and possibility, desires and intentions, knowledge and belief, appearance and actuality, and feelings and affects.

Findings indicated that 68% of Rogers's utterances contained at least one instance of a subjective elaboration. In fact, a full 40% of his utterances contained two or more such instances, and 19% contained three or more. The more specialized speech, geared at specific corrections in thinking (à la Ellis) contained significantly fewer subjective elaborations. This finding was corroborated when using a different analytic strategy (Collins, Day, & Russell, 1992). Rogers' speech was found to be more tightly organized around the disclosive expression of subjectivity than around claims to objective truth or to socially sanctioned rights. Moreover, this organization was more characteristic of Rogers than of Ellis's discourse, which was more organized around claims to truth. Note, however, that in both studies, all therapist speech was at least partially and systematically organized around the subjective elaboration of the meaning of objective events. Such findings provide suggestive evidence that one intervention strategy in therapy is to provide clients with models of, or repairs in, the ways in which events are elaborated subjectively.

This claim that "subjective elaboration" is implicitly, and should perhaps become more explicitly, an intervention strategy gains some justification from two additional studies. Segments of therapy that had been independently coded for the depth of client experiencing using a standardized and widely used scale (i.e., the Experiencing Scale; Klein, Mathieu, Gendlin, & Kiesler, 1969) were assessed for the degree of subjective elaboration in them using the Essig and Russell system described earlier (Lord, Castelino, & Russell, 1990). Results indicate that segments of therapy judged to contain the deepest levels of client experiencing (Levels 6 and 7) were comprised of utterances 80% of which had one or more indicators of a subjective elaboration. Segments of therapy judged to contain the most shallow levels of experiencing (Levels 1 and 2) were comprised of utterances, only 55% of which had one or more indicators of a subjective elaboration.

In the second study (Russell, van den Broek, et al., 1993), an expert child therapist's narrative speech, and the children's narrative speech to which it was a reaction, were again assessed on subjective elaboration and on levels of perspective taking and self-awareness. The therapist's speech contained significantly more subjective elaborations and significantly higher levels of perspective taking and self-awareness. In addition, such subjective elaborations figured more often in causal statements in the therapist's narratives than in the children's. "Thus, the therapist's retellings explicitly portrayed the psychological or motivational structure of the action that had been initially portrayed in concrete terms in the children's narratives. . . . Here it seems that the therapist's narrative invites the child to consider the internal, intentional, or motivational character of conduct from several points of view" (p. 353).

These studies suggest that there is something special about the elaboration of subjectivity—of belief and desire, possibility, necessity, appearance and actuality in the intervention strategies of therapists. In fact, in a recent study (Russell, Catelino, Wandrei, & Jones, 1995), the extent of the therapist's elaborations of subjectivity in the earlier narrative study (Russell, van den Broek, et al., 1993) was compared to that of a sample of lay individuals when presented with the same child story to elaborate under three conditions—exactly as told, as a helpful parent would, and as a therapist might. Findings indicated that lay subjects provided more elaborations than the children had, but lagged far behind the amounts provided by the therapist. In other words, the therapist may indeed be using a somewhat specialized, exaggerated style of discourse that emphasizes the elaboration of subjectivity in order to model or repair defects or distortions in the client's discursive repertoire.

Is there a link between this therapeutic strategy and tasks in normal development? We believe that the elaboration of subjectivity in child therapy promotes the acquisition and development of "theories of mind," a cognitive achievement that is critical for adaptive social functioning. Theories of mind enable us to distinguish between "a world of thoughts, beliefs, intentions, [emotions], and knowledge from the world of mere bodily presence [and movement]" (Johnson & Wellman, 1982, p. 222). Critically, these theories are used to provide organization and structure to behavioral expectations, self-understanding, and perspective taking. They seem to be acquired with such rapidity and to be so crucial to human functioning that it has been argued that "the perception of intention, like that of causality, is a hard-wired perception based not on repeated experience but on appropriate stimulation (Premack, 1991, p. 39). Lack of the development of a normative theory of mind has been empirically associated with childhood psychopathology, most consistently in autism, but in conduct and oppositional defiant disorders as well, in which cognitive and emotional perspective-taking deficits are commonly encountered (Baron-Cohen, 1991; Baron-Cohen et al., 1986; Eisenmajer & Prior, 1991; Selman, 1980). Deficiencies in explicating internal states in narratives told to a variety of prompts have also been demonstrated to predict significant amounts of depressive, anxious, and cognitive difficulties in late adolescents and young adults (Hambleton, Wandrei, & Russell, in press). This makes good sense, since without the normative means to account for and understand one's own and others' conduct, adjustment to the normative culture that depends on such understandings would be difficult.

Research has revealed that at a very early age there is a progression from behaving in ways suggesting that very young children have an understanding of other people's internal states, to using explicit linguistic terms to denote mentalistic operations or internal emotions in themselves and in others descriptively, and in causal sequences of explanation. Later development ushers in the capacity to comment upon their own and others' internal states that have come to be topics of discourse (see Bretherton, 1991). This development of a theory of mind goes hand in hand with other very important developments, such as the development of perspective taking, empathy, and the moral emotions of shame and guilt, along with the growing awareness of standards and the ability to provide "altruistic" comfort or help to others in distress (e.g., Bretherton & Beeghly, 1982; Brown & Dunn, 1991; Hay, 1994; Lamb, 1991; Miller & Aloise, 1989; Zahn-Waxler & Radke-Yarrow, 1990). Although the relations between these achievements have not been empirically established, we should note generally that by the middle of the elementary-school years, these prosocial functions are mediated and communicated in discourse, and that the normative adult relies on discourse and symbolic gesture predominantly to carry them out.

When we ask the question of how these theories of mind are acquired or what kinds of interaction promote their acquisition, there are some suggestions in developmental psychology that are very intriguing. Beyond the most general description of the caregiver's provision of the linguistic and interactive scaffolding to facilitate their acquisition by the child, we will briefly focus on three types of interaction that seem to promote their acquisition, namely, a particular type of topic–comment sequence, the use of narrative and storytelling, and engagement in pretend or symbolic play.

Feldman (1988) begins by assuming that "if we want to know what objects a person has constructed, then we can look at the topics he has created, and if we want to know how the new world version [i.e., a new object] was created from a previous one, then we can look at how a new topic was made and from what" (p. 127). She notes that very early, between the ages of 2 and 3 years old, children can use mental-state verbs such as "think," "believe," "doubt," and "know"; and such epistemic adverbs as "maybe," "actually," "probably," and "sort of"; and such modal auxiliary verbs as "would," "could," "should," "might," and "may," along with others and their contractions. These appear in children's speech, marking their subjective attitudes mainly toward events and things and people outside themselves. For Feldman, acquiring a theory of mind is not just to be able to use these mental attitudes in describing and evaluating the world "out there," but must also entail being able to use these selfsame attitudes in describing and evaluating mental attitudes themselves. What this means is that the world of mental attitudes must somehow come to replace the world "out there" as the topic that will be elaborated upon by further use of mental attitudes. This is, in fact, what adults do in conversation and in storytelling quite naturally. We seem most interested in our own and other's subjective reactions to concrete events and elaborate and comment upon them with the use of our own favorite set of linguistically marked attitudes.

Obviously, we have now left the lived, prereflective plane of existence in social life and have now turned to a reflective or metalevel of discursive activity. Feldman proposes the well-known dialectic or procedure of taking the new and stipulating it as a given about which something new can be said. This given–new or topic–comment structure seems fundamental to reflection and to discursive expressions of thoughts about thoughts or other mental entities in conversations. "The irreducible unit of both language and cognition are two-term expressions. They are composed on the first hand of topics, of that which is known, taken for granted, or stipulated as given, and on the other hand, of comments, of the new, of that which can be predicated or thought of the given" (p. 37). This same topic–comment structure can be extended to discourse. In fact, the topic–comment of discursive exchange may be the precursor to its internalization as a cognitive structure for reflection.

Feldman (1988) goes on to show how children in dialogue with their mother and father learn between the ages of 2 and 3 how to turn comments of their parents into topics that they elaborate, apparently with the model of their parents' sensitive use of the procedure first, followed by those of the young children. This procedure that gets first worked out mostly as concerns the world "out there" then lays the groundwork for the development of turning subjective attitude comments about old topics into new topics for further subjective attitude comment. Here we would have the subjective attitudes as topics and as comments. We would move from taking the world as the target of our conversational transformations to taking aspects of our theories of mind as our targets of conversational transformation. We move from transforming our attitudes about the world to transforming the attitudinal stances that define who we are.

If we look at therapeutic discourse closely, especially that comprised of reflections, as in client-centered theory, we can see that it is exactly these types of recursive topic–comment sequences that comprise many of the exchanges. In effect, therapists, in using reflections, are attempting to provide the means, the scaffolding, to repair or to augment clients' theories of mind. Of course, with children, especially the younger ones, it is the acquisition of the appropriate use of the mental attitudes that is first a focus of work; that is, every therapist will recognize procedures to help children correctly label their feelings, thoughts, and attitudes. In fact, the work is often concentrated in the attempt to get children to verbalize their subjective experience rather than to act it out. The ability to use the mentalistic terms precedes the ability to reflect on them, naturally. But with older children and with advancing younger clients, the work progresses to a new level. Here the hope is, of course, that the reparative work that is accomplished in collaborative topic–comment sequences can be internalized and carried out by the client in reflection.

This may all sound very abstract, but the following sets of utterances will indicate just how central this strategy is to therapy. To a child slumping in the chair, looking dejected, a therapist might say: "You seem sad today, [and perhaps to further qualify the impression], but I can't tell for sure." If the child picks up on the sad theme, we can be sure there has been some chaining of topic and comment: "I feel down in the dumps because Mom is away again." And we would be pleased. But here the talk sequence is still mostly rooted in the world "out there," even if there is elaboration of the event that has caused the sadness. But if the child picks up on the "seem" (appearance vs. reality) or on the epistemic uncertainty (can't tell [know] for sure), then a very different quality emerges: "Maybe I only seem sad because I am really not all sad;" or "I am trying not to be too sad"; or, "I really want to be less sad than I really am." Here the work has shifted from the world to the subjective attitudes and how they may or may not be consonant with the child's experience or hopes or desires, on which the therapist may now offer another comment. As such, these topic–comment exchanges not only accentuate the basic structure of communicative exchanges and its social suppositions, but they also serve to impart, enhance, or repair the child's theory of mind.

It is interesting to consider a traditional psychodynamic *linguistic* intervention—interpretation—in this context. Historically, interpretation has been equated with making the unconscious conscious (Freud, 1949); that is, interpretation is a form of communication that promotes insight by drawing attention to and building links between current emotions and behavior and thoughts, wishes, and fantasies that are outside of awareness. In fact, in traditional psychodynamic theory, interpretation is the cornerstone of the treatment of internal conflicts (Sandler et al., 1980). Therapeutic change through the resolution of internal conflict rests on the assumption that there is a causal connection between the expansion of self-awareness and the modification of maladaptive emotions and behaviors. Interpretation functions to increase children's awareness of the conflicting determinants of their behavior.

A close examination of the process of interpretation suggests that one of the major consequences of this intervention may be the modification of the child's theory of mind. As Levy (1963) has noted, interpretation "consists of bringing an alternative frame of reference, or language system, to bear on upon a set of observations or behaviors" (p. 7). And according to Kennedy (1979), interpretations "repeatedly introduce a sequence of cause and effect and suggest the need to look for motivation" (p. 16). Interpretations go beyond overt behavior and introduce psychological processes such as wishes, conflicts, and intentions into the child's self-understanding (Shirk, 1988a). In essence, they orient the child to his or her psychological interior and focus on mentalistic concepts. Thus, interpretations function to make the child more "psychologically minded," or put another way, they elaborate the child's developing theory of mind.

Narratives and Narrative Change Processes

There is an extensive theoretical literature on the importance of narrative and narration in human culture, in cognition, in development, in attaining self-knowledge and moral character, and in the conduct of science. Stories have been key tools for the work of enculturalization from as long ago as we have records and are evident across all cultures. There is also an extensive theoretical literature on the importance of narrative and narration in psychotherapy. The stories that we tell not only describe and redescribe what we have done but also help to construct the lives that we live. It has been argued that who we are and who we hope to become are intricately tied to the stories that we tell and hear, whether in everyday life or in therapy. In fact, our narrativity has been argued to be the defining feature of our species (e.g., Bruner, 1986, Cohler, 1982; Fisher, 1984; Franzke, 1989; Labov & Fanshel, 1977; Russell, 1991; Schafer, 1981; van den Broek & Thurlow, 1991; White, 1980).

Are narratives important in clinical treatment and assessment? First of all, it must be recognized that narratives have long been used implicitly in clinical assessment of children. Both the Thematic Apperception Test and the Children's Apperception Test (Bellack, 1986; Henry, 1973) require children and adolescents to create stories. Moreover, children's characteristic narrations are used to assess a wide range of psychological constructs, from motivation to perspective-taking capacity. More specific assessment instruments also rely on clients' narrative abilities, such as the Means–Ends Problem-Solving Task (Platt & Spivak, 1975) and some tests of neuropsychological functioning, as in Wechsler Memory Scale and the Babcock Memory test (Wechsler, 1945; Babcock & Levy, 1940). Note that here cognitive reasoning abilities and memory abilities are assessed using narrative stimuli and the scoring systems based on the narrative productions (see Russell & Wandrei, in press). Even very young children (between ages 4 and 5) are prompted to tell stories to narrative stems, and their productions lead to valid assessment along such dimensions as emotion regulation, internal representation of relationships, and early moral development (Buchsbaum et al., 1992).

These formal assessment tasks are almost always accompanied by informal clinical assessment via interview. Here the clinician bases many of his or her judgments about the type and severity of the presenting problem on the basis of clients' narrative productions. Clients tell stories about their problems and about their daily lives, and clinicians use their everyday narrative competencies and their general clinical training to assess their narrative productions along many content and noncontent dimensions. In fact, if a client cannot string together a coherent story about an episode in his or her life, then this is almost always a cautionary flag indicating the possibility of severe pathology.

In therapy, the case for the relevance of narrative is even stronger. For example, in some of the early process studies, a storytelling or narrative category was included, and it was found to have the highest number of instances among all categories (e.g., Lebo, 1952). Moreover, when child therapists were surveyed, 32% of the respondents indicated that storytelling as a technique was at least occasionally useful, and 12% indicated that it was often useful (Koocher & Pedulla, 1977). There are also several techniques (such as the Mutual Storytelling Technique, Hero–Heroine Modeling, Folktale Analysis) that explicitly use storytelling in a highly structured way with young children and even adolescents (e.g., Costantino, Malgady, & Rogler, 1986; Franzke, 1989; Gardner, 1971; Malgady, Rogler, & Costantino, 1990). Although these are specialized uses of storytelling, one can be sure that narratives, as part and parcel of our everyday communicative competence, play a very large role in almost every type of therapy and at almost every age level. As Russell, van den Broek, et al. (1993) note:

Given that narratives are (a) deemed essential for our functioning as human beings, (b) considered theoretically important by psychotherapy theorists, (c) used routinely in standard assessment batteries, (d) recognized by practicing psychologists as useful, and (e) incorporated into the clinical treatment armamentarium, it is surprising that little clinical research on narratives has been undertaken. (p. 339)

The explanation for this is at least partially supplied by the fact that clinical psychologists and psychotherapists have just not been very interested in language or communicative processes generally. However, there is ample reason why this should change, just as there was ample reason for considering how central the exchange structure and the theory of mind are to therapeutic change processes when considered from a cognitive and communicative perspective.

Perhaps the first and foremost reason for considering narrative as both a primary target for intervention and for focusing attention on narrative exchange or discourse as a change process is because narrative is a primary means by which episodes in everyday life are represented cognitively. In other words, narrative is a form, if not *the* form, in which everyday episodes are cognitively represented. Moreover, even some of our schemas and scripts may take narrative form, in that they contain temporal information about how episodes unfold in time and how the numerous events that comprise the episode are causally related. The narrative representations that we have of repeated events and traumatic, novel, or peak experiences must affect how we engage new episodes and events (van den Broek & Thurlow, 1991). In brief, narratives entail the implicit cognitive structures that affect our interpretation of new events, and accordingly, our emotional and behavioral reactions to such events. As such, we propose that narrative change is an important pathway to *schema transformation*.

The structure of narratives provides a frame for organizing the ongoing flow of action as we live it, and this type of narrative categorization helps us reduce our uncertainty about what we can expect and when. Knowing that stories and events in the world can be usefully parsed into settings, initiating events, internal responses, goal attempts, consequences, and ending, moralistic or other appraisals provide means with which our social-cognitive processing can proceed efficiently. If events or recollections are jumbled and helter-skelter, then we can impose our internal narrative template on them to achieve a more satisfactory sense of coherence. But perhaps even more importantly, narrative competencies allow us to engage others in discourse and ourselves in a type of reflection that builds a sense of personal identity.

Russell and van den Broek (1988) have provided a sketch of the developmental and cognitive findings about the acquisition of narrative understanding among children. It is surprising how early children begin to tell and comprehend narratives (or proto- or minimal narratives), which occurs soon after they have acquired just the rudiments of language at around age two. By age 4, children are able to understand the thematic structure of brief narratives and can apply such understanding in selecting similar narratives. Two-year-olds seem aware of the referential relations of noun phrases in short narratives, and preschoolers are aware of the temporal ordering of events from beginnings to endings in narratives (e.g., Bennett-Kastor, 1983; Fivush & Slackman, 1986; Stein & Glenn, 1979). Even when we look at more complex structural relationships in narratives, such as the causal relationships between event categories, or the hierarchical structure of narrative episodes, it is surprising how much children know and use in their storytelling. First graders, for example, are sensitive to causal factors in the structure of narratives, as they appear to perform better on recall tasks and on question–answer tasks with events that have many causal connections in the narrative, or if the narrative itself is tightly organized causally.

These latter aspects of narrative concern structural or abstract features, ones that are involved in everyday reasoning. In fact, some have viewed narratives as a primary problem-solving strategy. This functional view of narrative maps nicely onto other structural features: Narratives involve obstacles, or at least potential obstacles, that the protagonist's action and strategies attempt to overcome. Being able to tell stories about problematic events in everyday life, or listening to stories in which other protagonists succeed over obstacles to meet their goals, is a way children and adults alike can learn better and different ways to solve problems.

We have focused so far primarily on structural features of narrative—basically on how narratives help us to categorize the ongoing flow of events, and how to organize these events in time and in hierarchical and causal relations. Here we are dealing almost entirely on the plane of activity—what has been termed the "landscape of action." But in addition to this landscape, which we could certainly deal with in other forms of representation, such as propositional networks or by use of scientific covering laws or generalizations, there is another landscape which is said to be at the heart of narrative and narration. This landscape—called by Bruner (1986) and Genette (1980) the "landscape of consciousness"—allows us as human beings to place action or activity into relief and to focus on what makes us who we are: individuals interested in and importantly defined by our motivations, needs, desires, quests, and so forth. In fact, only when we place this second landscape in the foreground do we know how to interpret our own or another's behavior.

Consequently, it will not be surprising to learn that narratives are seen as a way to help children acquire theories of mind. In fact, their perform-ance in understanding the presuppositions of factive sentences, including the verbs "know," "remember," and "forget" have been shown to improve when children as young as age 4 were provided with story context (Abbeduto & Rosenberg, 1985). In addition, exposure to narrative is exposure to multiple points of view, even in the most basic stories, as there is almost always a change in state in the protagonist from the beginning to the end of the story, even if there is only one character. From this basic change in point of view or feeling over time, one can progress to stories that have multiple protagonists and multiple points of view that are themselves part of the obstacle or conflict in the story. Learning about propositional attitudes and theories of mind is now contextualized in the interpersonal conflicts and actions of the scores of actors that one learns to identify with and to imaginatively experience. The exposure to the diversity of points of view and of means to bring them to satisfactory resolution or compromise in endings here, too, must be seen as a way in which individuals learn a diversity of perspectives and options for them-selves.

What we have said so far should alert us to the therapeutic value of not only assessing our child client's narrative competence but also to the value of targeting distorted or impoverished narrative representations for therapeutic change. How would we get narrative representations to change if we wanted to? First, there is a powerful argument against trying to change narrative schemas or scripts piecemeal, as one does in other cognitive interventions. In the more traditional cognitive interventions, logical or other problems in the relationship between statements are challenged, or they are critically assessed for their empirical warrant. It is as if the goal is to change the overarching script or schema or narrative on the basis of a bottom up procedure, whereby the whole is progressively changed or challenged by falsification or correction of its part. But such a procedure has even been questioned in the realm of science, where paradigm changes are not understood to have been brought about by such piecemeal attacks on bits of evidence or bits of poor reasoning.

Instead, we should remember that it is oftentimes the case that the whole gives meaning to its parts, and not the other way around. In fact, MacIntyre (1980) clearly indicates that it is narrative processes taken in a more holistic manner that is crucially involved in scientific change:

> The criterion of a successful theory is that it enables us to understand its predecessor in a newly intelligible way. It, at one and the same time, enables us to understand precisely why its predecessor has to be rejected or modified and also why, without and before its illumination, past theory could have remained credible. It introduces new standards for

evaluating the past. It recasts the narrative which constitutes the con-
tinuous reconstruction of the scientific tradition. . . . What a scientific
genius such as Galileo achieves in his tradition, then, is not only a new
way of understanding nature but also and inseparably a new way of
understanding the old science's way of understanding nature. It is
because only from the standpoint of the new science can the inadequacy
of the old science be characterized that the new science is taken to be
more adequate than the old. (p. 69)

Interestingly, this model of change in science relies on an understanding
of how narratives change in our everyday life, when we are in a time of
personal crisis.

Consequently, if we are to find a strategy of intervention that targets
narrative representations—the representations that give meaning to their
subparts—we should focus on the narratives as wholes, and fashion a
top-down manner of intervention. In an article on achieving narrative
change in psychotherapy, Russell and van den Broek (1992) proposed
several therapeutic strategies that could be used to better organize cognitive interventions along the lines suggested by MacIntyre (1980). Three
basic tasks were defined: (1) the differentiation of rival narratives, (2) the
evaluation of one of the rival narratives as better on the basis of its
"coherence, personal accuracy, and wider developmental range of applicability," and (3) "the subsumption of the inferior narrative within the
superior narrative" (p. 348) so as to provide an explanation of the former
in terms of the latter.

Basically, the cognitive change is achieved by first eliciting a narrative
from the child client, opportunistically getting the child to tell or entertain
a rival more developmentally appropriate or reasonable version, and to
proceed in engaging the child in the task of evaluating the two versions.
Here there are a number of dimensions to focus on, in addition to the
provision of new information in the rival narrative. For example, one can
help the child assess the temporal, or causal, or hierarchical structure of
the rival stories. One could also engage the child in the assessment of levels
of theories of mind that the protagonists seem to have in each story,
perhaps concentrating on perspective-taking levels, on modal concepts
(shoulds, coulds, cans, musts, etc.), or on levels of self-knowledge and
degrees of certainty.

Similarly, the rival narratives can be assessed for their subjective sense
of personal accuracy, that is, how true they ring for the current and virtual
self that the client may want to be. "Thus, a subjective sense of accuracy is
attained not solely with respect to the relation of the narrative to objective
and subjective circumstance [that are referentially true], but also with
respect to potentialities prefigured in the client's narrative and relationship

with the therapist" (Russell & van den Broek, 1992, p. 350). Finally, the rivals can be assessed with respect to their comparative levels of developmental applicability; that is, their structure and contents can be compared for their developmental or normative appropriateness, with one or the other having a more or less advanced range of applicability.

Notice that this is problem solving, but of a slightly different variety than is commonly studied in child treatments. Here, a focus on learning a method of problem solving is secondary to dealing with narrative construals, their landscapes of action and of consciousness per se. The focus on the latter is justified, because it is these forms of narrative that serve as representations of the episodes that comprise everyday life. In other words, this form is the fundamental form of problem solving that we use in daily life, and it is this that may be most in need of repair, refinement, augmentation, and so forth. The acquisition of another, secondary and more formal method of problem solving, as all children are exposed to in the schools in one form or another, and that some children are exposed to in more common problem-solving therapies, may be missing the point.

Finally, the work of subsumption begins, wherein the child client is helped to use the more highly evaluated narrative as the means for explaining the merit that the less highly evaluated narrative once had, but can have no more. Because the narrative is the child's own, we will have heightened the chances that the child's own internal representation will have undergone modification. "The acquisition of new knowledge from the new narrative provides the criteria that allows the old story to be newly understood and evaluated. The new narrative also provides exemplars of the types of action or activities that would satisfy the emerging criteria" (Russell & van den Broek, 1992, p. 351). Having been exposed to different ways of telling his or her life, or episodes therein, and in comparatively judging the results of each story, the stage has been set for the new representation to propel the child into new conceptual and, it is hoped, behavioral possibilities. Here, the change in behavior should follow in the same way that changes in particular types of attributional biases tend to change behavior.

In all of these tasks, from the provision of a rival narrative to the work of subsumption, the therapist needs to be guided by knowledge about the client's current level of narrative competence and what is more or less normative for same-age children on all of the structural and other constituents of narratives. This knowledge is required because the therapist, like the sensitive parent, will have to attune each of his or her interventions in a way that will maximize the chances that the child will engage in progressive changes. Luckily, Vygotsky (1978, 1936/1986) has articulated a developmental theory of learning that has been shown to be effective in facilitating learning. Basically, this theory stipulates that if the child is engaged in active, cooperative learning efforts on tasks that just minimally outstrip their current levels of competence, but which can be successfully solved with hints and pointers from a teacher or therapist, change can be maximized.

The target for such activity has been termed the "zone of proximal development," and its use in teaching contexts and assessment has been shown in research to be a highly effective strategy (Brown & Ferrara, 1985; Stone & Wertsch, 1984). Translated into the current context, use of the zone of proximal development would require therapists to provide rival stories that are just beyond the child's current levels of narrative competence. This means that the structural form of the story, the levels of theories of mind evidenced by its characters, the types and number of emotions in them, the types of games or play that are represented, and the language used could each be adjusted so that it would present a solvable problem for the child, with the collaborative work of the therapist. Moreover, in each of the evaluative tasks and subsumption, therapists should strive to keep the work at a level that is both accomplishable by the child and transformative in terms of its cooperatively achieved level of developmental advance. The work achieved in this cooperative zone, then, can be internalized by the child and can restructure the narrative schemas that have been judged to impede adaptive functioning.

Symbolic Play Interaction

The line between play and nonplay, and between play and games, is blurred somewhat when we begin to discuss narrative techniques in therapy, since the latter have often been used to construct imaginative situations and characters. But there is no intrinsic reason why narrative change processes as depicted earlier cannot be enjoyable, even if they involve problem solving in game-like or play-like exchanges. Therapy with children or with adolescents is hard to conceive without at least some portions of them being enjoyable, and for younger clients, play may be an especially important component, given their frequent unwillingness to talk for long periods of time. But play per se and learning how to participate appropriately in games are also important cultural means whereby infants, toddlers, and children try out and master behaviors that will later serve them well in their attempts to adjust to the literal, nonplay contexts, of school, work, and much of adult life.

This importance of play is well documented not only in human society but also in primates and even other animals lower down on the philogenetic scale. For humans, involvement in play and games is associated with many sorts of later intellectual and social achievements, and has been linked to the development of a sense of self as well. There have been several different proposals for the developmental stages through which the form of a child's play progresses, from rudimentary physical play without the use of symbols or rules, to complex social games that involve language, cognitive planning, and the awareness of sets of abstract rules. Probably the two most famous divisions of the stages of child's play are oriented respectively to the cognitive underpinnings or the social form of the play.

Piaget's system can be divided, as is well known, into primarily three stages of play. In the sensorimotor period of play from birth to about the second year, the child's play is oriented to mastering the physical world, manipulating concrete things in novel ways that seem to be pleasurable to the child. In the second stage, symbolic play, from about the second year until kindergarten, the child's play progresses into the area of make-believe and role taking, in which their play actions begin to represent or symbolize literal interactions but now in nonliteral contexts. Here, too, children are observed to use language in nonliteral ways and to be able to speak as if they were others, or as if they were assuming different roles. In the third stage, in which play gives way to organized social games in kindergarten and on the playground, children now must have internal representations of sets of rules that define not only different roles in the game but also what is and is not permissible as an appropriate action within the game context.

The other common way of dividing types of children's play that is also developmental in orientation concentrates on its social form. Several different schemes have been proposed, but most are relatively minor variations of that proposed by Parten (1932). Her scheme consisted of unoccupied play, solitary play, onlooker play, parallel play, associative play, and cooperative play. As with most developmental stage theories, current thinking and research do not provide unqualified support for such qualitative divisions along the developmental path.

For example, we have already seen how very early games, both physical and vocal, between parents and infants have an implicit rule structure pertaining to turn taking. Games such as peekaboo also have an implicit organization that clearly defines roles and appropriate reactions to fill in the various slots. Thus, even these very early types of games have rudimentary organizations that can be seen as the precursors of the much more complicated, rule-governed games that play such a significant role in the beginning school years. In fact, if we look at what is most striking about play and games, it points to the acquisition of another plane of reality in which to participate and in which to experiment symbolically in new roles and with new behaviors, without worry about literal sanctions. It is in this new, nonliteral context that a child can acquire symbolic rules that function to define all of the roles of the players and the meaning that their various behaviors will have (see Garvey, 1977, for an informative view of the development of play).

What we are interested in when we think of play as a strategy of intervention in psychotherapy is the question of whether play functions to facilitate development. Fisher (1992) conducted a meta-analysis of 46 studies of different types of play that included some type of outcome variable, such as cognitive–linguistic competence, or role-taking ability. The upshot of his review is that if you envision play as a technique, "play enhances the progress of early development from 33% to 67% (e.g., by reducing failure rates in academic/adjustment functioning due to non-achievement, language problems, or socioemotional difficulties from 67% to 33%)" (p. 168). These figures are "on average" and represent both maximal and minimal effects of all types of play on all types of outcomes. The magnitude of these affects is comparable to those achieved by many types of psychotherapy.

If we look closer at particular types of play and particular types of outcomes, what becomes clear is how facilitative play is in enhancing development in key areas of cognitive functioning. The type of play that has the biggest impact on later development is sociodramatic play among children, followed by free play among peers. Adult-directed play training and structured thematic play also had an impressive impact on outcomes, but to a lesser extent than that achieved by play when participants are childhood peers. The three areas that appeared to be most strongly affected by variations in play were children's perspective-taking abilities, ideational fluency, and reading readiness, all three areas clearly cognitive or socio-cognitive in character.

One of the conclusions to be drawn from this review is that an often overlooked goal of therapeutic play is to enable the child to participate in the play and games that occur among childhood peers, for they seem to have a greater impact on cognitive development than play with adults. The work of Selman directly exploits this and Vygotsky's principle by conducting peer therapy in which two children, one higher and one lower in the development of key adaptive functions, are engaged in cooperative activities. A therapist oversees their play and other activities and intervenes when necessary to solve interpersonal problems. The advantages that accrue from involvement in play and games with peers, however, are often not an option for disturbed children. For example, it is not uncommon for both undercontrolled and overcontrolled children to be rejected by their peers and to be excluded from play and games. They thus revert to solitary play as an alternative. As in other areas of functioning, the goal is to enable the child to return to a level of functioning that would allow him or her to participate in the normal developmental tasks and activities that confront the child's cohort. Thus, when we ask what can play or games achieve as a strategy of intervention in therapy, one answer is to increase the likelihood that the child will participate in more and higher quality play and games in his or her everyday life.

This, obviously, is not the only goal of play as an intervention strategy. In therapy, thematic, sociodramatic, or puppet play can help the child and the therapist understand and correct problematic scripts or schemas, or difficulties in perspective taking that hinder adjustment generally. In play, the child can take risks that have little literal cost, and can conceive and act in a virtual world that he or she could choose to try to bring about in the future. For very young or regressed clients, play may be the most appropriate way to symbolize their internal struggles, emotions, fantasies, and other scripted representations of interactions. In other words, symbolic play may be the best communicative medium for the child's expression and for the therapist to gain access to the linguistically underdeveloped inner world.

The value of play as an intervention strategy has been cogently summarized by Russ (1995). She explains why play is and has been a major intervention strategy regularly used by child clinicians: It is useful as a means of emotional discharge or catharsis, can help to provide corrective emotional experiences and insight, can be a form of problem solving, and can help to develop internal structure (pp. 368–369). Divergent and creative thinking have also been associated with quality play. In our view, each of these accomplishments both contributes to and is made possible by the development of the child's symbolic capacities within therapeutic discourse contexts.

INTEGRATING LANGUAGE PROCESSES IN CHILD PSYCHOTHERAPY: A CASE EXAMPLE

A case vignette will provide an example of a way communicative exchange, narrative, and play can be integrated into the very same intervention strategy aimed at changing an internal episodic representation of a traumatic event. As such, this case presents the use of language processes as interventions for the transformation of internal representations.

A 10-year-old girl, "Amy," had been seen for some time in individual therapy for problems with risk taking, oppositional and antisocial behavior, and inappropriate sexual acting out. She had over the past 4 years been moved from foster home to foster home, because in each case her behavior had become intolerable. In particular, she would either act out sexually in a manner that put other children in these homes at risk or she would be so extremely oppositional and defiant that the parents felt that they could not adequately cope with her.

Her mother had committed suicide when she was 6 and her father had abruptly abandoned her shortly thereafter. The mother's death, traumatic enough in itself, involved circumstances that were particularly unfortunate. Apparently depressed, and alone with her daughter in her home, the mother asked the child to retrieve for her particular medicines from the medicine cabinet in the bathroom. Upon doing this, the mother ingested enough pills of various sorts to cause her to convulse and die in her daughter's presence. She stayed alone with her dead mother for several hours until the father returned and discovered his wife's death and the circumstances leading to it. Hysterically, and perhaps brutally, he proceeded to blame the 6-year-old and to verbally abuse her for the mother's death. He left shortly thereafter, and neither social services nor the police could locate him.

Previous therapy had had a limited degree of success in improving the child's conduct, mood, or dangerous risk-taking behavior. Amy had been unable to talk about the traumatic circumstances of the death or the impact of the loss of both of her parents, or the losses of the foster parents along the way. At the time the new treatment regimen began, she had been placed in a foster family hoping for adoption, but she had continued to be problematic in her usual ways, and everyone involved in the case was holding his or her breath, afraid that she would succeed again in doing something in the near future that would lead to her rejection by the otherwise nearly perfect adoptive family.

It was felt that Amy's behavior was driven by an undisclosed feeling of guilt and terribly low sense of self-esteem. The traumatic episode of her mother's suicide, father abandonment, and his rage-filled blame, had been internalized and functioned as a sort of blueprint of what she could expect of herself and from others. In fact, her acting out seemed to be a way of confirming this schema, as well as a means to externalize some of her overpowering feelings of responsibility and sense of personal blame. This, then, became the target for therapeutic intervention, even though, or rather, precisely because she had as yet been able to tolerate literal discussions of her experiences or the impact that they had had on her behavior.

Following the usual period of building rapport and establishing a "good enough" bond, the child was engaged in benign doll play, wherein she seemed to enjoy grooming the dolls and taking a part in their pretend dialogues. After this initial period of familiarization with pretend doll play "in therapy," which was a new experience for her, the therapist opportunistically constructed parallel homes, each with two foster parents and one child, one slightly older than the other, along with a third cottage that housed an old wise man. After initial play periods, in which Amy was induced into playing all the roles in her family, and in which all the characters had interacted around benign topics, the therapist's older child doll began to ask specific questions of Amy's child doll.

Questions were formulated to involve the child in talk about her past. "Are those your real Mommy and Daddy, or are they foster parents like mine?" "I don't like to talk about what happened to my real Mommy and Daddy, do you?" "I have a secret about what happened back then, and I haven't told anyone. Could I tell you? Promise not to tell?," etc. Here we see the use of the question–answer sequence, a fundamental exchange structure, to help to involve the child in specific contents of discourse (a fundamental rule of discourse, learned very early in life, is that questions require replies). These questions prompted a series of dialogues wherein Amy's doll learned that the therapist's doll had had very similar experiences. In fact, they were quite parallel except for incidental detail. Eventually, both dolls told extended stories about the circumstances surrounding the loss of their biological parents, with the therapist's doll taking the lead where necessary. Amy's doll even went so far as to claim that she had been responsible for her mother's death, which was, surprisingly, the same reaction that the therapist's doll had experienced. Amy's initial reactions were a combination of slightly heightened anxiety and surprise, but also of some relief, to learn in the realm of play that there had been other children with similar experiences to her actual ones.

The therapist's doll, however, had another story, the rival narrative. It contained the same factual content as his original story but had been corrected in terms of who was and was not responsible for the death and abandonment. In other words, the causal and the moral and intentional structure of the original story had been transformed. This doll explained that he had told the first story over and over to himself, but only until he had learned some surprising new things in the adventures he took when venturing up the block into the old wise man's neighborhood. And, of course, Amy's doll was persuaded to go on this adventure too, with the older doll as a guide.

Over several sessions, the two dolls then interacted with the old wise man, who recounted what he had told the therapist's doll about the limits of childhood responsibility and its relation to culpability. Such discussions took the form of comparative evaluation of the child's original and transformed version of the story. In these discussions, Amy often seemed deeply involved in thought and periodically seemed as if she would bubble over with flashes of insightful relief. The therapist's doll and Amy's doll would continue their discussions of the two sets of narratives even after leaving the old wise man's house. Here, the goal was to achieve subsumption, how the new narrative could both succeed and explain the old narrative and in so doing prove its superiority.

The play culminated with Amy's doll telling her parents about her adventures and about her two stories, one she had once believed and one she now believed. This narrative play took about 8–10 sessions to work through. There were lulls and fits and starts, as in all therapies. However, something very important seemed to be happening. Acting out diminished measurably at home and at school. Of more surprise to the foster parents was Amy's increasing warmth and affection toward them, and her appropriate nonverbal requests for comforting and verbal requests for attention. At night, to her foster mother, she began to disclose how much she often thought about her biological mother and was saddened by her memories. Her risk-taking behavior had abated at school and in the neighborhood, and Amy was even spending more time with same-age peers. Happily, she was adopted later in the year into this family.

Presumably, the distorted narrative schema of the events leading and following the mother's suicide had generalized in such a way as to provide maladaptive expectations of the process and outcomes of social interaction. Included in this overgeneralization was a distorted self-schema that was biased in the negative direction, and that predisposed Amy to the type of negative behavior that would confirm her naughty, guilty, unlovable status. The narrative play was aimed at providing the child the opportunity to revise the underlying narrative schema of the suicide episode, and to transform the negative view of the self that had been its upshot. The nonliteral symbolic play, which allowed Amy to formulate and observe thoughts, feelings, and behaviors like hers from a distance, functioned to change the literal underlying narrative schema, and through such change, the child's literal experience of self and other. This seemed to lead to changes in conduct that transformed the habitual organization of the social world around her.

CONCLUSION

In conclusion, we have stressed in this chapter change processes that rely most heavily on symbolic functioning. Here we have focused on structures (the exchange, topic–comment sequences, narrative, play), content (most notably, theories of mind), and process (as in the rivalry between narratives, their comparative evaluation, and their subsumption). In each, we have refrained from repeating what has elsewhere been covered under the rubric of cognitive-behavioral intervention (e.g., self-instructions, thought stopping, or social problem solving), not because we think that they can be understood better from points of view that do not seriously look at them as types of discourse or language interaction, but because we felt that they are basically specialized versions of the essential strategies canvassed here. In other words, they are embedded in the communicative exchange structure underlying social interaction, in the narratives that we have of our lives or of episodes therein, in our theories of mind, and they are embedded in literal or nonliteral play frames of meaning making. In this sense, it seemed useful to concentrate our discussion of cognitive change processes at these more molar and perhaps deeper constitutive levels that coalesce to define our experience.

III

⌣

CASE FORMULATIONS IN CHILD PSYCHOTHERAPY

P ART III CONTAINS three chapters. The primary aim of the first two is the development and elaboration of a case-formulation approach to the selection of interventions for childhood emotional and behavioral problems. The final chapter summarizes the core themes of the book, and places the case-formulation approach in the broader contexts of development, family, and culture.

Intervention into childhood psychopathology has moved well beyond the "one size fits all" model of treatment. The current quest for prescriptive treatments for specific disorders is based on the assumption that different types of emotional and behavioral problems will not be equally responsive to all forms of treatment. One major problem with the current search for prescriptive treatments is that disorders are defined, almost exclusively, in terms of shared diagnoses that are based on phenotypic similarities among cases. Developmentalists have long recognized that similar manifest behaviors do not necessarily share the same underlying substructure, and that similar developmental outcomes can be reached by way of different pathways or processes (Werner, 1957). The same can be said about maladaptive outcomes. Consequently, children with the same overt constellation of symptoms may be far from homogeneous in terms of the underlying processes that produce or maintain their manifest problems. The tendency to equate phenotype and genotype, that is, to assume that there is an invariant relation between developmental outcome and underlying developmental process commits what Werner (1957) has called the "behavioral constancy fallacy." In this section, we propose that in order to avoid this fallacy, the search for prescriptive treatments must move beyond the classification of treatment cases in terms of phenotypic similarities, that is, psychiatric diagnoses.

In contrast to current trends in the classification of childhood psychopathology, especially as reflected in the DSMs, we recommend the reintroduction of formulations of pathogenic processes as an integral feature for grouping cases. It is maintained that such formulations are essential for the design or selection of psychosocial interventions. However, in contrast to early diagnostic systems, such as DSMs I and II, formulations of pathogenic process are not restricted to psychodynamic conceptualizations. Instead, multiple basic-level formulations of pathogenesis are proposed. In brief, we contend that in order for the current taxonomy of childhood disorders to be maximally useful for treatment selection, it must include not only manifest symptomatology but also formulations of *classes* of pathogenic processes.

The idea that intervention strategies follow from formulations of pathogenic process is by no means new. What is new in our approach is the identification of what we call *basic-level* case formulations. It has often been argued that case formulations, by virtue of their specificity, are too idiosyncratic to provide a reliable framework for the classification of cases. Drawing on prototype theory, we propose that it is possible to identify formulations at an intermediate level of abstraction that distinguish different classes of pathogenic process and hold promise for reliable classification. In addition, we provide a set of principles for the development of case formulations. These issues are the main focus of Chapter 8.

In Chapter 9, we provide a set of case studies that illustrate the selection and implementation of treatment strategies on the basis of case formulations. The aim here is to offer clinical examples of a case formulation approach to the treatment of child psychopathology. In the final chapter, our focus on the psychological interior of child psychotherapy is expanded by a consideration of some of the contexts in which child treatment occurs. Of central concern are the contexts of development, family, and culture. We close the volume with the recognition that successful child psychotherapy cannot be reduced to matching promising treatments to accurately identified childhood disturbances. Instead, we offer a reminder that the procedures of child psychotherapy come alive through the person of the therapist, and suggest that the revitalization of this tradition could benefit from an examination of the characteristics of effective child psychotherapists.

8

~

Treatment Selection:
Formulations
of Pathogenic Processes

O UR REVIEW OF the child psychotherapy literature has revealed a complex set of therapeutic change processes. Within the interpersonal, emotional, and cognitive domains, multiple treatment mechanisms have been identified. Table 8.1 lists the major change processes by domain. Each has been described in some detail in the preceding three chapters. By no means do we assume that specific change processes are exclusively cognitive, emotional, or interpersonal in character. Instead, virtually all of the identified change processes involve elements from each domain. Nevertheless, cognitive, emotional, and interpersonal components are differentially prominent in each change process; consequently they have been grouped on the basis of the relative prominence of each component.

The classification scheme itself is of less importance than the fact that the table shows that practicing child clinicians are presented with a myriad of potential change mechanisms. The problem, then, for child therapists is not the lack of treatment alternatives, but how to select the most useful therapeutic strategy for a particular case.

Thus, the main aim of this chapter is to provide a conceptual framework for the *selective application* of specific change processes. The basic premise of this volume is that current models for treatment selection are based on a conceptualization of "matching" at an inappropriate level of analysis. In brief, the elements in the matching equation have typically been

TABLE 8.1. **Change Processes by Psychological Domain**

Cognitive	Emotional	Interpersonal
Schema transformation: Change produced through the modification of implicit assumptions/expectations embedded in narrative representations.	*Abreaction/release:* Change produced through the expression or discharge of feelings.	*Interpersonal validation/support:* Change produced through the provision of social–emotional support and validation of the child's worth.
Symbolic exchange: Change produced through recurrent participation in the structure of communicative exchanges.	*Emotional experiencing:* Change produced through the integration of emotional experience with an understanding of its personal meaning.	*Supportive scaffolding:* Change produced through coparticipation with the therapist in situations that exceed the child's functional capacity.
Interpersonal/insight: Change produced through the reorganization of the meaning of experiences or through expanded self-awareness.	*Affective education:* Change produced through teaching children to recognize, label, and talk about their own and others' emotions.	*Corrective relationship:* Change produced through modification of repetitive relationship patterns through alternative or discrepant relationship experiences with the therapist.
Skill development: Change produced through learning adaptive or compensatory cognitive skills, e.g., social problem-solving, self-monitoring, or verbal mediation.	*Emotion regulation:* Change produced through the development of coping strategies or the modification of psychological defenses.	

constituted as *therapeutic orientation* (e.g., psychodynamic or cognitive-behavioral) and *diagnostic entity* (e.g., conduct disorder or dysthymia). As an alternative, we have proposed that *change processes* (e.g., interpretation, cognitive skill remediation, or emotion expression) and *case formulations* of pathogenic process (e.g., cognitive distortions or self-esteem deficits) represent the most useful components for a matching equation. To this point we have identified a set of therapeutic change processes; now our task is to provide a framework for developing case formulations.

At the heart of the case formulation approach is the simple idea that prescriptions for therapeutic action are linked to formulations of pathogenic process (Persons, 1991). The core assumption of child psychotherapy is that children's behavior problems and emotional difficulties are mediated by internal psychological processes that represent the key targets for clinical intervention. Child maladjustment is understood in terms of distortions, deficits, or compromises in these internal psychological processes. Such distortions, deficits, and compromises constitute what we have referred to as "pathogenic processes."

In practice, this means that child therapists must move beyond the assessment of presenting problems to a formulation of the psychological mechanisms that create or maintain children's overt difficulties. In essence, a basic tenet of the case formulation approach is that clinical cases must be conceptualized at two levels: at the level of overt, observable problems (focal problems) and at the level of psychological processes (pathogenic mechanisms). Conversely, according to this approach, a differential diagnosis based on an evaluation of overt problems alone—typical of current diagnostic systems—will be insufficient for the development of -specific treatment plans.

Consider the following case example. "Jack" is a 10-year-old boy referred by his single mother for outpatient therapy. In the intake interview, Jack's mother reported a number of problems. She was especially concerned with Jack's temper and his inability to handle frustrating situations. As she put it, "Jack doesn't have a *short* fuse; he has *no* fuse." She noted that it was often a struggle to get Jack to do his chores at home, and that his teachers reported missing homework assignments on a regular basis, despite Jack's above-average scores on intellectual and achievement tests. Periodically, Jack would come home with a bruise or scrape, the result of some physical altercation with a peer. On the Child Behavior Checklist (Achenbach & Edelbrock, 1983), Jack showed a clinically significant elevation on externalizing problems. Diagnostically, the pattern of hostile, negativistic, and noncompliant behavior suggested that Jack was a budding oppositional defiant disorder, perhaps on his way to more serious conduct problems. Among Jack's more prominent problems was the increasing frequency of peer conflict and aggression. Not surprisingly, this problem was worrisome to both his mother and his teachers.

How, then, should the child therapist plan for the treatment of Jack? If we use the diagnosis as our guide for treatment planning—in this case, a disruptive behavior disorder—clinical research suggests that Jack should be treated with a cognitive-behavioral intervention; that is, evidence exists that cognitive-behavioral procedures are relatively effective for children with problems involving disruptive and aggressive behavior (Lochman, White, & Wayland, 1991; Weisz et al., 1987). In essence, treatment selection would be based on matching Jack's disorder with a "brand-name" therapy. Although the existence of empirical evidence for treatment effectiveness is a good basis for treatment selection, the task of treatment planning for a specific case is not so simple.

First, like most therapeutic systems, cognitive-behavioral therapy involves multiple treatment procedures. Which would be most appropriate for the treatment of Jack—anger control training, social problem-solving training, restructuring of interpersonal expectations? The answer to this question is not evident from the list of overt problems, that is, from the diagnosis. Second, children with externalizing disorders are far from a homogeneous group. Research has indicated that there are multiple developmental pathways to disruptive behavior problems (Loeber, 1990). Consequently, despite empirical evidence linking this disorder with social-cognitive deficits or information-processing biases (Lochman & Dodge, 1994), not all children with this disorder share the same underlying pathogenic process. For some, aggressive behavior follows from pervasive gaps in affect regulation; for others, the problem is rooted in underdeveloped problem-solving skills; and for still others, aggressive behavior is linked to schematic assumptions about the exploitive or manipulative nature of social relationships. Consequently, associations (i.e., correlations) between disorder and deficit should not be confused with confirmation that all children who present with disruptive behavior problems do so because of the same underlying psychological processes. Quite simply, it is unwarranted to assume that all individuals with the same disorder manifest similar problems for the same reason (Persons, 1989). Such an assumption may be a "first cousin" of the old uniformity myth of psychotherapy and might be dubbed the *homogeneity myth* of child psychopathology. In fact, like Persons (1991), we would argue that the "disorder-based" approach to child treatment planning and much of contemporary child psychotherapy research is founded on this myth; that is, when disorder or diagnostic entity is the unit for matching child to treatment, substantial variability in developmental pathways and corresponding pathogenic processes is ignored. Standardized treatments, the goal of much current child therapy research, can, at best, be expected to fit the needs of only a subset of children within a diagnostic grouping. In this context, it is interesting to consider the fact that child treatments often increase within-group variability at outcome, perhaps in large part because children with the same diagnosis do not share the same pathogenic processes. Thus for some, treatment remediates the underlying problem, whereas for others, it misses the source of the disorder or, in fact, aggravates it.

To return to Jack's case, the initial presenting problems pointed to difficulties with aggressive behavior. Given evidence for social problem-solving deficits among aggressive children, it was reasonable to focus treatment on the development of these social cognitive skills. However, Jack quickly demonstrated that he could execute the component skills of self-monitoring, consequential thinking, and generating response alternatives. In fact, an initial period of therapy that focused on the consolidation of these skills did little to reduce Jack's aggressive behavior with peers. The point here is not that social cognitive interventions are clinically ineffective for oppositional and aggressive children; in fact, a growing body of evidence suggests otherwise. But in Jack's case, social-cognitive deficits did not appear to be responsible for his problems. The clinical error in this case—the offspring of the homogeneity myth—is the assumption that overt problems bear a one-to-one correspondence with underlying pathogenic processes. Although there may be probabilistic relations between diagnostic entities and underlying pathogenic processes, as in the case of aggressive behavior and social problem-solving deficits, one-to-one correspondence is likely to be the exception rather than the rule for most disorders. Thus, knowledge of the diagnosis is not equivalent to understanding the pathogenic mechanisms responsible for the disorder. Of equal importance, differential diagnosis cannot be equated with clinical assessment. In contrast to differential diagnosis, clinical assessment involves the development and evaluation of hypotheses regarding the pathogenic processes that give rise to specific disorders. In Jack's case, a different treatment plan would have been pursued had alternative hypotheses been entertained and an initial assessment of his social problem-solving skills been conducted.

In fact, a review of Jack's developmental history pointed to an alternative formulation for his case. Jack's early years had been marked by high levels of marital conflict. His mother described it as one of the most difficult periods of her life. Although she currently presented as energetic and nondepressed, she acknowledged that she felt anxious and preoccupied during the period of marital demise that coincided with Jack's first 2 years of life. Jack's father, now only episodically involved, had been physically abusive toward Jack's mother, although she was unsure how much of this violence Jack had witnessed. The degree to which either parent had been available to Jack during those early years was certainly a question. Thus, one clinical hypothesis is that Jack's early relationships with his caregivers had been disrupted by marital turmoil, and that his early care was, at best, unpredictable, and at worst, colored by violence. This, in turn, led to the development of core beliefs about what to expect from others, and given Jack's early history one could reasonably hypothesize that such expectations were tipped in a negative direction.

In support of this hypothesized formulation, Jack appeared to be primed to respond to provocative situations in a hostile or aggressive manner. In interview, Jack portrayed relationships, like many oppositional defiant children, as "me versus you." For example, when we played football, we were not on the same team, running pass patterns, or devising clever plays. Instead, the game was one-on-one, full competition, and Jack showed a desperate desire to defeat me. More directly, some of his offhand comments were quite revealing: About his teachers, he said, "They're unfair; they don't know what's going on"; about his baseball coach, "He plays favorites; I should start all the time, the fool"; about his mother, "She's always on my case, but all she wants is for me to look good to her boyfriends"; and about his therapist, "You just see me because my mom pays you." In summary, Jack's representations of others tended to be rather negative. His core interpersonal expectation seemed to be that others would be disinterested, unresponsive, and unfair. Given this implicit schema for interpersonal interactions, it was not surprising that Jack often responded to minimal provocation with hostile and aggressive behavior. Thus, his problem with aggressive behavior was not the result of social problem-solving skill deficits, but appeared to be attributable to representational factors—and their associated emotions—that interfered with the *utilization* of adaptive social skills. Jack's negative interpersonal expectations primed him for hostility, which in turn increased the likelihood of aggressive behavior. With this alternative formulation of the underlying pathogenic process, skills training was not the treatment of choice; rather, interventions aimed at transforming his schematic beliefs would become the focus of treatment.

In many ways Jack's case is a good illustration of the potential tension between "nomothetic" versus "idiographic" models of clinical practice. The former approach emphasizes universal processes characteristic of people in general or typical of an identifiable subgroup, whereas the latter highlights individual differences and emphasizes the uniqueness of each case (Silverstein, 1988). On the one hand, a substantial body of evidence indicates that *as a group,* aggressive children evince more social problem-solving deficits compared to nonaggressive children. Statistically, their mean performance on problem-solving tasks is significantly different from their nonaggressive counterparts. But Jack, or for that matter, any disruptive child, is not captured by the average performance of the group to which he has been assigned diagnostically. Nevertheless, the nomothetic approach to clinical practice, in general, and to treatment planning, in particular, tends to treat specific cases as instances of the group mean; that is, characteristics of the individual case tend to be equated with the characteristics of the group as a whole. Consequently, it becomes tempting to move directly from diagnosis to intervention without an adequate assessment of the individual characteristics of the specific case. The logic goes something like this: If aggressive children have been shown to be deficient in problem-solving skills, and a child is identified as aggressive, problem-solving therapy is often judged to be the treatment of choice. Such a pattern typifies contemporary psychotherapy outcome research, in which a shared diagnosis or comparable scores on overt symptom scales (e.g., depression inventories) are the exclusive criteria for inclusion in a treatment group (Persons, 1991). In turn, a standardized treatment protocol is applied without assessment of the underlying processes that may be contributing to the disorder.

In contrast, the idiographic approach emphasizes the uniqueness of each individual case. From this perspective, what is important to know about Jack or other clinical cases cannot be derived from the mean performances of a category of individuals. Treatment planning, then, must be based on an understanding of the unique history and characteristics that distinguish Jack from other clinical cases. In essence, no two cases are alike; therefore, treatment plans must be tailored to the unique features of each specific case. If we take this perspective to its extreme, then clinicians who successfully treat one case will not learn much about what might be effective for the treatment of another case. Thus, a potential pitfall of the idiographic approach is that practicing child clinicians will be overwhelmed by uniqueness, and will be forced to "start from scratch" with each new case. In order to avoid this potentially paralyzing problem for practitioners, a method for clustering similar clinical cases is essential.

We have argued that grouping by diagnosis typically fails to account for substantial within-group variation in pathogenic processes, that it is an error to equate the average characteristics of a diagnostic group with the presentation of each member of the group. However, this position should not be viewed as an endorsement of the idiographic perspective that child cases are so unique they cannot be meaningfully classified. In fact, we believe that progress in child therapy is predicated on the establishment of a system that allows us to detect important differences and similarities across cases. Such a system would enhance clinical efficiency and reduce the amount of "trial and error" in treatment selection. But from the perspective of *psychosocial treatment planning and intervention*, the classification of cases on the basis of overt symptoms and problems is simply inadequate. Psychotherapeutic interventions are not typically directed toward the symptoms themselves—be they depressive, aggressive, or anxious—but are aimed at the psychological processes that create or maintain such symptoms. Therefore, it is our proposal that it is clinically more useful to classify cases on the basis of similar *formulations of pathogenic processes* rather than on the basis of overt symptoms or problems. In turn, treatments can be selected on the basis of their goodness of fit with the hypothesized or identified pathogenic processes, and treatment generalizations can be made to cases that share pathogenic mechanisms.

A major question, and challenge, for this perspective is: *Are there meaningful clusters of case formulations or does uniqueness prevail?* To this question the idiographers are likely to respond that infinite variability rules when we turn to individual histories and underlying processes. The differential diagnosticians are likely to join them in an unusual alliance, and to assert that such variability raises the titanic problem of reliability in clinical judgment and must be avoided if we are to preserve some semblance of order. In fact, they will note that for this reason, etiological and process dimensions were largely purged from recent versions of psychiatric diagnostic systems (Shapiro, 1989).

To these challenges we offer counters on two fronts. First, in response to the diagnosticians, it is important to note that the current major system for diagnosing childhood disorders has serious reliability problems of its own. As Achenbach (1985) notes, even when very broad categories of disorders were used as the criteria for agreement—in contrast to requiring precise agreement about specific diagnosis—reliability was not good (the overall kappa for child and adolescent disorders was only .52). Moreover, reliability for child and adolescent diagnoses dropped from an early version of the DSM-III-R to the final draft in field trials (Achenbach, 1985). Although it is possible that DSM-IV will show better results, high levels of interclinician reliability have not been attained with the elimination of etiological and process dimensions.

Second, there is emerging evidence that case formulations can be made at a comparable, if not better, level of reliability (Barber & Crits-Christoph, 1993). For example, the Core Conflictual Relationship Theme Method developed by Luborsky and Crits-Christoph (1990) describes relationship conflicts in terms of three components: wishes and needs, expected responses from others, and responses to the expected reactions of others. Although all of these dimensions are processive and inferential, level of agreement among clinicians who judged patients' descriptions of their interpersonal relationships was reasonably good (kappas in the .61–.70 range). Other approaches that assess underlying dynamics and pathogenic processes (e.g., Perry, Augusto, & Cooper, 1989; Weiss et al., 1986) have shown that interclinician reliability, although difficult to attain without substantial training, can be established at a reasonable level. Thus, when clinicians share a common conceptual framework, agreement about pathogenic processes increases. One possibility, then, is that reliability will be improved with the development of a set of prototypical case formulations.

In response to the idiographers, we turn to the insights of cognitive psychologists who have tackled the problem of human categorization of the object world. When one considers the vast array of stimuli we confront on a daily basis, the task of bringing cognitive order to the potentially infinite differences among objects seems overwhelming. Yet over the course of development, we parse the world into manageable proportions. The diversity of the perceived world becomes organized. One of the most useful models for how this task is accomplished is found in prototype theory (Rosch, 1973, 1978).

In contrast to the classical view of categorization, which holds that a set of "necessary and jointly sufficient" conditions define category membership, prototype theory maintains that most categories used in everyday cognition are best conceptualized as "fuzzy sets" that lack sharp boundaries. A "fuzzy set" is defined not by a fixed set of features (such as even numbers), but by a *prototype* that represents the conceptual ideal for the category (McCloskey & Glucksberg, 1978). In other words, a prototype is an abstract image or set of features that is most representative or typical of a particular category. Thus, categories can be viewed in terms of their clear cases (Rosch, 1978). To use one of Rosch's examples, a kitchen chair is far more prototypic of the class of chairs than is a chaise lounge or beanbag chair. Similarly, a robin typifies the category bird better than a penguin or chicken. As Rosch has noted, "Subjects overwhelmingly agree in their judgments of how good an example or clear case members are of a category, even for categories about whose boundaries they disagree" (p. 36). Thus, in classifying objects, in order to determine category inclusion, individuals compare specific instances with the prototype or clear case. Rosch refers to this aspect of categorization as the *horizontal dimension*.

Prototype theory has been applied to the problem of psychiatric diagnosis (Cantor, Smith, French, & Mezzich, 1980; Horowitz, Post, French, Wallis, & Siegelman, 1981). For example, Horowitz, Post, et al. (1981) showed that the closer a description of a depressed individual matches the prototypic ideal for depression, the stronger the impression that the description (individual) was a member of the category. When the description included only a few features of the prototype, there were higher levels of disagreement among judges about the degree of depression. Of particular interest, in a different series of studies, Horowitz et al. showed that experienced staff members at a child residential treatment program could generate featural prototypes for the three most common childhood disorders treated in the program—aggressive–impulsive, depressed–withdrawn, and borderline–disorganized. Although some features were shared across prototypes, two of the three disorders—aggressive–impulsive and depressed–withdrawn—were characterized by a large, unique set of prototypical features. In other words, ideal or prototypical cases were consensually defined by experienced clinicians. They concluded that this conceptual procedure for deriving clinical prototypes could be useful in the identification of the major features of childhood disorders.

The question, then, is: Can prototype theory be applied to case formulations of pathogenic processes? One might expect that such processes are extraordinarily diverse, perhaps even idiosyncratic to particular cases, and thereby defy meaningful clustering. Consider, for example, the underlying processes found in the treatment of several depressed children. One child's depressive symptoms reflect pathogenic beliefs that high achievement is the principle criterion for self-acceptance, whereas a second child harbors the belief that he or she is essentially unlovable and will be rejected in close interpersonal relationships. A third child, equally depressed as the first two, shows no signs of maladaptive interpersonal assumptions, but responds to the arousal of sad feelings with withdrawal and passivity. A fourth depressed child presents as far from passive; in fact, when sad feelings are aroused she strikes out against the people closest to her and finds herself isolated and miserable. Finally, a fifth depressed child appears to be caught in loyalty conflicts between his divorced parents, and his preoccupation with this conflict interferes with his ability to muster the energy to engage in scholastic activities or to participate in close peer relationships. Now clearly, the pathogenic processes in these cases are quite different, at least at one level of analysis. And here lies the crux of the problem. Pathogenic processes, like virtually all objects or events, can be viewed at multiple levels of analysis, what Rosch (1978) refers to as the *vertical dimension* of categorization.

For example, at the most specific level, the subordinate level, one can identify specific types of chairs, such as kitchen chairs or high chairs. One level above this is what Rosch calls the "basic" level of categorization; in this example, it would include the category of all chairs. At the highest level of inclusiveness, the superordinate level, is the broadest category, in this case, of furniture. Research has shown that the middle level of categorization—the basic level—is special in several ways. Most relevant to our discussion are findings that basic-level categories are accessed most quickly when a relevant stimulus is encountered and are the most abstract categories that can be represented with a single visual image (Mervis & Crisati, 1982; Rosch, Mervis, Gray, Johnson, & Boyes-Braem, 1976). In essence, basic level categories convey more specific information than superordinate categories but are better than subordinate categories in the degree to which they highlight major distinctions between categories (Rosch, 1978).

Let us now transpose this framework to our example of pathogenic processes. Consider the first two cases. At the subordinate level, one child's depression appears tied to beliefs about self-acceptance, whereas the other's is yoked to expectations about social rejection. The contents of these pathogenic beliefs are clearly different. However, these two children share an important pathogenic feature, namely, maladaptive assumptions, or pathogenic beliefs underlie their depressive symptoms. In contrast, the third and fourth cases, although quite different in terms of the content of their maladaptive coping strategies, both involve problems with affect regulation. The final case is distinctive in that conflict appears to be at the heart of the child's depressive presentation. Thus, if we focus on the specifics of each of these cases, that is, at the subordinate level, they all appear to be different in the same way that kitchen chairs, high chairs, and bar stools are different. However, at the *basic* level of categorization, meaningful groupings are evident. Two of the cases fit the pathogenic category of maladaptive beliefs or expectations, another two involve affect regulation deficits, and the last involves internal conflict.

As suggested by these examples, it is our proposal that a set of *basic-level* case formulation can be identified. Moreover, it is our assumption that these basic-level formulations represent the fundamental building blocks for treatment planning; that is, the selection of an intervention strategy (change process) will be contingent on clinical judgments about the degree to which a specific case matches the prototype for one of the basic-level case formulations.

BASIC-LEVEL CASE FORMULATIONS

As we discussed in the first chapter, methods of intervention tend to be derived from models of etiology, such that theories of psychopathology and intervention come in "matched sets" (Cowan, 1988, p. 6). Our review of the child therapy literature reveals that specific change processes such as interpretation, skills training, or interpersonal validation are coordinated with models of pathogenic process. For example, skills training is based on a model of psychopathology that emphasizes deficits in adaptive capacities, whereas interpersonal validation is linked with models that emphasize vulnerabilities in self-esteem.

Our review also suggests that the early practice of child therapy suffered from the uniformity myth of psychotherapy, such that a single type of change process was often applied to widely diverse childhood problems. For example, early dynamic therapies typically attempted to promote insight into unconscious conflicts as their principal method for facilitating change. Eventually, however, it was recognized that such a procedure was not suitable for a large group of children whose symptoms and problems did not stem from internal conflicts. With the evolution of an alternative model of pathogenesis, the ego deficit model, interpretation and insight were replaced by validation and scaffolding as the principal mechanisms of change. Similarly, early client-centered therapy emphasized the role of unconditional regard or support as the primary vehicle of therapeutic growth for all child cases. Eventually, this model of intervention evolved with the development of other conceptualizations of pathogenic process (e.g., emotional blockage). In turn, supportive processes were supplemented with methods that emphasized the expression and understanding of feelings. And within the cognitive-behavioral tradition, the exclusive focus on skill deficits has given way to a comparable concern with cognitive distortions. In turn, some treatments attempt to promote the acquisition of compensatory skills, whereas others focus on schematic change. The point here is that both within and across therapeutic orientations, models of pathogenic process have become increasingly differentiated over time. As these examples suggest, it is no longer possible to equate a treatment orientation with a unitary model of pathogenesis. However, our review of the major systems of child psychotherapy point to a set of *basic-level* formulations of pathogenic process. These basic level formulations are presented in Figure 8.1 along with their theoretical origins.

Figure 8.1 is presented for heuristic purposes, that is, as a starting point for differentiating basic models of pathogenic process. Although our review of the child therapy literature supports the theoretical lineage portrayed in Figure 8.1, it is most certainly the case that versions of these models can be found in a number of theoretical orientations. For example, some contemporary dynamic theorists (e.g., Tolpin, 1978) emphasize vulnerabilities in the child's sense of self as the primary source of psychopathology; similarly, experiential therapists have recognized that emotional interference can be the result of internal conflicts (Wright et al., 1986). Thus, not only is it the case that more than one model of pathogenic process can be found within a theoretical orientation, it is also the case that different therapeutic orientations endorse similar models of pathogenesis.

What, then, are the core descriptive characteristics of these basic formulations? The *internal conflict formulation* posits that overt emotional or behavioral problems are a function of conflicts between aspects of the child's personality, for example, between desires and prohibitions, between antagonistic feelings, or between contradictory needs and wishes. Dynamic theory has offered a number of classic conflicts, including struggles between autonomy and dependency, hostility and guilt, and impulse and internalized constraints. Symptoms are understood as compromise solutions to unresolved internal conflicts.

Traditionally, the *ego deficit formulation* holds that emotional and behavioral problems reflect pervasive deficits in critical psychological functions such as frustration tolerance, impulse control, reality testing, and emotion regulation. Basic problems with the organization of interpersonal relationships are often evident. Consequently, this model often has been applied to understanding children with more severe forms of psychopathology. Typically, such children evince multiple symptoms and deficits across a range of functional domains (e.g., school, peer relations, and self-care). The *skills deficit formulation* clearly bears some relationship to the ego deficit model in that "deficits" in psychological processes are viewed

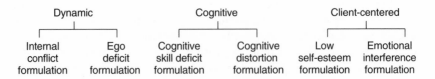

FIGURE 8.1. Basic pathogenic formulations by theory of origin.

as the source of overt problems. In contrast to the ego deficit model, this model conceptualizes psychological functions in terms of skills that can be analyzed into component elements. For example, problems with social judgment are recast as deficits in social problem solving and are analyzed in terms of limitations in component processes such as self-monitoring, generating alternative solutions, or consequential thinking.

It is not clear whether the skills deficit formulation simply represents a more specific characterization of functional deficits than is portrayed by the ego deficit formulation, or if "ego" deficits represent something more than component "skills." The fact that the ego has been conceptualized as a system of regulating mechanisms and that many skills deficits involve regulating processes suggests substantial overlap in these formulations. Thus, it is possible that an ego deficit formulation differs from a skills deficit formulation in quantitative rather than qualitative ways, that is, in terms of breadth or pervasiveness of deficits.

The *cognitive distortion formulation* maintains that maladaptive assumptions, expectations, or beliefs result in distortions or biases in social appraisal processes that, in turn, give rise to problematic behaviors and emotions. Although there is some disagreement about the degree to which these schema operate outside of awareness, it is assumed that these cognitive representations influence emotional experience and interpersonal behavior. For example, research with aggressive children has shown that they tend to overattribute hostile intent in ambiguous circumstances (Dodge, Price, Bachorowski, & Newman, 1990). Such attributions appear to be based on implicit expectations that others are likely to respond to the self in a malevolent manner. Thus, in contrast to the cognitive deficit formulation, the underlying problem does not reside in cognitive skill deficiencies, but in dysfunctions in cognitive processes (Kendall, 1991).

The *low self-esteem formulation* proposes that emotional and behavioral problems are markers of underlying vulnerabilities in self-esteem. Deficits in self-esteem translate into observable problems with motivation, emotion, and behavior. Although there are multiple developmental pathways to low self-esteem, problems with self-worth are not viewed as mere consequences of other pathogenic processes, but are conceptualized as both mediators and moderators of emotional and behavioral adaptation (Shirk & Harter, 1996). For example, Harter (1986) has demonstrated that self-worth mediates between the children's experience of social support and competence and their motivational and affective orientation in scholastic contexts. Similarly, research on risk and resilience has revealed that self-esteem is one of the most important buffers (moderators) of psychosocial stressors (Garmezy, 1985). Thus, low self-esteem is viewed as a contributor to maladjustment, and not just an indicator of it.

Finally, the *emotional interference formulation* frames childhood psychopathology in terms of the disruptive influence of emotion on children's adaptive functioning. According to this perspective, the smooth and efficient operation of children's functional capacities (e.g., social judgment, concentration, peer engagement) are undermined by poorly regulated emotional processes. The basis for interference is conceptualized in a number of ways, including (1) the inadequate processing of emotional experience such that the child is preoccupied with emotionally charged material; (2) the blockage of emotion expression, such that the child redirects emotion, often unconsciously, in a manner that disrupts other processes (e.g., the child expresses anger toward parents through school underachievement); and (3) the ineffective control of emotion, such that the child is overwhelmed by feelings and therefore unable to deal effectively with task demands. In all three variations, emotion dysregulation is viewed as the source of overt problems.

Consistent with the notion of "fuzzy sets," these basic formulations lack sharp boundaries. In fact, it is possible that these formulations could be reduced to a smaller set of core formulations corresponding to the psychological systems that have been disrupted, for example, *cognitive problems* in which distortions in meaning or problems with information processing (reality testing) predominate; *emotional problems* in which the varieties of affect dysregulation are pivotal; and *interpersonal problems* in which maladaptive patterns of relating or the lack of supportive relationships prevail. Alternatively, these groupings could represent the superordinate level of pathogenic processes.

Two factors support the use of the proposed basic level formulations. First, these formulations have been prominent in the major theories of child psychotherapy; consequently they have provided a conceptually meaningful way of differentiating types of cases. What distinguishes the current model from other formulation-based approaches is the inclusiveness of our basic level formulations. For example, Strayhorn (1988) argues quite cogently for a formulation-based approach to child treatment, but limits his formulations to the skills deficit model. *It is our proposal that the major systems of child psychotherapy have evolved multiple formulations of pathogenic process, and that the diversity of child cases demands a conceptually inclusive framework.*

Second, the basic level formulations presented earlier seem to convey more specific information about a case than the alternative (superordinate) categories. Although the distinctions between these basic-level formulations may not be sharp—only empirical evidence will ultimately determine the breadth and number of these categories—they do lend themselves to case descriptions; that is, abstract and prototypic features of the formulations can be captured in case presentations.

Some might argue that the set of basic-level formulations is not broad enough (i.e., that a number of basic formulations have been omitted). For example, there has been growing recognition of the role of trauma in the genesis of childhood psychopathology (Shirk & Eltz, in press). In fact, "traumagenic" models have been proposed for victims of child sexual and physical abuse (cf. Strauss, 1988). However, whereas trauma may be the *etiological* source of the child's presenting problems, treatment does not aim at undoing the traumatic *history,* but instead is directed toward the *sequelae* of the traumatic past (Eltz, Shirk, & Sarlin, 1995). These sequelae, or consequences of trauma, can be understood in terms of one, or in many cases, more than one of the formulations of pathogenic process. For example, a child who has been exposed to recurrent episodes of family violence may lack the capacity to regulate his or her feelings. In such a case, the emotional interference formulation would apply. Alternatively, a child who has been repeatedly victimized may have developed assumptions about the danger inherent in interpersonal relationships. Although these assumptions may be accurate in relation to the original victimizing relationship, they often become overgeneralized and therefore maladaptive in relation to significant others (e.g., potentially benign teachers). Consequently, the child is unable to feel safe at school, and academic achievement suffers. Again, whereas trauma is the etiological source of the problem, the pathogenic process is captured by the cognitive distortion formulation.

As these examples suggest, a distinction must be made between the etiology (causal origin) of the child's difficulties and the pathogenic process that currently accounts for the child's focal problems. For example, one can contract an infectious disease through an insect bite. Thus, whereas the etiology is exposure to an infected insect, the pathogenic process for the ensuing fever or rash is the underlying infection. Treatment would not consist of wearing mosquito netting but instead would involve efforts to eliminate the infection.

Two other basic-level formulations were considered for inclusion. Common to both is a maladaptive reaction to immediate or relatively recent environmental stressors. The first formulation might be called the "enduring adversity model." In such a situation, the child is exposed to ongoing turmoil, threat, or disruption. Children who are living in actively abusive situations represent clear case examples of this formulation, as do refugee children or children in war zones, or perhaps even children who live in violent neighborhoods where personal danger is a fact of everyday life. Although such circumstances touch the lives of far too many children, from an intervention standpoint, the source of the problem resides in the environment, and the primary intervention must be to ensure the safety of the child by altering the environment or locating the child in a less disruptive situation. The second, and related formulation, appears to be captured by the notion of "adjustment reaction." Here the child's emotional or behavioral problems are reactions to *past* psychological or environmental stressors. But like the "traumagenic" formulation, this model focuses on etiology rather than pathogenic process, and in most cases of adjustment reaction, the ongoing focal problems can be understood in terms of one of the basic level formulations for example, emotional interference due to overwhelming anger about parental divorce.

Thus, for heuristic purposes, we will begin with a set of six basic-level case formulations. Empirical research will be needed to determine whether these conceptually derived categories adequately represent the variations in child clinical cases. Other investigators (e.g., Horowitz, Wright, et al., 1981) have shown that experienced child clinicians can reach consensus regarding common types of childhood disorders. Certainly, a demonstration of consensus among child psychotherapists regarding common case formulations would be an important starting point for the validation of this approach.

CASE FORMULATION PROTOTYPES

According to prototype theory, categories are defined in terms of their clear cases (Rosch, 1978). Classification of a specific case is made on the basis of its similarity to the clear case or prototype. Thus, in an effort to facilitate the classification of specific cases in terms of pathogenic processes, what follows is a set of cases that typify each of the basic-level case formulations. The cases were selected as prototypes or clear cases of each formulation.

The Internal Conflict Formulation: The Case of Corine

Focal Problems

"Corine" is a 12-year-old girl who was referred to the psychology clinic for psychotherapy following a neuropsychological evaluation. The initial evaluation revealed that Corine was of average intelligence but had a significant nonverbal learning disability that manifested itself in problems with spatial and mathematical reasoning. Consistent with this finding, Corine struggled with math, art, and geography. In addition to the cognitive findings, the neuropsychologist noted that Corine appeared to be very inhibited, despite the fact that her mother reported troubling episodes of mother–daughter conflict. During the testing feedback session Corine expressed sadness about her school situation. She felt that she was disappointing her mother, who wanted her "to get the chance in life she'd never had." And to add to her troubles, she disclosed that she "just didn't fit in" with the other girls at school. In addition to remedial and compensatory recommendations for her learning problems, the neuropsychologist noted concerns about possible depressive trends that could be obstructing Corine's social development. Thus, psychotherapy also was recommended.

In the initial intake with Corine's mother, a disparate set of focal concerns were presented. On the one hand, Corine was described as inhibited and socially immature. Her mother noted that she preferred to play with younger children, resisted participating in school activities such as sports or various clubs, and had refused to attend a day camp the previous summer. On the other hand, Corine was described as willful and noncompliant. Although the school had offered tutoring in math, Corine was often only superficially compliant and occasionally flatly refused to attend. Her mother was extremely troubled by this situation because she had worked very hard to get the school to provide special services for her daughter. As she put it, "Corine told me she couldn't do the math without help; then when I finally got them to provide a tutor, she turned around and made me look the fool." Last, but by no means least, Corine's mother expressed concern that their relationship was deteriorating. Over the last year, Corine had increasingly "challenged her mother's authority" with a lot of verbal back talk. The mother found these battles to be especially stressful, in part, because she was so easily drawn into them. She noted that she needed to "own up" to getting "entangled" in these conflicts, but felt, as a single parent, that she needed to maintain firm control over her preadolescent daughter. What was so puzzling to the mother was the fact that after these "blowups" Corine would feel guilty for upsetting her and would attempt to make reparations by doing special "nice" things for her mom.

In her initial interview, Corine presented as a rather thin, pale child, who appeared somewhat young for her age. Her affect was rather flat, and one could readily understand the neuropsychologist's concern about possible depressive trends. When asked about her understanding of the referral, Corine said that she was doing poorly in school and that she got into fights with her mom. When asked how these situations made her feel, she turned her attention to a set of farm animals on one of the shelves. Without responding verbally, she began to set up a farm scene. She placed two colts in a corral along with the larger horse. For a period of time the larger horse was "teaching" the colts how to jump over barrels, drink from a trough, and find "sweet grass" on the other side of the fence. Suddenly one of the colts bolted from the corral by jumping the fence, coaxed the other to come along, and together they galloped across the floor of the office. From a high cliff—atop a desk—the colts looked down upon the lone horse now lying in a corner of the corral. In a flash they returned to the corral but stopped short and asked the larger horse to open the gate. The larger horse promptly got up, opened the gate, and the three returned to their earlier activities. Just as quickly as she had started the play, Corine abruptly stopped and asked if she could go to the bathroom. When she returned, she spent the remainder of the session talking about her plans for summer and about how happy she was that the school year was coming to an end.

Corine's initial presentation was remarkable in a number of ways. First, the ease with which she moved into symbolic play seemed to be more typical of a younger child. Although she showed some awareness of the reason for her referral, her capacity to verbalize her feelings seemed limited. In contrast, her symbolic play was rich and appeared to parallel some of the conflicts expressed by her mother; that is, in this thematic episode the youngsters broke away from their caregiver only to find that it left the caregiver lifeless. As a result, they returned home and asked for the help of the caregiver (to open the gate, when only a short time earlier they had jumped over it on their own). Although only a fragment, the theme of Corine's play involved a conflict between autonomy and responsibility. On the one side was the wish to be free and independent, but on the other were fears about the impact of such strivings on her caregiver. In fact, this brief episode turned out to be a "preview" of one of the recurrent themes of Corine's play, namely, how to separate without doing damage to the one who has cared for you.

Developmental History

Corine's developmental history was noteworthy in several respects. First, she had experienced anoxia during delivery, which probably accounted for her learning disability. It had been necessary for her to be in the intensive-care unit, on oxygen, for the first week of life. Throughout her early childhood, Corine's mother had her evaluated repeatedly by neurologists, neuropsychologists, and school psychologists, despite consistent feedback that Corine's condition was stable. Corine's father had "abandoned" his wife and daughter when Corine was 2 years old. Her mother reported that she had been moderately depressed for an extended period of time following the separation, had "bounced" from one job to another, and had attempted to return to college to complete her degree. She had given up this goal about 2 years prior to Corine's referral. She had not been involved in a "serious" relationship since her husband's departure and was not currently dating. Much of her energy was directed toward providing for Corine and working to ensure that she received the services she "deserved." Corine had not seen her father since she was a toddler, although she had substantial contact with a maternal uncle. In addition, Corine and her mother lived a great distance from the maternal grandparents. Her mother described her own childhood as "problematic," and felt that it was essential to maintain distance from her parents.

Case Formulation

Prominent among the disparate list of focal concerns was recurrent and moderately intense mother–daughter conflict. An increase in such conflict is not uncommon during the transition to adolescence. Thus, it is tempting to characterize Corine's difficulties as "normal problems" of development. However, given the apparent depressive trends, her refusal to make use of remedial help that would facilitate school success, and evidence of social immaturity, Corine was showing greater than expected difficulty with the developmental task of increasing autonomy and self-reliance.

In this case, the developmental history provides a frame for formulating the focal problems. First, based on the early medical difficulties, it was evident that Corine's mother viewed her daughter as a "vulnerable" child. Throughout her early years she had sought reassurance that her daughter was medically stable and worked diligently to ensure that she received the medical and school services that she "deserved." Her mother's own development had been disrupted by the sudden termination of a marriage that left her depressed for an extended period of time. In fact, at the time of the referral, she was still experiencing difficulty with sustained employment and schooling, and was uninvolved, in fact, disinterested in developing intimate relationships. The mother's identity was almost exclusively defined as Corine's caregiver and advocate. This relational experience appeared to create a core conflict for Corine.

As a preteen, Corine was faced with the developmental press toward increasing autonomy and self-reliance. Not surprisingly, there was evidence of her desire to be independent and to make decisions for herself. However, this wish resulted in conflict on two fronts. First, Corine appeared to have absorbed the message of her vulnerability as evidenced by her avoidance of age-appropriate challenges and her preference for younger children. Thus, the wish to be self-reliant conflicted with an image of herself as vulnerable. Second, the desire to be independent conflicted with her sense of obligation to her mother, who wanted her to "get the chance in life she never had." It appeared that Corine recognized her mother's own vulnerability, as evidenced by her guilt and attempts to please following episodes of conflict. Thus, Corine was caught between the age-appropriate wish to be more separate from her mother and the fear that such separation could be damaging to her mom.

This core conflict casts new light on the focal problems. On the one hand, Corine is drawn to less mature activities (e.g., playing with animal figures and dolls, preferring to associate with younger children, and refusing the help that would make her more competent in school). In brief, she behaves in the manner of a younger child who needs her mother's involvement; consequently the fear that her strivings for autonomy will hurt her mother is kept in check. However, the desire for greater autonomy and self-reliance is not satisfied by this arrangement. As a result, she is increasingly defiant toward her mother, refuses tutoring as a way of asserting her autonomy, but then feels guilty for disappointing her mother. In the end, she is stuck on the path of development. She is unable to participate in age-appropriate activities and relationships, lacks more mature methods for expressing her feelings, and appears to be moderately depressed. As is typical of the internal conflict formulation, the resolution of this conflict is equivalent to removing an obstacle in the path of normal development. As long as Corine remains caught between her wish and her fear, the normative processes of maturation will be obstructed and she will increasingly appear to be out of step with her age-mates. Of course, as is often the case with internal conflicts in *children,* their resolution depends on collateral interventions that alter current relational contributions to the conflict.

The Ego Deficit Formulation: The Case of Sam

Focal Problems

"Sam" is a 10-year-old boy who was referred to the Day Treatment Program from the public schools. According to school reports, Sam showed significant problems with self-regulation. He had a limited capacity to remain on-task in class, and his "silly" behavior was highly disruptive to other students. He was typically isolated from peers, although he was able to attract considerable attention from classmates with his artistic talents. Unfortunately, the content of his drawings were often graphic depictions of aggressive acts or highly sexualized renderings of human figures. Sam actually had made a small profit from his classmates selling these pictures. He often appeared to be preoccupied in class, although in the context of academic tutoring—a one-to-one situation—he demonstrated a much higher level of academic competence. Sam was not typically aggressive, but could become "wild"; that is, he would tantrum and scream when demands for participation were made or firm limits were placed on his behavior. At such times he could "lash out" at a teacher. Emotion regulation was a serious problem for Sam. As mentioned, he often engaged in "silly" disruptive behavior, and evidenced affect that was clearly incongruent with situations, for example, laughing when presented with "serious" subject material, or showing signs of heightened fear when another child was accidentally hurt on the playground. He showed little capacity to engage in age-appropriate games such as kickball and often spent his time during recess hunting for insects. Thus, on several fronts Sam presented with significant problems, including difficulties with regulating emotion, sustaining attention in the absence of substantial adult support, containing fears and primitive preoccupations, and relating to peers in an age-appropriate manner. He did present with several strengths, including average intelligence, a desire to relate to adults, and artistic talent.

In his initial interview, Sam readily joined the therapist and showed substantial interest in the toys and games in the office. Without comment, he began to set up the "playhouse" with family figures. After spending a brief time, he surrounded the family with army figures and played out an attack. All family members were mortally wounded. After completing the thematic play, Sam was asked about his current school situation. His answers were brief but were peculiar. He said he did not get along with the kids there, and wondered what the kids were like at this school. In particular, he was concerned about whether they would be mean and whether the teachers would be nice. Near the end of the session he was asked to complete a human figure drawing. He readily complied; however, the drawing itself was a grotesque depiction of a pirate whose flesh had been torn away from one leg, who had a sword thrust through his stomach, and a crab claw for one hand. Thus, in his play, his drawings, and his conversation, Sam showed an intense preoccupation with aggressive themes.

Developmental History

Sam's developmental history was remarkable for its level of family instability and disruption. Sam's father had been a polysubstance abuser who eventually had been imprisoned for an assault on a police officer. His mother attempted to raise Sam and his two siblings in the home of the maternal grandparents. There was a high level of conflict between Sam's mother and grandmother who, according to mother's report, "had never given a damn about me." After a short period, the family was "kicked out" of the grandparents' home and briefly lived in a shelter. Sam was 18 months old at the time. While at the shelter the mother's harsh disciplinary practices were brought to the attention of the Department of Social Services. With the help of their caseworker, the family moved into a small apartment, and the mother was assisted with parenting skills and with finding a job. During the preschool period, Sam's mother had a series of romantic relationships that appeared to absorb much of her time and energy. Social service reports indicated that the children may have been frequently exposed to adult sexual activity. Day-care reports indicated that Sam often came to school dirty and hungry. There was one case report of suspected physical abuse; however, the report was not substantiated. Sam's behavior deteriorated badly during kindergarten; he was aggressive and "uncontrollable" both at home and at school. As a result, he was briefly placed in a therapeutic foster home. He was returned to his mother's custody after 6 months. Throughout the elementary-school years, he received tutoring and therapy in school. A case report alleging neglect was filed on behalf of Sam and his siblings when he was 8 years old. This report was verified, and the sibling group was placed in foster care. At the time of his referral, Sam remained in foster care but had frequent visitation with his biological mother.

Case Formulation

Sam's presentation is characterized by pervasive self-regulatory problems. Common to his difficulties with peer relations, emotion control, and cognitive focus are deficits in regulatory capacities. It is noteworthy that Sam functions best in a one-to-one relationship in which he can draw on the functional capacities of an attentive adult to manage his emotions, cognitions, and behavior. Left to himself, Sam shows sharp decrements in his level of functioning. In addition, there is clear evidence of problems with regulating cognitive processes. Sam often appears preoccupied to the point of distraction by images of danger, sexuality, and violence. In brief, he has substantial difficulty "neutralizing" his social experience; that is, interactions are strongly colored by his intrusive preoccupations. Given the highly disruptive, overstimulating, and neglectful early environment, such preoccupations are not surprising. His inability to contain such preoccupations interferes with his social judgment, results in isolation from peers, and represents another example of deficient internal regulatory structures.

In addition to these pervasive regulatory problems, Sam's developmental history is highly consistent with the ego deficit formulation. Clearly Sam's early developmental needs were not met by an "expectable environment." There were serious lapses in Sam's early caretaking, and he lacked a stable base from which to construct internal controls. As a result, he presented with multiple functional deficits. In this respect, Sam appears to be prototypical of the ego deficit formulation.

The Cognitive Skill Deficit Formulation: The Case of Tommy

Focal Problems

"Tommy" is a 7-year-old boy who was referred to the child psychology clinic by his parents. Among their primary concerns were Tommy's aggressive behavior with peers and his tendency to "act without thinking." When asked to provide examples of these difficulties, his parents noted several incidents. In the first, Tommy threw a rock at a school recess monitor after she had reprimanded him for misbehavior (roughhousing with younger children). Although he appeared quite angry when this behavior led to additional negative consequences—an afterschool detention—he later expressed remorse for his deeds and with little prompting apologized to the monitor. Tommy's father noted that on several other occasions his son had been involved in physical fights with older peers. Usually these episodes were prompted by teasing and took place on the playground or while riding the bus after school. Unfortunately for Tommy, because of the size differential, he usually sustained the "worst of it" in these fights. Despite such outcomes the frequency of these bouts was not decreasing.

In contrast to these difficulties, his relationships with his parents were described as "close" and "loving," although there were occasional episodes of age-typical noncompliance. His level of school achievement was on target for his age; however, he periodically would refuse to complete an assignment and on one occasion had told his teacher that her class was stupid. In terms of focal problems, Tommy's appeared to involve difficulties with impulsivity and aggressiveness. Although the intensity of these problems was by no means severe, the increasing frequency of such episodes had prompted the school to encourage the parents to seek psychological consultation.

In his initial interview, Tommy readily joined his therapist and eagerly explored the consultation room. When queried, he acknowledged that he had a hard time staying out of trouble. When pressed to elaborate, he mentioned that he sometimes said "bad" things and that he hated to be teased. During the session, he engaged the therapist is a game of checkers, played by the rules, and maintained composure when he did not win each round. At the end of the session, he helped with cleanup and asked the therapist if he would see him again.

It was noteworthy in Tommy's case that he demonstrated significant competencies in a number of domains. First, he had a number of age-appropriate interests (sports and collecting coins); second, he did reasonably well in peer interactions with adult supervision (he was an active and well-liked member of his T-ball team); third, he seemed oriented to and invested in forming relationships; and finally, he was able to perform in school at a level commensurate with his intellectual abilities. In brief, although Tommy presented with clinically significant behavior problems, by no means did he show a pattern of pervasive functional deficits.

Developmental History

Tommy's developmental history was unremarkable, with the exception of frequent family moves during the preschool period. As a result of these moves, Tommy had been enrolled in five different preschools. His parents described this as a difficult period for Tommy, who was often isolated in his preschool classes. As a result, his early peer relations were frequently disrupted, and his parents noted that his preschool teachers described him as "clingy" and overdependent on their support. Tommy briefly showed signs of school avoidance at the beginning of first grade, but this problem dissipated as he became attached to his first-grade teacher who was, as the parents put it, "very grandmotherly."

Case Formulation

Although Tommy showed a pattern of moderate behavioral difficulties involving impulsivity and aggressiveness, he also exhibited a number of significant strengths. As reported by his parents the developmental history was largely unremarkable with the exception of frequent moves during the preschool period. However, it is possible that these moves, and the associated disruptions in peer relationships, interfered with the development of self-regulatory skills, particularly in the context of peer interactions. Prominent in Tommy's presentation were difficulties with "acting without thinking," despite above-average verbal skills. As a result, Tommy responded to provocative situations impulsively and later regretted his behavior. What appeared to be missing in Tommy's social repertoire was the capacity to "stop and think" before acting, that is, the ability to inhibit an immediate response and apply verbal problem-solving or self-regulating strategies before acting. Thus, underlying his focal problems of impulsivity and aggressiveness were specific cognitive skill deficits. Although skill deficits may take many specific forms, and can vary in intensity and pervasiveness, Tommy's case typifies the cognitive skills deficit formulation.

The Cognitive Distortion Formulation: The Case of Darren

Focal Problems

"Darren" is a 10-year-old boy who was referred to the child psychology clinic by his social worker at school. Although Darren had been in group therapy at school for 2 years, he had shown little progress in forming relationships with both peers and teachers. Darren was described as a "loner" who had difficulty relating to other children and working collaboratively in study groups. His worker said that the children in the therapy group thought he was "weird" because he often told stories that were "gross." As a result, they avoided him or excluded him from activities. From his social worker's perspective, Darren did not appear depressed, but she noted that he was the kind of child who "rarely showed his feelings." Occasionally, however, he would have a "temper flare-up." Such flare-ups usually were precipitated by demands to participate in group activities. At such times Darren would contend that he would rather be left alone, and if given the choice, he would invariably work in isolation. Efforts by teachers to work with him on a one-to-one basis often resulted in "control struggles." Similarly, he often "bent the rules" when it came to his homework assignments. Although he typically completed assignments, he would "add his own mark" on tasks by altering some aspect of the assignment (e.g., he would print a story rather than write it in cursive, or he would work out math problems in crayon rather than pencil). His teacher was somewhat at a loss to explain this behavior, but noted that attempts to get Darren to fully comply only resulted in "power struggles."

Darren's mother reported that her relationship with her son was "distant," and that she wished they could be closer. She noted that Darren was happiest playing computer games, and that he rarely associated with other kids in the neighborhood. She, too, noted that she and Darren would get involved in "power struggles," particularly around the completion of chores. Overall, however, she said that Darren was not a "major behavior problem," that he rarely violated important family rules. Occasionally they enjoyed watching videos together. She also mentioned that Darren was a "talented baseball player," but that he had trouble getting along with the other kids on the team. Instead he would spend hours throwing the ball against a wall and fielding the rebounds. Recently he had quit the team because he felt like the coach was "ordering him around." The mother was very surprised by Darren's account, insofar as she found the coach to be an easygoing man who "didn't push the kids." The incident reminded her of other times when Darren would "lash out with a sharp tongue even before I got a word out of my mouth." She said that the same thing happened with Darren's uncles. They would be playing ball together, and suddenly Darren would "break things off," taking offense at some minor comment.

In a series of interviews, Darren was very cautious and difficult to engage. For much of the first session he played alone and responded minimally to the therapist's inquiries. His main concern involved the number of times he needed to come to the clinic. Although he seemed somewhat less detached over the next few interviews, his style of relating was highly competitive. He opted to play "Crossfire," a game whose primary goal—at least for Darren—was to push his opponent's pieces away from his "safety zone." He had difficulty accepting defeat, even though he usually won, and when he lost, he would protest that the therapist had "cheated." At the end of each session, Darren would leave without saying good-bye and showed little interest in returning. His therapist reported that she had never felt so "disconnected" from a child.

Developmental History

Darren is the only child of a marriage that was characterized by repeated separations and failed reconciliations. According to his mother, when Darren was about a year old, she began to experience medical problems that left her exhausted much of the time. She was later diagnosed with "chronic fatigue syndrome." As a result of these problems, she had given up her job as a nurse and became the full-time caregiver for Darren. She acknowledged that her condition made it difficult to care for Darren, that she was stressed by his high level of activity as a toddler, and that the loss of income placed added strain on the family. Her relationship with her husband also suffered, and there had been several separations during Darren's preschool years. The parents attempted to reconcile several times, and according to the mother's report, Darren was "deeply disappointed" when his father would leave after the failed reunions. Eventually the parents divorced, and Darren was caught in the middle of a custody dispute. As the intensity of the custody battle increased, conflicts around visitation mounted (e.g., his father would not return him to his mother at the appointed time, and she would retaliate by attempting to block future visits). The father remarried when Darren was 7 and had a baby with his new wife. Unfortunately for Darren, his father's new wife thought Darren was "disturbed" and restricted contact with the family because she "didn't want him around the baby." Although Darren's mother had been on disability for several years, her medical condition had improved, and she had returned to work on a part-time basis.

Case Formulation

Darren presents with significant problems with social relationships—he is described as a loner, someone who not only has difficulty relating to others, but also actively engages in behaviors that push them away. At a global level, one might describe his basic interpersonal orientation as mistrustful. Seemingly benign interactions often deteriorate into control struggles. An important trigger for these struggles appears to be misperceptions of others' intents; that is, attempts to involve, help, or guide Darren are frequently misconstrued as efforts to control or manipulate. In brief, Darren's capacity to differentiate benign and potentially supportive interactions from malevolent or overcontrolling interactions is extremely poor.

In light of Darren's developmental history, his behavior and cognitive processes seem to be biased by a number of maladaptive assumptions about relationships. At the core appear to be deep suspicions about the responsiveness, dependability, and tolerance of autonomy of significant others. One could hypothesize that these assumptions take a conditional form such as "If I rely on others, I'll be disappointed or manipulated," or "If you can't count on others, then you have to fend for yourself." In essence, Darren's early relationship experience, characterized by inconsistent parental care, manipulation in the context of a custody dispute, and repeated disappointment, appears to have evolved into a self-protective or avoidant interpersonal style. Thus, underlying Darren's focal problems are cognitive distortions that are grounded in maladaptive assumptions about social relationships. His judgments about others' intentions are strongly colored by concerns about manipulation and reliability. Although these assumptions may have been accurate in the context from which they developed, they are maladaptive in the sense that they are overgeneralized and lead to biased information processing in the context of new relationships.

The Low Self-Esteem Formulation: The Case of Colin

Focal Problems

"Colin" is a 9-year-old boy who was referred to the psychology clinic by his parents, who are divorced. Both parents described Colin as a very lovable and affectionate child who typically was eager to please both parents and teachers alike. They had become increasingly concerned about Colin's mood and behavior during the last year. At times he appeared to be disinterested in activities that he had previously cherished—Little League baseball and computers—and on several occasions he had "torn up" his homework, saying that "it wasn't good enough" to turn in. Since kindergarten Colin had shown a keen interest in school, and his parents were concerned by recent reports from teachers that he was "just doing the minimum required in class." Such a presentation was atypical for Colin in that he had always worked hard in school and took pleasure in the teachers' praise and approval. Although he was not disruptive in class and usually completed assignments, he seemed less motivated to take on new academic challenges. In addition, he had told his teacher, "No one really likes me," which came as a surprise since Colin seemed to have several "pals" with whom he played at recess. Although his parents felt that he eventually would overcome this "down period," they were prompted to seek consultation following a suicidal gesture. While on a weekend visit, his father found him in his bedroom with the dog's choke chain around his neck. Although it was evident that Colin had not injured himself, he told his father that "they'd be better off without him."

Colin was seen for an extended set of interviews to assess his level of suicidality. In these sessions Colin was quite open and was willing to talk about the episode with the choke chain. Although he acknowledged that he had thought about killing himself on several occasions, he denied that he really wanted to die. In fact, it was evident that he had not thought through a suicide plan (he had not planned to suspend the choke chain in a manner that would result in hanging), was oriented to future events (e.g., to an upcoming vacation with his grandparents), and did not appear to be impulsive (which was confirmed by his parents and teachers). In addition, it was clear that he enjoyed the evaluation sessions; not surprisingly, he readily complied with the evaluation tasks and expressed a desire to return for more meetings. Nevertheless, there were indications that Colin was feeling very down about his parents' divorce, and that he was having a difficult time maintaining positive feelings about himself. When asked to "draw a person," he made several attempts, erased, and reworked the drawing numerous times, eventually concluding that he could not make one that was "good enough." When asked to tell a story that went along with the picture, Colin presented a tale about a boy who went sailing on a lake, encountered a storm, was tossed overboard, and eventually feeling lost and hungry was washed up on a remote shore. Consistent with the theme of this story, his responses to the Self-Perception Profile (Harter, 1985) revealed both depressed mood and low global self-worth. In summary, Colin presented a number of focal problems, including suicidal thinking, decrements in academic motivation, and lowered interest in activities that he once found engaging. His tattered self-image was also quite evident.

Developmental History

Colin was the middle child of three siblings. His parents described him as a boy who was always eager to please others, and who had never been a behavior problem. The most noteworthy feature of the family history was the demise of the parents' marriage. They described their separation and eventual divorce as the result of "drifting apart" rather than the outcome of overt conflict and acrimony. Both parents were involved in their own careers, possessed a sense of self-sufficiency, and believed that the "romantic bond" that had drawn them together had dissipated over time. In their words, they were "going through the motions of marriage," and had jointly decided to "end the charade." They felt they had worked out a "reasonable" joint-custody arrangement that enabled the children to spend significant time with both parents. However, since the divorce had been finalized, both parents were actively involved with new romantic partners, and access arrangements were not working as smoothly as they had originally hoped.

Case Formulation

Colin's presentation is characterized by a set of focal problems that might be labeled "reactive depression." Of serious concern is the presence of

suicidal thinking, decreased motivation, and loss of interest in once-plea-
surable activities. It is also evident that Colin is feeling very poorly about
himself. He portrays himself as "lost and hungry," and shows signs of
feeling that he is not "good enough." The developmental history reveals
that Colin has always been "eager to please," and has been highly invested
in the approval of others. Consequently, he worked hard in school and
showed few, if any, problems with conduct. It is likely that this social
orientation secured Colin's feelings of self-worth; that is, by being a "good
boy," he received ample external support and approval from others that
served to maintain his self-esteem. With his parents' divorce, and more
importantly, their diminished emotional availability to their children, Colin
suffered a significant blow to his self-esteem. Unable to maintain a positive
sense of self in the face of decreased parental approval and support, Colin
feels inadequate and unlikable. As a result, he shows decrements in
motivation, loss of interest in activities, and self-destructive thinking.
Although the proximal cause of Colin's focal problems appears to be the
loss of parental availability and support, the underlying source of Colin's
difficulties are vulnerabilities in his capacity to maintain a positive image
of himself. Thus, while intervention would most assuredly aim at restructuring the parents' relationships with their children, an equally important
goal would involve decreasing Colin's overreliance on external approval as
the principal source of his feelings of self-esteem. In the interim, it is likely
that he would benefit from a supportive alliance with an empathic therapist.

The Emotional Interference Formulation: The Case of Sarah

Focal Problems

"Sarah" is an 11-year-old girl who was referred for a psychological evaluation by her parents. Their primary concerns centered on Sarah's academic
"underachievement." Although cognitive testing at the school had indicated above-average intelligence with no clear evidence of a reading
disability, Sarah was receiving very poor grades, including F's in two major
subjects. Although Sarah spent little time studying, she often performed
well on tests. However, she rarely turned in homework assignments, even
when she had completed some of them. Periodically she was disruptive in
class, made jokes at the expense of other students, and occasionally
"ditched" school altogether. Her relationships with peers in the neighborhood appeared to be better than at school, and she was a talented member
of the community soccer team. However, her parents noted that rather
minor incidents on the soccer field could unleash a torrent of "foul
language." Typically her outbursts did not involve physically aggressive

behavior, although such problems were a source of concern earlier in her development. Not surprisingly, family interactions were marked by episodes of angry exchanges. Both the mother and father were equal targets for her outbursts, which usually followed the setting of limits that Sarah perceived as unfair.

In her initial interview Sarah was virtually mute. When asked what she had been told about the reason for the consultation, she simply shrugged her shoulders. She asked how long she would have to stay and quickly noted that she knew plenty of other kids who "were a lot more screwed up" than she was and that they did not have to see "a shrink." After an extended period of silence, the therapist mentioned that he had heard that she was involved in soccer and that he was curious about what she enjoyed about the game. Much to the therapist's surprise Sarah began to talk at length about an upcoming state tournament and her team's chances at taking the title. When the therapist noted that soccer could involve some "hard knocks," Sarah grinned and said that it was her "escape valve." Unfortunately, she refused to elaborate on what she needed to escape.

Developmental History

Sarah's developmental history was remarkable for a number of reasons. During the preschool period, Sarah's mother and biological father had gone through an acrimonious divorce. Her mother noted that there had been one episode of physical violence but did not think Sarah had witnessed it. She was certain, however, that Sarah had heard numerous "vicious" arguments. Her parents separated when Sarah was 5, and her mother remarried when Sarah was 8. She described Sarah's relationship with her stepfather as one of "mutual toleration," although she noted that her second husband had made numerous efforts to spend time with Sarah, and in fact, had gotten her involved in community soccer. Sarah's biological father currently lived out of state, and Sarah spent 2 weeks with him in the summer and visited on alternating holidays. She noted that Sarah tended to "put her father on a pedestal." Her biological father was a prominent reporter for a major newspaper and had numerous acquaintances in the sports and entertainment fields. However, in part because of professional demands, he was often inconsistent in maintaining contact with his daughter. Consequently, Sarah was frequently disappointed when he failed to follow through on plans and promises. During the early elementary-school years, Sarah had exhibited more serious problems with physical aggression toward peers. Her aggressiveness often increased after changes in visitation plans. However, this problem seemed to diminish with maturation and increased regularity in visitation.

Case Formulation

Anger and hostility were prominent in Sarah's presentation. Consistent with parental report, over the course of the initial phase of therapy, Sarah seemed to oscillate between avoiding her feelings and expressing them in a passive–aggressive manner. Her developmental history was noteworthy for the presence of early dysregulation of anger—both her biological father's and her own. Eventually in interview, Sarah acknowledged that she spent a good deal of energy attempting to keep her angry feelings in check. It also appeared that Sarah's school underachievement was related to her difficulties with anger. On the one hand, she appeared to be preoccupied with controlling her anger, and on the other, she appeared to have found a means for expressing her anger, albeit indirectly, by failing to complete homework assignments. The indirect expression of anger elicited strong reactions from her parents, particularly from her biological father, who as a professional writer, valued academic success. Perhaps it should not be surprising that Sarah's greatest school difficulties were in English composition! Thus, in addition to indirectly expressing the anger aroused by the inconsistent relationship with her biological father, her school underachievement served the function of engaging her father, albeit in a negative manner.

In summary, Sarah's academic underachievement—the focal problem—can be readily understood in terms of the emotional interference formulation. First, emotions that had been insufficiently processed remained a preoccupation with Sarah and interfered with her ability to focus on academic tasks; second, unexpressed feelings of anger seemed to lower her threshold for tolerating frustration, which resulted in angry outbursts; and third, her inability to express anger in a modulated manner resulted in indirect expressions of hostility (underachievement) that functioned to engage her parents but also perpetuated a cycle of family conflict. Thus, at the heart of Sarah's case were problems with the experience and expression of emotion.

CASE FORMULATIONS AND TREATMENT SELECTION

The foregoing cases were selected as relatively clear examples of each of the basic case formulations. Like most child therapy referrals, these cases are by no means "pure." Instead, the cases are prototypical rather than stereotypical; they embody core characteristics as well as unique features. In clinical practice, cases are often not pure types. Such a situation parallels the "problem" of comorbidity at the diagnostic level, that is, at the level of observable symptoms. Children often meet the criteria for more than one diagnosis. Similarly, children may present psychological processes that are consistent with several basic-level case formulations (e.g., children who lack adequate emotion regulation strategies may also show serious problems with self-esteem). Thus, one challenge for the child clinician is to determine which pathogenic process is either most central to the child's focal problems or most accessible to treatment. Case formulations, then, must be viewed as guiding hypotheses that may require revision as knowledge of the case unfolds.

As hypotheses, basic-level case formulations orient the therapist to different approaches to treatment. Thus, if a case approximates the prototype for the skills deficit formulation, then a program of remedial or compensatory skills development would be the treatment of choice. In contrast, if emotional interference is viewed as the primary pathogenic process, then interventions that emphasize emotion expression or affect regulation procedures will be the focus of treatment. Thus, treatment selection is based on the "goodness of fit" between change processes and formulations of pathogenic processes. Although the selection of treatment strategies on this basis is by no means new, in fact, it is common among clinical practitioners (Persons, 1991), it is our belief that the practice of child psychotherapy is often based on a restricted set of basic case formulations, particularly among therapists with strong allegiances to specific therapeutic orientations. Therapists aligned with a specific therapeutic orientation (e.g., cognitive-behavioral or psychodynamic) are likely to consider the basic formulations that have developed within their theoretical system. For example, cognitive therapists typically divide cases into two types—skills deficits or cognitive distortions. Interventions, then, typically take two forms—skills remediation or schema transformation (Persons, 1993). However, we propose that the diversity of child therapy cases requires a more inclusive framework for case formulation, and that a restricted range of basic case formulations can attenuate the effectiveness of child psychotherapy, in part, because it results in mismatches between change processes and pathogenic processes.

Our review of the child psychotherapy literature has yielded six basic-level case formulations. These basic-level formulations are intended to provide a manageable set of conceptual frameworks for specific cases, and an alternative method for clustering similar cases. By drawing attention to underlying psychological mechanisms that create or maintain overt problems—the target of psychotherapeutic interventions—these basic formulations orient the child therapist to different treatment strategies.

As a starting point we have presented a set of cases that typify the basic case formulations. Judgments about the degree of similarity between a specific case and a formulation prototype would undoubtedly be enhanced by the derivation of *featural* characteristics of basic-level case formulations.

For example, Horowitz, Wright, et al. (1981) have shown that experts could generate a consensual set of features, including the typical thoughts, feelings, and behaviors of common childhood disorders. Similarly, it should be possible to derive features that typify basic-level case formulations. The extraction of such features from clear case examples would enable clinicians to judge the degree of similarity along multiple dimensions. Although typical thoughts, feelings, and behaviors (i.e., psychological processes) represent potential candidates for such a featural analysis, it is also possible that developmental histories and family processes are important components of case formulation prototypes.

In fact, as is evident from the foregoing case examples, a critical element in the construction of a case formulation is the child's developmental and family history. Formulations are not typically apparent from the focal problems alone, but emerge when these problems are considered in the broader context of the child's developmental and family history. It is this historical perspective that provides essential clues about underlying pathogenic processes. For example, in the case of Darren, the plausibility of maladaptive assumptions and cognitive distortions increases in probability when his focal problems are viewed in light of his developmental history. Similarly, the formulation of low self-esteem in the case of Colin increases in conceptual coherence when his focal problems (depressed mood and suicidal ideation) are viewed in the context of his developmental history (long-standing need for approval) and current family situation (parental unavailability). Thus, the construction of a case formulation involves the integration of information about focal problems, developmental history, and family functioning with basic knowledge of psychological processes.

It would be misleading to conclude that case formulations typically emerge after a single parent or child interview. Although it may be possible to pin down focal problems through structured diagnostic interviews, formulations about pathogenic mechanisms are constructed from a thorough developmental and family history, and from opportunities to assess the child's functional capacities and central concerns. The latter often requires the utilization of psychological test data, for example, to evaluate coping strategies or thematic issues. In summary, multiple sources of information must be integrated in order to develop a case formulation. The presentation of basic-level case formulations is intended to provide an organizational framework for evaluating case-specific information.

It has been our contention that differential diagnosis based solely on an evaluation of symptom covariation is insufficient for the development of case-specific treatment plans. Instead, we have proposed that intervention strategies follow from formulations of pathogenic processes, that is, from an understanding of the psychological mechanisms that create or maintain the child's presenting problems. This idea is by no means new; in fact, it is a perspective that has been advocated by both psychotherapists and behavior therapists (cf. Shapiro, 1989; Turkat, 1985). What *is* new in our approach is the identification of a set of basic-level case formulations that provides an inclusive framework for conceptualizing child treatment cases. These basic-level formulations were derived from a review of the major systems of child psychotherapy and thus provide a broader range of basic formulations than is found in any single approach to child treatment. Furthermore, we assume that these formulations are not just rival conceptualizations of similar pathological phenomena, that is, different perspectives on the same problem, but reflect the diversity of child therapy cases.

Of equal importance, therapeutic procedures have developed in conjunction with formulations of pathogenic processes. In fact, there is some evidence that technical advances in the field of child psychotherapy have been prompted by *failed* applications of specific change processes to new populations of children. For example, in the dynamic tradition, interpretation did not appear to be helpful in the treatment of more seriously disturbed child patients. This technical failure eventually led to a new formulation of pathogenic process (the ego deficit model). In turn, new therapeutic procedures (supportive scaffolding) were developed in response to the new understanding of pathogenic process. Similarly, within the cognitive tradition, skills training procedures proved insufficient for children who did not present with skills deficits, but who showed other types of cognitive dysfunctions (cognitive distortions). As a result, an alternative approach to treatment that "fit" with the new formulation of pathogenic process needed to be developed.

Treatment selection, then, should be based on the "goodness of fit" or conceptual coherence between change process and formulation of pathogenic process. For example, to return to the case of Sarah, emotional dysregulation was hypothesized to underlie her focal problems of academic underachievement, conflict with parents, and anger outbursts; that is, her case typified the emotional interference formulation. Emotions that had been insufficiently processed remained a preoccupation; unexpressed feelings of anger lowered her threshold for tolerating frustration; and her academic underachievement appeared to be an indirect, but maladaptive, form of emotional expression. This formulation orients the therapist to change processes that emphasize the expression and processing of Sarah's emotional experiences. One would expect change in her focal problems to be a function of the degree to which Sarah is able to express feelings of anger in therapy, connect them with their source, and develop alternative strategies for managing anger arousal.

Although conceptual coherence or "goodness of fit" between change process and case formulation represents a reasonable method for selecting treatments for troubled children, this approach to child psychotherapy must be supported by empirical evidence. However, empirical validation of the proposed framework will require a new approach to child psychotherapy research. To reiterate an earlier argument, much of existing child therapy research, particularly comparative outcome research, is predicated on matching "brand-name" treatments with diagnostic entities. Although some dismantling studies (in which component procedures are specified and controlled) come closer to the type of research needed to evaluate this model, the vast majority of treatment outcome studies, including dismantling studies, group children on the basis of a shared diagnosis without regard for variations in underlying pathogenic process. Not surprisingly, controlled treatments often have the effect of increasing variability in the treatment group. We suspect that one of the reasons for this well-documented phenomenon is the substantial within-group variability in pathogenic processes among children who share the same diagnosis. Minimally, then, investigators must attend to subgroups of children within diagnostic groupings, who vary in terms of underlying pathogenic processes. This means that children will need to be classified or selected on the basis of shared diagnosis or focal problems *and* basic-level case formulations. In essence, a valid evaluation of the foregoing model would require *both* the specification of change processes and the classification of patients on the basis of case formulations.

CONCLUSION

In summary, a basic tenet of the case formulation approach to child psychotherapy is that the coordinating link between a child's presenting problems and a treatment plan is the case formulation. Case formulations represent hypotheses about the pathogenic processes that underlie the child's focal problems. For the child psychotherapist, these pathogenic processes are the target of clinical intervention. A review of the child psychotherapy literature has revealed a set of basic-level case formulations. Given this basic set of formulations, cases that typify each formulation have been presented. Based on prototype theory, it is hypothesized that the establishment of a set of case formulation prototypes will provide a method for classifying specific cases in terms of shared formulations. It is assumed that the presentation of prototypical case examples represents a starting point for this classification procedure, and that the derivation of featural characteristics will advance this approach. Finally, it has been proposed that treatments are selected on the basis of the "goodness of fit" between change process and formulation of pathogenic process.

Historically, therapeutic procedures have evolved with formulations of pathogenic process. One of the most common "errors" in clinical practice has been to ignore this evolution, and to extend therapeutic procedures that were developed in relation to one formulation of pathogenic process to cases that involve a different type of pathogenic process, for example, using interpretive techniques with children with skills deficits or applying skills training procedures to children with internal conflicts. Although the uniformity myth of psychotherapy represents an extreme form of this clinical "error," interventions based on the consideration of a limited number of basic-level case formulations is a variation of the same problem. Consequently, a broader set of basic-level case formulations has been presented in an effort to account for the diversity of child treatment cases. In the next chapter, the integration of change processes with formulations of pathogenic processes will be considered in greater detail through a set of case studies.

9

~

Formulation-Guided
Child Psychotherapy:
Case Studies

T HE PRINCIPAL AIM of this chapter is to provide case examples of formulation-guided child psychotherapy. Although the focus will be on the development of case formulations and their translation into clinical practice, it is assumed that this process occurs in the context of an ongoing emotional relationship with the child and parent(s). Thus, the child therapist is faced with dual tasks as therapy begins: the development of a formulation-based treatment plan and the cultivation of a working alliance.

There are many routes to the child psychotherapy clinic, but one well-worn path is the referral call from a distressed parent who can no longer accept, tolerate, or ignore the child's problems. Typically, a number of adults are involved in the presenting picture: Teachers or school psychologists have raised the issue of "counseling" at an end-of-the-year staffing; the child's pediatrician no longer comforts the parents with the phrase, "It's only a phase"; or members of the extended family have "shared" their concerns either directly or indirectly. And although the substance of the referral calls varies widely, it is not uncommon to find that the child's problems have developed over a period of time and that the parents were "hoping" that they would spontaneously remit or would respond to informal changes made at home or at school. Not surprisingly, then, the child clinician is faced with a parent who is distressed, not just by the presence of the child's problems, but also by his or her intransigence. Thus, parents or other caregivers who contact child therapists are often feeling a range of emotions, including frustration, helplessness, and demoralization. These feelings can have an important bearing on the way caregivers present the child's focal problems and account for their origins.

In contrast, the child patient may or may not be upset by the presence of problems. For many children, especially those with externalizing symptoms, the major source of distress is the adult reaction to their problems. Such reactions have resulted in recurrent conflicts, undesirable consequences, or constraints on their freedom. In the extreme, therapy is viewed as another attempt to coerce or control, or perhaps somewhat more optimistically, a chance to "get my parents off my back." Other children, in contrast, may be as distressed, or even more distressed, about their difficulties than their caregivers. Such children often openly disclose their problems, directly play out their difficulties, or show a great deal of sadness in the initial interview. Therapy is seen as an opportunity to find relief from vexing problems, upsetting feelings, or impediments to personal relationships.

Thus, presented with this complex matrix of information *and* emotions, the child therapist is faced with dual tasks. On the one hand there is the challenging cognitive task of developing a case formulation that will guide the course of treatment. Yet the presented material is by no means emotionally "neutral," neatly linear, or devoid of meaningful omissions. Consequently, the task of organizing and integrating the material places a rather substantial burden on the therapist's processing capacities. And as if this were not enough, the child therapist is simultaneously confronted with an equally challenging emotional task. In order to successfully launch the treatment process, the initial interview cannot be reduced to a highly technical, cognitively neutral, information-gathering process. Instead, the therapist must attend to the parents', the child's, and his or her own affective response to the referral problems in order to begin to build a working alliance. In fact, the therapist's attunement to the parents' and child's emotional presentation during this initial phase of information gathering is probably one of the best predictors of early dropout or continuation. Just as treatment requires a formulation for direction, continuation in therapy is predicated on the establishment of a relational bond or alliance with both child and caregiver. And given the predictive power of the therapeutic alliance, the cultivation and maintenance of a working relationship is essential for the efficacy of all change processes. The neglect of either aspect of this clinical process–case formulation or alliance formation–constitutes a serious threat to successful treatment outcome. Thus, although a major goal of this chapter is to demonstrate the *coordination* of change processes with case formulations, it is understood that child psychotherapy cannot be reduced to technical procedures, but instead rests on the foundation of a working relationship.

TREATING EMOTION DYSREGULATION: THE CASE OF MELINDA

"Melinda" is a 9-year-old fourth grader who was referred for psychotherapy by her mother, Carla. Carla was concerned that her daughter might be depressed. She noted that she was often very "sluggish" and periodically cried for no reason. She was particularly troubled by Melinda's "clinginess." Carla felt frustrated by her daughter's difficulties, in part, because she had overcome serious problems of her own and was upset that her daughter could not do the same.

Initial Assessment

In the initial interview Carla presented a very mixed picture of her daughter. On the one hand, she seemed genuinely concerned about Melinda's emotional difficulties, but on the other, it was evident that she was very frustrated by her problems. For example, after describing her worries about Melinda's low energy and depressed mood, her tone shifted and she stated that she was "sickened" by her daughter's fearfulness. She described Melinda as a child who was very uncertain of herself and who approached new situations with considerable anxiety. Carla was very candid and stated quite simply that she was "tired of dealing with her clinginess." She compared Melinda to her sister, Louisa, who was "more independent" even though she was 3 years younger than Melinda. As Carla put it, "Louisa and I are survivors, but Melly (her nickname) doesn't have the same toughness." Although she reported relatively few behavior problems on the Child Behavior Checklist, Carla was also upset by Melinda's periodic noncompliance at home. She seemed confused by this mixed pattern of emotional and behavioral problems and expressed surprise that a child who could be so sad and fearful could also be so willful.

Despite her low energy and emotional distress, Melinda was doing well in school. Her teacher reported that she worked hard on her assignments and usually participated in classroom activities. Her academic achievement levels were on target for her age. However, she, too, noted Melinda's sad demeanor, particularly during unstructured time. Occasionally, Melinda would appear "distant" to the teacher, and when attempts were made to reengage her in classroom activities, she would appear "sad and moody." The teacher also reported that Melinda had a small group of friends with whom she played during recess. In contrast, she seemed to have more difficulty participating in large group activities. At such times she seemed somewhat shy.

In her first meeting with her therapist, Melinda presented as rather shy and cautious. She rarely smiled and her listless behavior suggested dysphoric mood. Although she gradually engaged in unstructured play, she did not involve the therapist. In reply to a question about the purpose of her visit, Melinda responded, "Are you going to help me be happy?" When asked if she was feeling unhappy, Melinda became very quiet, returned to her play, which appeared to lack direction, and then sat looking out the window. Although she had not responded directly to the therapist, her behavioral response indicated emotional distress. Attempts to engage her in a conversation about things that made her happy or sad were largely unproductive. She did, however, mention that she liked school but provided little elaboration. Over the next few sessions a similar pattern emerged: Melinda would cautiously join her therapist, engage in solitary play but show no signs of wanting to leave the session, appear sad but then be unable to talk about her feelings. In general, it appeared that Melinda was experiencing significant internal distress, consistent with both maternal and teacher reports, but was unable to acknowledge or express it. In fact, her rather flat presentation suggested that she had a great deal of difficulty expressing any affect at all.

Thus, Melinda's focal problems appeared to center around dysphoric mood. Emotionally she appeared sad or flat, and she approached her therapist with great caution. Her play lacked vitality and tended to be rather repetitive (e.g., drawing pictures of houses with only minor variations). Maternal report indicated depressive symptoms that had been evident for over a year, along with "clinginess" and "fearfulness" in new situations. School appeared to be an island of safety, although even in that context Melinda seemed sad and moody at times. From a diagnostic perspective, Melinda's presentation was consistent with dysthymia; however, when her symptoms were viewed in the context of the family history, an alternative diagnosis seemed probable.

Developmental and Family History

Melinda's early development had been greatly disrupted by marital violence. During the preschool years, her father's violence had increased toward her mother, possibly exacerbated by cocaine abuse. Over a period of 2 years, beginning when Melinda was 3, her father battered her mother on multiple occasions. During this period there were numerous marital separations and reconciliations, and Carla and the girls frequently lived with friends or other family members. Following an extremely violent episode, during which Melinda's father threatened her mother with a loaded gun, Carla decided to terminate the relationship and press charges. Unfortunately, both girls had witnessed many violent interactions, although given Louisa's young age, it was difficult to know how much she had observed or processed. The fact that she was not presenting with notable symptoms and appeared to be making a smooth transition into school suggested that these early events had not had the same effect on both sisters. In contrast, Melinda had been hiding in the room during the loaded-gun episode, and later "scolded" her father for his "bad" behavior. Despite the high level of marital violence, Carla reported that her husband had not been abusive toward the children. After an investigation and trial, the girls' father was jailed for a year and Carla feared that he might seek revenge. Consequently, she and the children moved several times over a 3-year period without leaving any forwarding address for family or friends.

Carla recalled that the period of frequent moves had been difficult for the children, in part, because she was often so upset that she could barely attend to their needs. In addition to losing connection with members of their family, the girls would reexperience loss with each new move. Relationships with preschool friends and teachers were disrupted by changes in residence. Fortunately, the family had remained in the same residence for the last year, and Carla was beginning to feel that she had "better footing" and could devote more time to the children's needs. As a result, she contacted the clinic for an appointment for Melinda. It should be noted that after learning the family history, Louisa was also seen for a course of time-limited psychotherapy, in part, to make sure that her outer presentation did not belie underlying difficulties that the mother failed to notice.

In many ways, the family's experience resembled the plight of refugees. They had been dislocated, not by the impersonal violence of war, but by the intimate violence of marital strife. And although they were now out of the "war zone," for years they had lived in fear–particularly Carla–and had suffered the absence of a safe haven. In light of this history, Melinda's sadness, fearfulness, and clinginess could be viewed as posttraumatic symptoms.

Case Formulation

When Melinda's focal problems–depressed mood, emotional flatness, fearfulness, clinginess, and noncompliance–are considered in the context of the family history, the disruptive impact of intense and unresolved emotional experiences emerges as a central pathogenic process. First, her exposure to high levels of marital violence at an early age, which undoubtedly overwhelmed her resources for adaptive coping, appears to have resulted in significant restrictions in her capacity to acknowledge and express emotion. Consequently, Melinda's emotional range was quite limited, and dysphoric feelings appeared to predominate. Her solution to the problem of overwhelming emotion had been to restrict access to a broad range of feelings through avoidance and denial. Her orientation to emotional experience was further complicated by the fact that her mother has been victimized, living in fear, and was preoccupied with her own emotional stability. Consequently, Carla has not been responsive to Melinda's expressions of distress. In fact, Carla showed little tolerance for Melinda's distress, probably because such expressions kindled similar emotions in her mother, who had been struggling to attain "better (emotional) footing." As a result she was "sickened" by Melinda's fearfulness and clinginess, and provided little, if any, emotional support to her daughter. In order to secure her relationship with her mother and not provoke rejection or rebuff, Melinda sealed over her emotional distress as much as possible. Thus, Melinda experienced highly disruptive emotional events and had little opportunity to express her reactions to them or process their meaning. In fact, the expression of distress was potentially dangerous for Melinda in that it threatened the security of her relationship with her mother. Her minor episodes of noncompliance may have reflected an indirect expression of anger toward her mother for the lack of maternal responsiveness.

In addition to the experience of marital violence, other experiences contributed to her difficulties with regulating emotion. First, it is likely that Melinda continued to "reference" her mother's emotional reactions for cues about her own emotional experience. Given Carla's experience of fear and preoccupation with safety, it is not surprising that Melinda presented with apprehension and clinginess. Second, the experience of marital violence set into motion a series of events that were far from emotionally neutral. Central among them was the dislocation of the family and the recurrent experience of loss. Not only had Melinda lost her relationship with her father, but also she had lost contact with members of the extended family and with preschool friends and teachers who were potential sources of comfort and support. Given the recurrent experience of loss, it is not surprising that depressive symptoms were prominent in her emotional presentation.

Finally, Carla's response to the experience of marital violence had been to "bury" the events and to "put the past in the past." She expressed reservations about "digging things up," and was very reluctant to talk about the family's traumatic history. Instead, she presented the events as matters of fact and described herself as a "survivor" who had managed to endure this terrible period of her life. Although this resolve allowed Carla to manage the demands of daily living, and in that respect her method of coping had been adaptive for both herself and her children, it did not provide a narrative or story frame that might have enabled the children to encapsulate or organize their emotional experiences. Instead, Melinda, in particular, appeared to be overwhelmed by disorganizing emotion. In response to these disorganizing feelings, she restricted her emotional experience and presented as listless and dysphoric.

In summary, the emotional interference formulation appeared to provide the best integration of Melinda's focal problems with her developmental and family history. At the center of her presenting picture were inadequately processed emotional experiences that resulted in maladaptive strategies for emotion regulation. Her highly restrictive defenses limited the range of her emotional experience, left her listless and with low energy, and made her vulnerable to periodic disruptions in emotional control. Specifically, she showed a very limited capacity to acknowledge, express, or talk about feelings. However, at times she was overwhelmed by strong emotion, as reflected in her dysphoria, crying, and fearfulness. Yet Melinda lacked *both* the social support that could help her manage these feelings and a framework for understanding and organizing her emotional experience. Thus, by no means could therapy be reduced to facilitating the expression of emotion (i.e., to catharsis). Although increasing Melinda's capacity to experience and express her feelings was most certainly an important goal for her therapy, it was evident that other changes must accompany this aim.

First, Melinda had experienced rejection or rebuff when she expressed emotional distress. Consequently, it is likely that she harbored beliefs about the potential danger of expressing her feelings to caregivers. Thus, an initial goal of therapy would be the provision of an emotionally accepting relationship that demonstrates to Melinda that it is safe to show her feelings to others. This corrective experience could promote changes in her emotion regulation strategies by increasing the likelihood of utilizing others for emotional support. Second, as Melinda developed a greater capacity to express and flexibly regulate her feelings, she would need help in understanding the source of her strong emotions. In part, this aspect of therapy would involve the construction of a narrative or story that would encompass important aspects of her emotional experiences. Finally, but by no means of least importance, collateral psychotherapy with Melinda's mother was clearly indicated. From the standpoint of Melinda's treatment, changes in Carla's responsiveness to her daughter's distress and in her willingness to help the children integrate their current emotions with past traumatic events were critical elements of the treatment plan. Melinda could not be expected to give up her restrictive regulation strategies as long as the expression of distress threatens the security of her primary caregiving relationship. By no means were these goals incompatible with the overall aim of psychotherapy with Carla, namely, to help her process and integrate the traumatic experiences she had suffered.

Course of Treatment

The goal of the initial phase of treatment was the development of a trusting relationship that would enable Melinda to experience and express her emotions without fear of rebuff or rejection. She was told by her therapist that the purpose of therapy was to "help her feel better" and that in order to accomplish this goal they would work together on "helping Melinda deal with her feelings." Melinda's initial reaction was to appear somewhat panicked, and her therapist assured her that she would not have to talk about feelings until she was ready. Given her initial reaction to the stated aim of treatment and her lengthy learning history of emotional avoidance, a decision was made to follow Melinda's lead during the initial weeks of treatment. This decision was based on the belief that, in light of the uncontrollability of many of her past experiences, the development of an alliance would be enhanced by increasing her sense of control in the therapy relationship. Her therapist would not "push" emotional activities or topics, but instead would remain closely attuned to even the faintest emotional expressions presented by Melinda. Her task would not be to interpret expressed emotion, but rather to acknowledge and accept it (or from Melinda's perspective, to demonstrate that it was tolerable). Thus, while the initial phase of therapy was largely child directed, her therapist remained focused on Melinda's direct and indirect expressions of feelings by providing verbal labels and demonstrations of validation when possible.

For example, if Melinda presented as depressed and listless, her therapist would comment on her sadness; if she engaged in thematic play with doll or animal figures, she would observe and label the presented emotion (e.g, "The lion mother is scared, she's hiding"). During this initial phase of treatment, the therapist did not seek elaborations from Melinda, for example, by probing for the causes of feelings. Instead, she simply reflected Melinda's feelings–hoping to give the implicit message that emotions could be expressed without rebuff and without the danger of their becoming overwhelming. Because of Melinda's emotional constriction, it was necessary to utilize this reflective approach for several months. With children who have been traumatized and have developed ingrained means of coping with emotional experiences and interpersonal relationships, alliance formation cannot be rushed. Efforts to press children into therapeutic *work*–a realistic concern, given the current fiscal emphasis on time-limited treatments–are often counterproductive in that they confirm underlying maladaptive beliefs, for example, that caregivers are essentially manipulative. In Melinda's case, pushing her into emotionally charged activities would probably have overwhelmed her fragile coping resources, thereby solidifying her restrictive defenses and increasing her sense of the uncontrollability of emotional experience.

Typically, Melinda engaged in relatively "neutral" activities such as board games, but over time she began to share some of her experiences from home and school. In addition, she began to engage her therapist in "playing school"–an area of competence (and safety) for Melinda. As self-disclosure and her willingness to engage her therapist in thematic play increased, her therapist (and supervisor) viewed this shift as a signal to test Melinda's capacity to tolerate more emotionally evocative material in therapy.

At this point in treatment, Melinda's therapist introduced a puppet family and suggested that she and Melinda spend part of their time together "making up stories" with the puppets. Although her therapist said nothing about the content of the stories, or that the stories were going to be about family feelings, Melinda responded by exclaiming, "They remind me of my mom and dad," and fell face forward onto the floor. She covered her eyes with her hands and remained on the floor for some time. A great deal of soothing on the part of the therapist was required before Melinda could even sit up and look at her therapist. It was evident that Melinda's capacity to tolerate even a relatively remote reminder of her traumatic past was extremely limited. In fact, given the range of possible stories that could be composed with a puppet family, it was clear that Melinda's immediate construction of family life was imbued with overwhelming affect. Overwhelmed, her only recourse was physical avoidance.

Given her rather dramatic demonstration of her limited coping resources, the aim of the next phase of treatment was to increase Melinda's capacity to tolerate and regulate stronger feelings. Again her therapist reminded her that she would not be forced to talk about upsetting feelings, but that in order to feel better, it would be necessary for her to learn how to deal with her feelings. Melinda agreed that she wanted to feel better but was worried that she would be asked to do things she could not handle. In an effort to approach this problem collaboratively, the therapist asked Melinda if she had any ideas about how they might work on her upsetting feelings. Much to the therapist's surprise, Melinda suggested that the therapist could ask her one question about feelings each week, but added that she would not answer if the questions were too hard. Because of Melinda's feelings of competence in school, and her willingness to play school in therapy, her therapist suggested that they could treat the feelings questions like school assignments. Melinda responded very positively to this suggestion, particularly when she was given the option of responding to the therapist by talking, by writing some words or sentences, or by drawing a picture. For each session, a small portion of time was set aside for "feelings school." At Melinda's request, questions were initially presented by the therapist in written form. In turn, she would write or draw an "answer" to the question. Initially, the questions were rather general, including queries such as: "How have you been feeling in school?" "How are you feeling about your sister?" or "Tell me about how you felt about Christmas this year." Over time, the questions became both more specific and more directly related to Melinda's experience in her family (e.g., "Tell me about how you and your mom are getting along"). Usually Melinda would write several sentences in response to the question, but occasionally she would make a drawing that accompanied her sentences. In order to help her anticipate questions that might arouse strong reactions, her therapist would "warn her" by saying, "Now this might be a hard one, but I think you can handle it." Such phrasing provided an opportunity for Melinda to prepare herself before reading the question and offered support for her growing sense of efficacy. She began to look forward to "feelings school" and, in fact, gave the therapist permission to ask more than one question in each session.

In addition, the balance of activities in sessions shifted. Although Melinda continued to engage her therapist in board games and other activities, her thematic play involved much greater emotional elaboration, and she selected games with emotional content (e.g., emotion checkers). Most striking, she was increasingly open about significant experiences. She shared her distress about an episode of peer rejection and expressed upset about her mother's demands that she take on additional chores. Thus, in sharp contrast to her original presentation, Melinda expressed negative emotion with the therapist and appeared far less emotionally flat. In addition, there were signs of increasing vitality in her play. Of equal importance, she expressed anger, albeit somewhat indirectly, toward her therapist after the therapist mentioned that she was going to take a vacation. In summary, it appeared that Melinda was becoming increasingly comfortable with revealing her feelings and was beginning to anticipate a nurturing response to her expressions of distress.

This significant shift in emotional presentation was uniquely captured in an episode involving the experience of fear. Because of changes in her mother's schedule, Melinda needed to switch afterschool programs. In the past, such a change would have resulted in intense fear and heightened clinginess. She acknowledged to the therapist that she had been frightened by the prospects of attending the new program. When asked how she dealt with her feelings of fear, Melinda replied that she thought of her talks with the therapist, imagined what they would do together, and knew that she could handle the change. In essence, the soothing response of the therapist to Melinda's experience of distress was now becoming part of her own emotion regulation repertoire. She was beginning to treat herself as she was being treated by her caring therapist.

Simultaneously, after some initial resistance, Carla was increasingly involved in her own therapy. Over the course of 8 months of treatment, several critical themes had emerged. First, Carla was increasingly aware that the anger aroused by Melinda's distress was linked, in part, to the fact that Melinda reminded her (due to physical resemblance) of her ex-husband. She also was beginning to acknowledge that Melinda's fear and insecurity undermined her own stability and that she was terrified to "give in" to such strong emotions. Not surprisingly, the latter problem was complicated by a pattern of intergenerational repetition; that is, Carla felt that one "lesson" she had learned growing up was that "you can't count on others when you're down and out." Thus, her own history of attachment and receiving care were affecting her capacity to respond to Melinda. Interestingly, Carla's increasing utilization of her therapist as a source of emotional support suggested that she was learning a new "lesson" about the potential responsiveness of others. In essence, there were important parallels in the treatment of mother and daughter. Despite the fact that it was still a struggle for Carla to respond to Melinda's distress, she was determined to try to alter a pattern she now viewed as undesirable.

With these changes the timing appeared to be right to begin to address Melinda's experience of her traumatic family history. Melinda was more open to expressing her emotions, showed more flexible means of coping with emotional arousal, and clearly was utilizing her therapist as a source of emotional support. In addition, although Carla still struggled with responding to Melinda's distress, she believed that Melinda needed to deal with the events she had witnessed and supported her daughter in her efforts to overcome her fears and sadness.

The decision to address the traumatic past was a point of critical choice in therapy. On the one hand, Melinda had made significant gains in the area of emotion expression and regulation. There was even evidence of diminished fearfulness in other contexts. Why, then, move forward to address highly distressing experiences from the past that could potentially disrupt Melinda's functioning? The decision to move forward was based on two major factors, both of which were consistent with the emotional interference formulation. First, Melinda still showed significant vulnerabilities in dealing with strong emotion. Although she clearly had made some gains, in the absence of social support, her immediate inclination was to avoid or deny difficult feelings. It was hypothesized that this ingrained pattern of affect regulation had its roots in her attempts to contain the overwhelming emotion associated with her exposure to marital violence. Unfortunately, her method of regulating strong emotion had become overgeneralized, and because the experiences had been partially contained but clearly unprocessed, the basis for emotional overcontrol was still intact. It was expected that the opportunity to talk about these experiences under conditions of support, and with more mature means of coping, would offset the maladaptive overgeneralization of her coping strategies. Second, and of equal importance, the overwhelming quality of these experiences was not bounded by a narrative frame that could help Melinda master her traumatic experiences. Instead, her understanding of the violent episodes seemed quite limited and appeared to be strongly colored by affect with little coherent form. The combination of intense affect and limited cognitive organization is fertile ground for disruptive memories, repetitious behavior, and lapses in social judgment (misperceptions of new social relationships). Consequently, the next phase of treatment involved attempts to help Melinda address some of the strong feelings she had experienced in her early development.

Although Melinda had made gains in her ability to tolerate and manage strong feelings, her therapist anticipated that memories and feelings associated with her experience of violence and loss would be extremely challenging. Consequently, dealing with this material in an open-ended manner seemed risky. Melinda had clearly benefited from the structure of "feelings school," and the provision of an organizing framework seemed essential in order to help her approach this highly charged material. In an effort to provide a narrative structure, her therapist introduced the idea of creating a "life story book." Melinda would be free to choose any episode she wished to include in the book, and together she and the therapist would assemble the episodes into a story line. Although Melinda reluctantly engaged in this activity, it quickly became evident that she had little desire to include some of the most troubling episodes from her life. Her therapist pointed out some of the major gaps in the story and suggested that Melinda might need some help in remembering them. At this point, the decision was made to help Melinda address the traumatic events by soliciting her mother's assistance in reconstructing the past. Fortunately, the collateral therapy with Carla had progressed to the point where she was willing to talk with her children about the events they had experienced together.

Melinda was prepared for these joint sessions by her therapist. Her therapist acknowledged that some of the stories might be hard to hear, but that she and her mother would be there to support her if things got too tough. She also reminded Melinda that she had made a lot of progress in dealing with feelings and that this would be a good chance for her to use the things she had "learned in feelings school."

Four family sessions were planned to tell the family story. In order to titrate the intensity of these sessions, the therapists orchestrated a series of questions that evolved around the construction of a family tree. In fact, in order to gradually introduce the children (and their mother) to this task, the first session focused solely on filling in mother's side of the family lineage. Carla was asked to tell stories about each family member, and the girls were asked if they had any memories they wanted to add. As Carla related these stories, some of them with considerable humor, the girls filled in the names and "decorated" the family tree. After two sessions of describing her own family and her own childhood, Carla began to present material about her relationship with the girl's father. She began with a story about how the couple met and went on to describe their life together before the birth of the children. To her credit, and with the support of the therapist, she presented a relatively balanced perspective, noting that he had been affectionate toward the children. But with the therapist's prompting she explained that he could be "dangerous," and that he had hurt her very badly on several occasions. The girls were given the opportunity to ask questions and to relate any memories (or fantasies) they had about the traumatic episodes. Although much detail was left out, the basic outlines of the marital violence and its impact on the family's stability was clearly communicated. Melinda showed signs of heightened anxiety during the sessions and sought comfort from her mother and her therapist. As a reflection of the progress she had made in therapy, Carla was highly attuned to Melinda's anxiety and responded by comforting her. At one point she asked Melinda to sit on her lap and held her closely as she told the family story. The family sessions appeared critical for several reasons. First, material that had been avoided by Melinda was now in the open. Second, the outlines of a family story were now available to help Melinda organize her early experiences. And finally, but by no means least important, Melinda had the opportunity to experience her mother as responsive and supportive when she expressed distress.

Following the family sessions, individual therapy continued for several months. In the next session, Melinda announced that she no longer wanted her therapist to write "feelings questions," but instead wanted her to present them orally. Therapy quickly became more conversational in nature, even when emotional topics were discussed. Although Melinda had been making significant progress in her ability to tolerate and regulate emotion, the degree of change following the family meetings was dramatic. Melinda herself commented in one session, "I don't know why, but I feel different." It was certainly evident that she was feeling relief.

In hindsight, it appeared that the family sessions had provided Melinda with graded exposure to emotionally charged experiences, and that she had "discovered" that she could manage "tough feelings" without becoming overwhelmed. Moreover, she now possessed a narrative framework for organizing some of her most difficult experiences. In the ensuing sessions, she was able to talk with her therapist about some of the stories that had been told in the family meetings. Finally, consistent with her experience in individual therapy, the sessions also provided evidence that others could be used for support in times of distress. Consequently, Melinda did not have to resort to avoidance or denial, but could utilize others' support as a means of coping with strong emotion. Obviously, the durability of this defensive transformation would depend on the availability of responsive caregivers, and most importantly, on the continued progress of her mother in her own therapy.

In order to ensure the availability of support, arrangements were made at the end of therapy for Melinda to participate in a mentoring program through her school. In this program, older individuals volunteered as supportive "grandparents" to children from difficult backgrounds. It was hoped that the transition from formal therapy to an ongoing, supportive relationship would enable Melinda to sustain the gains she had made in therapy.

Treatment Outcome

Over the course of 15 months of treatment, Melinda had made significant gains in her capacity to experience, express, and regulate emotion. In session, it was evident that she did not rely on avoidance and denial to the degree she had at the start of therapy. Instead, she increasingly turned to others for support in times of distress and showed an emerging ability to comfort herself with self-calming thoughts. Of equal importance, she tended to express her feelings rather than sealing them over. Consistent with these changes in her approach to emotion regulation, her mother reported that Melinda seemed more robust and less fearful. It is not clear whether this change in maternal report primarily reflected actual emotional and behavioral changes or stemmed from changes in Carla's perceptions of and attitudes toward her daughter. Probably both factors were involved, but both represented positive changes. There was no doubt, however, that her persistent dysphoria had given way to more positive mood and greater vitality. Reports from school indicated a decline in moodiness and sustained investment in academics. At termination, Melinda appeared to be liberated from the constrictions of her maladaptive emotion regulation strategies, and evinced the playfulness of a typical school-age child.

Treatment Summary

From a diagnostic perspective, Melinda's persistent dysphoric mood was consistent with the diagnosis of dysthymia. Knowledge of the family history, along with her presentation of emotional constriction and fearfulness, suggested a more complex diagnostic picture involving posttraumatic symptomatology with depressed mood. When her focal problems–represented in the diagnoses–were considered in the context of her developmental and family history, the emotional interference formulation appeared to offer the best integration of the available information. Moreover, the formulation, with its emphasis on underlying pathogenic processes, provided direction for Melinda's treatment. Central to the formulation was evidence of maladaptive emotion regulation strategies that appeared to leave Melinda constricted and depressed. Her response to the early experience of overwhelming emotion (trauma) was to restrict access to a broad range of feelings through avoidance and denial. For Melinda, feelings, especially strong feelings, were construed as dangerous in that they could become overwhelming and disorganizing. The major aim of therapy was the transformation of Melinda's emotion regulation processes.

A number of factors appeared to contribute to Melinda's increased capacity to tolerate and express emotion and to utilize more adaptive regulation strategies. First, therapy provided her with graded exposure to emotional material. The structure offered in the therapeutic context enabled Melinda to experience and express emotion in a "titrated" manner and appeared to increase her sense of efficacy in dealing with emotion. In essence, emotions did not have to be dealt with in an "all-or-none" fashion but could be experienced and expressed in manageable ways. It is likely that this experience resulted in a more flexible sense of control over her own feelings. Second, over the course of therapy, Melinda also had the opportunity to learn, perhaps incidentally, that the expression of distress did not necessarily lead to rejection or rebuff by caring others. Although the focus of treatment was on Melinda's emotion regulation strategies, the transformation of her perception of others' emotional responsiveness reflects the importance of interpersonal processes in emotion regulation. As she learned that the expression of distress would not alienate her from caregivers, she showed greater comfort with emotion expression and could utilize others for emotional support. Obviously, the collateral therapy with her mother played an integral role in facilitating these changes in Melinda. Third, the original basis for her overrestrictive emotional controls was addressed and processed in the context of a supportive relationship. It is likely that this therapeutic experience demonstrated to Melinda that she could manage strong feelings with her newly developed capacities and the support of others. Given the dramatic response to this intervention, it is likely that this experience had a significant impact on Melinda's assumption that emotions are inherently dangerous and overwhelming. Finally, her traumatic memories, which appeared to be colored by strong emotion but unbounded by coherent form, were placed in the organizing context of a family story. Given Melinda's sense of relief following this phase of treatment, it is likely that the construction of a narrative framework for these disruptive experiences provided her with another means of organizing what had previously been fragmented and overwhelming.

In summary, the emotional interference formulation guided treatment toward multiple interventions aimed at transforming Melinda's experience, expression, and regulation of emotion. By directing treatment toward underlying pathogenic processes, in this case, maladaptive emotion regulation strategies, substantial changes were produced in Melinda's focal problems.

TRANSFORMING MALADAPTIVE SCHEMAS: THE CASE OF CHRIS

"Chris" is a 16-year-old high school junior who was referred for psychotherapy by his mother following an emotional episode during which Chris expressed a desire to kill himself. Over the previous 2 years, Chris, who was an outstanding student/athlete, had shown signs of social withdrawal and self-deprecatory thinking. There had been no overt suicide attempts, but he had informed his mother that he had thought about suicide on several occasions.

Initial Assessment

Chris was interviewed with his mother during the first session. It was very clear that he was overwhelmed by strong feelings. Initially, he was so choked with emotion that he asked his mother to talk. As she described her concerns, Chris began to cry. She reported that Chris was a "model son" who was near the top of his class academically, well-integrated socially, and a starter for the high school basketball team. She was both perplexed and concerned about "how hard Chris was on himself." During the last 2 years, she observed that Chris seemed to be driven by the idea that he needed to be "perfect." An A– on an exam would unleash harsh self-criticism and self-punishment. For example, when Chris failed to receive the highest grade on a physics exam, he did not permit himself to see his close friends for over a week; instead he spent much of the time sequestered in his room studying. Asked about the family's expectations for Chris, his mother noted that she and her husband would be happy with a solid B average. This had been the academic expectation they had applied to Chris's two older sisters, and they saw no reason to hold Chris to a higher standard. Chris acknowledged that the pressure he felt did not come from his parents; in fact, he felt that his parents, although proud of his performance, were primarily worried about the amount of time he spent studying and the pressure he was putting on himself.

In individual interview, Chris acknowledged that he had thought of suicide a number of times, but denied any "real" desire to be dead. In fact, he had not considered a plan. Instead, he expressed a wish to feel better about himself and said that he wished he could enjoy life more. On the Youth Self-Report (Achenbach & Edelbrock, 1983), Chris showed clinically significant elevations on several of the narrow bands, including depression. The most prominent feature of his presentation was self-criticism. Diagnostically, Chris appeared to fit the parameters of what Blatt (1974) calls introjective or self-critical depression. He set extremely high standards for himself and was sharply self-critical when he failed to attain them. On several occasions he had actually slapped himself on his face following what he perceived to be academic "failure" (not getting an A). Not surprisingly, he reported low self-worth on the Self-Perception Profile (Harter, 1985). In brief, his self-esteem appeared to be extremely fragile. Acknowledged achievements brought limited satisfaction, whereas perceived failures resulted in sustained self-reproach. Thus, the most prominent focal problems were his depressed mood and corresponding self-critical thinking.

Developmental History and Family

The family history was noteworthy in that Chris had been adopted at 3 months of age. Although his adoptive parents already had two biological children, they wished to expand their family and felt committed to "extending our love" to a child in need. Consequently, they sought an adoption through their church. Chris's biological mother, a teenager at the time of his birth, had attempted to raise him alone, but given her limited resources, including little family support, found the task to be overwhelming. For a brief period, Chris had been placed in foster care. According to his adoptive parents, social service records had not contained any suspicions of abuse or neglect. In fact, when Chris was placed with their family, they were impressed with his physical size and robust demeanor. Chris had been informed about his adoption at an early age, and his parents were open to talking about the circumstances of the adoption. However, given the "closed" nature of the adoption, he had no contact with his biological mother. In interview, he reported no desire to locate her and expressed a strong sense of being an integral part of his adoptive family. Other than Chris's adoption, his family and developmental history were rather unremarkable, with the exception of several family moves during the elementary-school years due to changes in his father's employment.

Case Formulation

Chris's focal problems and developmental history are compatible with a number of basic-level case formulations. On the one hand are striking problems with self-worth. The fact that less-than-perfect performances could lead to serious self-reproach suggested significant vulnerabilities in his self-esteem. Thus, there is evidence for the low self-esteem formulation. On the other hand, Chris's depressed mood appeared to follow from unrealistically high standards, misperceptions of "failure," and self-critical cognitions. From the perspective of pathogenic process, the initial assessment suggests that Chris's focal problems revolved around his unrealistic self-expectations and his tendency to utilize self-punishment as his primary method of self-regulation. The question, then, was whether these problems represented skills deficits (e.g., in standard setting, coping, and self-reinforcement) or reflected cognitive distortions that were rooted in maladaptive schemas. At this early point in treatment, both formulations seemed plausible, although the unrealistic nature of his thinking and his misperceptions of his own performance strongly suggested a cognitive distortion formulation.

However, the choice of an intervention strategy is not only based on "goodness of fit" between formulation and change process, but also on the degree to which the pathogenic process is accessible, that is, the degree to which the child or adolescent is willing to engage in the treatment procedures that address the underlying process. Although Chris seemed to be motivated to participate in therapy and expressed a strong desire to find relief from what he called his "inside pressure," his focus was on dealing with the ongoing demands of school. In fact, he asked if there might be some things he could *do* that could give him some immediate relief. Given his sense of urgency and his focus on immediate problems, we agreed to try some new "techniques" to see if they might help. However, I cautioned Chris that we might have to go "a bit deeper" to find the "relief valve." Our alliance was forged around a mutual attempt to find the "relief valve" for his "internal pressure." In essence, although it seemed likely that Chris's difficulties were most coherently conceptualized in terms of cognitive distortions that were rooted in maladaptive schemas, a cognitive skills approach was selected as a starting point for treatment because of his problem focus and desire to "do something" that might bring immediate relief. Therapeutically, the choice of this strategy entailed both potential risks and benefits. The major risk was that the skills-oriented approach, although plausible, would miss the fundamental source of his difficulties and result in demoralization. Premature dropout from therapy could be a potential consequence. In contrast, there were a number of benefits to taking such an approach. First, skills remediation might result in significant symptomatic change. Thus, there was the possibility that change could be produced through a relatively time-limited form of treatment. On the other hand, if the skills-oriented approach did not work, it could be used as "evidence" that we needed to go deeper to find the "relief valve." In order to increase the chances that treatment failure would not result in demoralization, but would provide us with useful information, the initial phase of treatment was framed as an "experiment." One might view this treatment strategy as following a "surface to depth" pattern; that is, the clinician attempts to bring about change through modification or remediation of skills and proceeds to a deeper level of intervention only if this approach fails to produce the desired results or if treatment maintenance calls for reworking less readily accessible processes, such as defense mechanisms or maladaptive representations.

Following the establishment of a contract around suicidal ideation, interventions were aimed at modifying Chris's self-standards and self-punitive coping strategies. As will be seen, the aims and methods of treatment evolved as therapy progressed, or more to the point, as the initial interventions failed to bring Chris sustainable relief and confirmed our initial hypothesis concerning the pivotal role of cognitive distortions.

Course of Treatment

During the first weeks of treatment, Chris and I explored his goals and expectations for himself. Consistent with the initial interview, his academic standards were extraordinarily high and somewhat at odds with his long-term goals–to attend a good state university and eventually become an architect. Neither goal required the level of perfection that Chris demanded of himself. To begin, Chris was asked to keep a log of his "inner pressure," noting any occasion when he acted punitively toward himself. He was an active recorder of his moods and thoughts, which typically included references to his "stupidity" and "worthlessness." At this point, I began to challenge his high expectations and his harsh self-criticism through role plays aimed at introducing a new perspective on his situation. After we clarified the connection between performance standards, self-reproach, and his inner pressure, I asked Chris if he held the same standards for his friends, and of equal importance, if he treated them so harshly when they failed to perform so perfectly. Not surprisingly, Chris was far more forgiving with his friends and certainly did not expect them to be perfect. We focused on this double standard for several sessions. During this time, I role-played one of his friends. In a typical scenario I would express disappointment in my performance. It was Chris's task to demonstrate how he would console or support a friend in distress. Again, Chris had little difficulty being supportive and had no trouble generating the type of calming statements that he consistently failed to use with himself. It was easy to see why Chris had a large network of friends. In relation to *others,* he demonstrated remarkable empathy and warmth, but in relation to himself, he was a harsh taskmaster.

From a case formulation perspective, the presence of effective coping strategies in his cognitive and behavioral repertoire was discrepant with the skills deficit hypothesis. He demonstrated a variety of strategies that could be effective in response to failure or disappointment, but he was unable to utilize them in relation to himself. However, before abandoning this approach, therapy was framed in terms of "skills transfer," that is, as an attempt to transfer the adaptive coping skills Chris demonstrated in relation to others to himself. Thus, the aim of therapy came to be defined as "teaching Chris to be a friend to himself." We began by recording the calming statements he used with his friends when they were disappointed (e.g., "Don't take it so hard, there'll be another test"; "So this one didn't go so well, think about everything else you have going for you"). In session we continued the role plays, but this time Chris was asked to recall episodes of disappointment and to practice the self-calming statements. During the week, he was asked to practice "being a friend to himself." At one point I prescribed "intentionally failing" an exam so that he could practice the self-calming strategies. With a wry smile, Chris acknowledged that he might consider studying a little less.

Unfortunately, despite his efforts in therapy, Chris continued to struggle with perfectionism and self-criticism. It was simply easier to be a good friend to others than to himself. Thus, given the presence of adaptive coping skills and the persistence of his focal problems, the original formulation for the case–the cognitive distortion model–became the guiding framework for treatment. The recalcitrant nature of the perfectionistic and punitive cognitive pattern appeared to be embedded in deeper assumptions about the self and others. Although the skills training approach had not been effective in providing relief from his "inner pressures," our preliminary work had revealed a number of noteworthy themes in Chris's thinking.

A recurrent theme was a link between "failure" (lack of perfection) and interpersonal rejection. For example, Chris made numerous comments suggesting that his interpersonal security was tied to outstanding performances across multiple domains (e.g., "They'll laugh at me if I make a mistake"; "I don't measure up, so I have to show them I'm better"; "No one wants to hang around a loser"). These expectations had all the hallmarks of cognitive distortions. First, they were overgeneralized and unqualified; second, they were incongruent with what I had learned about Chris's parents and friends; that is, Chris did not appear to be faced with an unsupportive social environment. One plausible hypothesis, then, was that the schema linking perfection with rejection had its roots in Chris's developmental history. As Leahy (1988) has observed, the problem is not that something happened in childhood, but from a cognitive perspective, the problem resides in the continued belief in the validity of the conclusions drawn from the early experience. Thus, with this new formulation, the aim of treatment became schematic change.

Given evidence that Chris's schematic expectation (imperfection = rejection) was not based on current interpersonal experiences, we began to look for the origins of this belief. I assured Chris that he must have good reasons for holding this belief, and that our new task was to discover how he came to believe it so fervently. Given the positive alliance that had developed over the initial phase of treatment—Chris seemed to sense that I was working with him to find a "relief valve"—he readily engaged in this process. Initially he focused on the anxiety he had experienced when he changed schools and peer groups during the elementary- and middle-school years. Not surprisingly, a salient theme in these memories revolved around anticipated rejection by new classmates and teachers. As we examined his experience more closely, it became clear that his expectation of rejection was rarely, if ever, confirmed. Instead, he had been relatively popular in most of the new school situations, possibly due to his athletic ability and sociability. Interestingly, the discrepancy between his expectation of rejection and his past peer experience (acceptance) did not trouble Chris. He discounted this evidence by suggesting that he had been "star player" and "top student," and that was why the kids accepted him. Given the fact that the peer experiences had not disconfirmed this core belief, but in fact had been assimilated to it, I suggested that his assumptions about himself must have deeper roots. Chris initially showed great difficulty with imagining other possible sources for his maladaptive belief, but clearly recognized that his assumption about perfection filtered into a lot of his thinking about himself and social relations. In an effort to identify other possible sources for his assumption, we began working on a time line of life events. Of course, our starting point was his early adoption.

Chris, and his parents, knew relatively little about the specific circumstances of his relinquishment; however, Chris was adamant that somehow he had played a role in the process. As we explored the possibilities, he alluded to being "too difficult," or "being a burden." Eventually, with a great outpouring of emotion, he said very softly, "Something must have been wrong with me." When asked "If nothing had been wrong, if you'd been perfect, what would have happened," Chris began to cry. It appeared that beneath Chris's self-critical stance was the implicit belief: "If I had been flawless (perfect), she would have kept me." This core assumption, undoubtedly constructed during childhood to make sense of his early experience, found expression in his current working assumption that "others will reject me (or I must reject myself), if I am not perfect."

The next phase of treatment involved gentle challenges to Chris's core assumption about his relinquishment. First, a series of joint sessions between Chris and his mother were held to review the known "facts" of his early placement. His adoptive mother emphasized the difficult situation of his biological mother and underscored the fact that Chris had been a "wonderful" baby when he joined the family. She brought along pictures that clearly depicted the family's joy around his arrival. In our individual sessions, we explored possible alternative accounts for his placement, noting that each was as likely as the "theory" that Chris had constructed. One of the aims of this phase of treatment was to help Chris attain some distance from his construction of his early experience, and to emphasize its hypothetical nature, given the absence of historical evidence; that is, the cognitive procedure of asking for supporting evidence was applied at the level of this core belief. Interestingly, this approach resulted in a marked change in his emotional presentation. For the first time, Chris directed anger not at himself, but at his birth mother whom he now regarded as "weak." In later sessions I noted that he was now directing his harshness in another direction, and although I was pleased to see him direct it away from himself, we needed to recall that his perception of his birth mother as "weak" was also only a theory. Although Chris initially directed anger at me for appearing to support his birth mother, this intervention seemed to open the door to the process of grieving his early loss. The strength of the emotions expressed during the ensuing sessions provided strong evidence for the intrinsic link between core schemas and intense emotion. Thus, while this phase of therapy had been guided by a cognitive distortion formulation and primarily involved an analysis of cognitive assumptions, it was evident that schema transformation also involved the expression of associated emotion. Over the course of several weeks, Chris began and ended his sessions with tears. It was clear that the cognitive analysis had provided access to feelings that had never been openly expressed. During this phase, I assumed a supportive role and validated Chris's emotional experience.

During the last portion of therapy, we revisited the parallels between his "theory" of his relinquishment and his drive for perfection. During this period of treatment, I offered a reframe for this parallel by suggesting that it was "one way of remaining connected with his biological mother." This intervention led Chris to reconsider other ways of acknowledging his adoptive heritage, including further conversations with his adoptive mother about his arrival and participation in a group for adopted teens. Near the end of treatment, Chris began to show signs of schematic change, albeit indirectly. For example, he talked about the challenges faced by teenage girls who got pregnant and how they would need family support. He wondered aloud whether, in fact, this would be best for a child. Simultaneously, his mood began to elevate and stabilize, and he showed increasing interest in nonachievement-related activities (e.g., serving as a peer counselor). In striking contrast to his teary initial presentation, he began to show a sense of humor about his tendency to drive himself so hard. It was clear that Chris was gaining meaningful distance from the core assumption that had caused him so much pain.

Treatment Outcome

It was evident that Chris had attained significant distance from his maladaptive assumption linking perfection to interpersonal security or acceptance. Maternal report indicated increased involvement in social activities and, for the first time, Chris began to date. The intensity of his achievement concerns and his drive for perfection were clearly in better balance with other age-appropriate interests and activities. More directly, Chris reported the cessation of suicidal thinking, and although he remained highly motivated in the academic domain with high standards, he did not show the self-punitive cognitive or behavioral pattern following disappointments. His tendency to construe the best grade as the only acceptable grade also diminished. Thus, one of his main cognitive distortions involving perceived failure had changed significantly. Perhaps of greatest relevance is the fact that at the time of termination Chris reported that his "internal pressure" had dropped, and that he was feeling more relaxed with himself.

Treatment Summary

Like many child and adolescent treatment cases, Chris's case involved characteristics that were consistent with a number of basic case formulations. Although the cognitive distortion formulation appeared to provide the best integration of Chris's focal problems with his developmental and family history, because of his orientation to his problems (action focused), interventions based on an alternative formulation guided the initial phase of treatment. The focus on developing adaptive coping skills, although unproductive in providing Chris with sustainable symptomatic relief, did uncover useful information, consistent with a cognitive distortion formulation. Treatment based on the latter formulation focused on explicating the assumptions that appeared to guide Chris's behavior and cognitions about himself. The treatment process moved from the identification of operating assumptions to a search for their developmental origins. The latter process was clinically useful in that it enabled Chris to reevaluate his assumptions in light of alternative perspectives, and more importantly, provided access to associated emotions that had been inadequately processed. Thus, although therapy was guided by the cognitive distortion formulation and primarily involved an analysis of maladaptive assumptions, it also provided a framework for processing emotion associated with core schemas.

CASE FORMULATIONS IN CHILD CLINICAL PRACTICE

A basic assumption of formulation-guided child psychotherapy is that case formulations link clinical interventions with the child's focal problems. By directing attention to pathogenic mechanisms that contribute to presenting problems, case formulations orient the therapist to change processes that can alleviate the child's difficulties. Thus, case formulations play a critical *functional* role in the delivery of child psychotherapy. Not only do they orient the therapist to intervention strategies, but they also provide a framework for evaluating treatment progress; that is, as clinical hypotheses, case formulations are tested through the application of treatment procedures. For example, in the case of Chris, the use of skills training procedures did not result in sustainable relief, thereby providing feedback that a skills deficit formulation was not the best conceptualization for the case. Similarly, case formulations highlight aspects of therapy process that can be used as in-session *markers* of treatment progress. For example, in the case of Melinda, the emotional interference formulation underscored the importance of changes in her capacity to tolerate and express emotion. With this formulation in mind, the therapist is cued to observe changes in emotion processing capacities. Of course, the therapist must attend to reports of changes outside sessions as well. It is interesting to note that subtle changes in underlying pathogenic process may be detected prior to symptomatic change, provided the therapist has developed a case formulation that orients him or her to the changes that would be predicted from the formulation. For example, in the case of Melinda, her report of dealing with a frightening situation by thinking of her therapist (by using self-calming imagery) suggested an important change in her emotion coping capacities. Such changes in psychological processes are likely to proceed clinically significant changes in overt symptoms. Thus, by directing attention to underlying psychological processes, the case formulation provides a framework for selecting treatment-specific indices of outcome.

Of equal importance, the case formulation offers the therapist a set of guidelines for decision making at critical choice points *within* sessions; that is, not only does the case formulation orient the therapist to an overall treatment strategy, it can operate as a frame for responding to the child's verbalizations or behavior within sessions. In this respect, the formulation can contribute to the coherence and direction of individual therapy sessions. As Strupp (1986) has observed, one of the factors that distinguishes the therapeutic efforts of well-intentioned college professors (untrained therapists) from trained therapists is the absence of a formulated theory that links the patient's problems with processes that could contribute to their perpetuation. Consequently, Strupp found that the college professors often ran out of material or were confused about what to do next during a therapy session. Conversely, the availability of a working formulation provides the therapist with basic parameters for the selection of in-session interventions.

In recent years, investigators have begun to examine the degree of correspondence between case formulations and therapists' verbal interventions, as well as the relationship between degree of correspondence and treatment outcome (Piper, Joyce, McCallum, & Azim, 1993). Most of this research has focused on the accuracy of therapist verbal interpretations (Crits-Christoph, Cooper, & Luborsky, 1988; Piper et al., 1993; Silberschatz, Fretter, & Curtis, 1986). For example, as mentioned in Chapter 8, Crits-Christoph and colleagues have utilized the Core Conflictual Relationship Theme Method to establish a working formulation of each patient's focal interpersonal conflicts. This approach distinguishes three interrelated components of the core conflict: (1) wishes, needs, or intentions expressed by the patient, (2) expected responses from others, and (3) reactions by the self to the expected responses by others. These components constitute the basic elements of the case formulation and provide the criteria for evaluating the accuracy or congruence of therapists' verbal interventions. According to Crits-Christoph et al. (1988), an "interpretation"–the verbal intervention of interest in their research–is defined as a statement that either explains possible reasons for the patient's thoughts, feelings, or behaviors, or highlights similarities between current interpersonal circumstances and other life experiences. Accuracy of interpretation, then, refers to the degree of correspondence between the therapist's interpretation and the components of the core conflictual relationship theme.

In a study of dynamic psychotherapy with 43 adult patients with diverse diagnoses, Crits-Christoph et al. (1988) found that interpretive accuracy, specifically for patient's wishes and expected responses from others, was significantly related to treatment outcome. Greater accuracy was positively associated with both changes in adjustment and self-rated benefits from therapy, even after controlling for the contribution of the therapeutic alliance. These results indicated that therapist's verbal activity that was congruent with the core dynamic formulation was related to positive treatment outcomes. Similar results have been obtained by other investigators who have operationalized case formulations in different ways (Piper et al., 1993; Silbershatz et al., 1986). If we extrapolate from these findings, it seems reasonable to conclude that therapeutic activity that is guided by a well-developed case formulation will yield beneficial therapeutic effects, assuming, of course, that the case formulation itself is on target. Therapist in-session behaviors, either verbal or interpersonal, which are inconsistent with the basic case formulation are less likely to be relevant to the child's problems, and in turn, less useful in facilitating therapeutic progress.

Consider, for example, the following choice point in the treatment of an 11-year-old girl, "Mary," who was referred for psychotherapy because of recurrent lying and stealing. Diagnostically, Mary appeared to be a budding conduct disorder.

It was not unusual for sessions to begin in the waiting room with Mary's mother telling her therapist about the most recent episode of stealing. For example, prior to one session, Mary's mother informed the therapist that she had discovered a small bag of cosmetics in her daughter's room. When asked how she had obtained them, Mary insisted that she had been given them by one of her friends. Later her mother discovered that the friend's older sister was quite upset by the disappearance of her cosmetics. In session, Mary initially told her therapist that she had been given the cosmetics, but when her therapist appeared puzzled by the divergent accounts given by Mary and her mother, she shifted her story and claimed that she "thought" her friend's sister did not want the cosmetics, so she kept them for herself. How, then, should the therapist respond to Mary's comments? Essentially, this will depend on how the therapist has formulated Mary's case.

One can imagine a number of possible options, including lines of inquiry that focus on Mary's social judgment ("How did you decide that she didn't want the cosmetics?"), on her perspective-taking ability ("How do you think your friend's sister felt when she discovered that her makeup was missing?"), or on her affect at the time of the episode ("How were you feeling when you took the cosmetics home?"). All of these verbal responses are clinically plausible, but which response is clinically most useful (i.e., has the greatest potential for producing change) depends on the case formulation.

When we examine Mary's focal problems in the context of her developmental and family history, elements of a case formulation become evident. First, Mary was removed from the home of her biological mother at an early age due to severe neglect. She was placed in foster care and later adopted by her foster mother when her biological mother's functioning deteriorated due to chronic substance abuse. Although Mary's adoptive mother provided a warm and caring home, Mary had experienced serious physical and emotional deprivations as a young child. In light of this developmental history, Mary's stealing takes on a new meaning; that is, the stealing appears to be linked to her early deprivation and represents an attempt to rework the difficult emotions associated with it. Severely neglected by her mother, it is likely that Mary had little control over access to emotional or physical supplies. The experience of lack of control, and the danger it entails, is not uncommon for traumatized children. Mary's recurrent stealing, then, did not appear to be the consequence of poor moral judgment or lapses in social reasoning, but was an attempt to gain mastery over a powerful, and incompletely processed, emotional experience. With this formulation in mind, the therapist is directed, not to questions about the morality of stealing, but to an exploration of the feelings associated with the episode and their connection with past experiences. In this session, the following exchange took place:

MARY: I thought she didn't want them, like she was going to throw them out.

THERAPIST: You mean you felt like they were castoffs.

MARY: Yeah, she wasn't going to use them, so I kept them.

THERAPIST: I guess you figured you could use them more than her. It sounds like you really wanted them.

MARY: Mom won't let me use makeup; it's stupid.

THERAPIST: Oh yeah, I remember that the two of you have had some fights about using makeup. It's something you really want, but she thinks you're too young for it.

MARY: She's really out of it; all the other girls wear something.

THERAPIST: So it feels like you're not getting something everyone else can have.

MARY: Yeah, it's stupid; she won't even let me wear eye shadow.

THERAPIST: It's like everyone else gets what they need or want, and you're stuck with waiting, maybe not even knowing when you'll be able to have what the others have.

MARY: It really stinks.

THERAPIST: I get the sense it really makes you mad.

MARY: Good guess!

THERAPIST: You know Mary, I think there's more going on here.

MARY: Here we go again.

THERAPIST: No really, I think that when you feel like you're not getting what you deserve, it makes you really mad, and you feel like you have to take things into your own hands.

MARY: So?

THERAPIST: Well, when you feel like things are being kept from you, it's a lot like it was when you were little. You couldn't get things for yourself then, but now when you feel that way, it just makes you want to take things, even if they're not your own.

MARY: How would you feel if you really wanted something, and you couldn't get it?

THERAPIST: I'd probably be pretty upset, especially if it had happened to me a lot when I was little.

MARY: I hate it when she won't let me have things; it does get me in trouble, but I don't care.

Throughout this exchange, the therapist, guided by a variation of the emotional interference formulation, focused attention on the emotions that prompted Mary's stealing and linked these feelings (in a general way) with her early experience of deprivation. Overall, her verbal interventions appeared to correspond with the parameters of the case formulation. Thus, as reflected in this example, a working formulation not only orients the therapist to an overall treatment strategy, but also provides a frame for responding to the child's *in-session* verbalizations and behaviors. One of the most common quandaries encountered by developing child clinicians involves such choice points within therapy sessions, and one of the most important functions of the case formulation is that it provides a reference point for in-session decision making.

Of course, "good" child therapy sessions involve more than correspondence with a case formulation. The functional utility of a case formulation depends on its validity, which in turn, directs the therapist to interventions that have the greatest potential for producing change. Let us now return to the development of case formulations and the selection of change processes. First, what do the foregoing case studies teach us about the construction of case formulations? As both cases illustrate, children often present with a complex array of focal problems and complicated developmental histories. The cognitive or technical task for the therapist is to organize this complex information into a formulation that accounts for the child's difficulties and provides direction for treatment. By no means is this a simple task. However, child therapists might benefit from a number of guiding principles for the development of case formulations.

Principles for the Development of Case Formulations

A reasonable starting point for formulating a case involves referencing the basic level case formulations. The basic level formulations provide a framework for considering a limited, but comprehensive, set of alternative clinical hypotheses, and thereby offer the therapist a method for organizing complex clinical information. Consideration of the case in relation to the basic-level formulations also ensures that rival clinical hypotheses will be entertained.

With the basic-level formulations as an organizing framework, we propose three guiding principles for developing a specific case formulation. First is the principle of *similarity*, that is, the degree to which the specific case matches one of the formulation prototypes. For example, if we compare Melinda's case with that of Sarah (the prototype for the emotional interference formulation), emotional regulation problems in the form of maladaptive coping strategies and difficulties with emotion expression are prominent. In fact, despite substantial differences in focal problems between these cases, difficulties with emotion regulation represent the leading edge in both cases, even though one involves undercontrol and the other, overcontrol.

The second principle involves the degree of *coherence* between the focal problems and the postulated underlying pathogenic mechanism. As Persons (1989) has suggested, it is useful to examine the focal problems in relation to the hypothesized pathogenic mechanism in order to determine which formulation most readily accounts for *most* focal problems. Although it is possible that some of the child's presenting problems will be difficult to explain with a single formulation, an adequate formulation should provide coherence to the diverse array of focal problems. For example, in the case of Melinda, seemingly disparate problems–emotional restriction and episodic experiences of overwhelming fear–could be explained by problems in her emotion regulation capacities.

The third principle is *narrative integration*. This principle involves the degree to which the hypothesized pathogenic process integrates the child's focal problems with the developmental or family history; that is, a good formulation of underlying pathogenic process should "fill the gap" between the child's life story and his or her presenting problems. Formulations are not typically evident from the focal problems alone, but emerge when these problems are considered in the context of the child's developmental and family history. For example, in Chris's case, the gap between his self-punitive behavior and his history of early adoption was bridged by considering maladaptive (distorting) cognitions. The cognitive distortion formulation integrated his focal problems with his early developmental history.

It is important to note that the degree of confidence in a formulation will vary across cases. Consequently, the child therapist must be open to revising a formulation with the acquisition of new information. In this respect, formulations are essentially clinical hypotheses, and like all hypotheses, it should be possible to confirm *and* disconfirm them. Thus, as Persons (1989) has suggested, one way of judging the adequacy of a formulation is to make predictions based on it. For example, in the case of Melinda, we might have predicted that reminders of her traumatic history–presented in play–would have overwhelmed her resources for emotion regulation and resulted in decrements in her functioning. With Chris, the skills deficit formulation predicted symptomatic improvement, with the acquisition of new coping strategies. The lack of significant progress following coping skills training suggests that the formulation was not on target. Thus, feedback from interventions and the acquisition of new information may lead to revisions in case formulations.

It has been our basic proposal that the best framework for selecting an intervention strategy is a formulation of the pathogenic processes that contribute to the child's focal problems. Implicit in this perspective is the assumption that therapeutic procedures are not equally effective for all types of pathogenic processes; that is, some change processes are better suited to alleviating symptoms resulting from certain pathogenic mechanisms than others. Returning to the case of Chris, it is unlikely that supportive or expressive techniques would have been sufficient to alter the underlying cognitive assumptions that fueled strong, self-punitive emotion and behavior. Similarly, with Melinda, it is not likely that interpretive interventions, which were developed to resolve internal conflicts, would have produced changes in her emotion regulation capacities. Instead, the selection of the most *direct* and, we hope, most effective approach to treatment follows from a formulation of the underlying pathogenic processes. In the case of Chris, this involved the use of cognitive procedures that uncovered the origins of his maladaptive assumptions; and with Melinda, the formulation pointed to the use of procedures aimed at increasing her capacity to tolerate and express emotion.

In many cases, the most appropriate change process is the one that was devised in conjunction with one of the basic-level formulations of pathogenic process. For example, interpretative procedures were developed in connection with the internal conflict formulation; similarly, social problem-solving training was devised in relation to the skills deficit formulation. In essence, these procedures were developed to fit with specific formulations of pathogenic process and may provide the most direct route to modifying the mechanisms that create or maintain the child's problems. A major problem in the history of child psychotherapy has been the overextension of change processes (therapeutic procedures) to cases that do not share the same underlying pathogenic mechanism, that is, the same basic case formulation.

Table 9.1 reflects historical linkages between basic case formulations and their associated change processes. The change processes that are underlined represent the primary method of intervention associated with each of the basic case formulations. These typically represent the interventions that were originally developed in connection with the basic case formulation. However, alternative methods of intervention, some of them closely related to the primary method, have been suggested in the literature for each of the basic formulations. These alternative methods are represented in regular type.

Obviously, historical primacy does not provide an adequate founda-

TABLE 9.1. Linkages between Case Formulations and Change Processes

Basic case formulations	Associated change process
Internal conflict	Insight/interpretation Emotional experiencing
Ego deficit	Supportive scaffolding Symbolic exchange
Cognitive skill deficit	Skill development Affective education
Cognitive distortion	Schema transformation Corrective relationship
Low self-esteem	Interpersonal validation/support Skill development
Emotional interference	Emotional regulation Emotional experiencing or abreaction

Note. Underlined change processes represent the primary methods of intervention.

tion for prescriptive treatments. Simply because interpretative methods were *first* applied to internal conflicts does not justify their primary prescriptive status. Instead, the selective application of change processes requires other forms of justification. The first is the conceptual coherence between case formulation and change process. In essence, the method of intervention should be "geared" to the parameters of the pathogenic process. For example, if limited self-awareness is the pathogenic culprit, then methods that expand self-awareness (interpretation or emotional experiencing) should constitute the primary method of treatment. If disruptive emotion appears to be the central pathogenic mechanism, then treatment procedures that promote emotion regulation, or new coping skills should take precedence. Again, the case formulation should orient the therapist to change processes that were developed to *directly* address the underlying pathogenic process.

However, the most important justification for the selective application of change processes to specific case formulations is empirical evidence that such matching produces positive outcomes. Although conceptual coherence represents a reasonable starting point for practicing clinicians, ultimately the conceptual justification must be supported by empirical findings. It is possible, although we think unlikely, that "goodness of fit" between change process and pathogenic process will prove to be a less valuable clinical guideline than we propose. However, the test of this framework awaits treatment outcome studies that select children on the basis of shared pathogenic mechanisms rather than (or in addition to) shared symptom patterns. Such research would also require the specification of change procedures and would not just rely on the application of "brand-name" therapies. In fact, our review of the child therapy process literature reveals few examples of this type of research, although a process–outcome study conducted by Truax and Wittmer (1973) that examines the impact of "confrontations" on adolescent "defenses" suggests that such a strategy is both feasible and informative.

It is also the case that "goodness of fit" between change process and pathogenic process is only one, albeit critical, criterion for the selection of a treatment strategy. Another important issue involves the *receptivity* of the child or parent(s) to the proposed treatment method. For example, in the case of Chris, although there was substantial evidence to support a cognitive distortion formulation and the use of cognitive procedures to examine maladaptive assumptions, his desire to "do" something that might relieve his "internal pressure" suggested an alternative starting point for treatment. As a result, a skills training approach was initiated in response to his "action" orientation and as a method for building a working alliance. Patient receptivity is closely related to the notion of treatment acceptability (Kazdin, French, & Sherick, 1981). Acceptability involves the degree to which the child or parent(s) views the proposed treatment procedures as appropriate, fair, and reasonable for the problem. As Kazdin and his colleagues have suggested, child and family involvement in treatment is likely to be related to their perceptions of treatment acceptability.

Another critical aspect of "goodness of fit" in treatment selection involves the degree to which the developmental demands of the treatment procedures are congruent with the child's developmental level. For example, with Chris, who was a bright adolescent, it was possible to utilize cognitive procedures aimed at uncovering the origins of his maladaptive assumptions. His relatively mature cognitive capacities enabled his therapist to explore possible linkages between early life events and current assumptions. With younger children, who tend to view their emotions and behaviors in terms of current, situational factors, potentially effective cognitive procedures could be compromised by their limited cognitive capacities. Thus, developmental level represents a potentially potent moderator of the effectiveness of specific change processes and must be weighed heavily in the selection of treatment methods.

CONCLUSION

In summary, the principal aim of this chapter has been to provide clinical examples of the *coordination* of case formulations and change processes.

Case formulations, by directing attention to the mechanisms that create or maintain the child's presenting problems, provide the therapist with a framework for selecting treatment strategies and for guiding responses at critical choice points within sessions. In addition, the formulation can orient the therapist to markers of treatment progress. Without a case formulation, the child therapist is vulnerable to disorientation and the process of therapy is likely to lack consistent direction. In essence, the case formulation is the rudder of child psychotherapy. Without it, treatment is likely to drift or possibly run aground.

10

Change Processes and Case Formulations: Conclusions

CHILD PSYCHOTHERAPY, in contrast to its behavioral counterpart, is based on the assumption that *internal psychological processes* are the source of children's overt emotional and behavioral problems. Maladjustment is understood in terms of deficits, distortions, or compromises in these psychological processes. Child psychotherapy aims to correct or compensate for these disrupted internal processes. This perspective does not deny the role of the social environment, especially the family environment, in the etiology of childhood disorders, but focuses, instead, on the residual effects of interpersonal transactions on the individual child. In essence, deficits, distortions, and compromises are viewed as mediators between pathogenic interpersonal histories and current expressions of maladjustment.

FROM DIAGNOSIS TO CASE FORMULATION

Our review of the major approaches to child psychotherapy has revealed multiple models of pathogenic process, even within traditional "brands" of child treatment. In part, the proliferation of models reflects the evolution of the field away from a "one size fits all" model of dysfunction (Kazdin & Kagan, 1994). The diversification of basic models of dysfunction, what we have called *basic-level case formulations*, undermines the notion of a unitary developmental pathway to maladjustment. Moreover, the abandonment of the "one size fits all" perspective entails a recognition of diverse pathogenic sources for childhood disorders, and of equal importance, the possibility of multiple pathways to the *same* disorder.

Ironically, the movement toward models of dysfunction that embrace multiple developmental pathways and diverse pathogenic processes has taken place during a time when diagnostic classification has divorced itself from underlying pathogenic processes. Instead, current diagnostic systems, especially the DSMs, have emphasized classification on the basis of observable symptom clusters. Disorders, then, are largely defined in terms of patterns of overt problems with only limited reference to pathogenic processes. Yet the recognition of multiple pathways to the same disorder mitigates against such a restrictive approach to classification. Within a phenotypically similar diagnostic group (e.g., dysthymic disorder), children may evince dramatically different pathogenic processes. By ignoring pathogenic processes, the current approach to classification fails to differentiate phenotype from genotype.

Unfortunately, the prevailing approach to outcome research in child psychotherapy is based on comparisons of treatments for children who are grouped primarily on the basis of shared symptoms. No doubt, such an approach represents an advance over earlier studies that paid scant attention to reliable inclusion–exclusion criteria and, as a result, included children with diverse problems in their treatment samples. But if one accepts the notion of multiple pathogenic pathways and processes, then the current approach to evaluating comparative efficacy is confronted with the same problem, only a step removed. Children may share the same diagnosis but not the same pathogenic processes. In other words, there may be substantial within (diagnostic) group variability in the underlying processes that contribute to the manifest disorder. Sample heterogeneity, then, occurs at a different, but no less important, level of analysis. Perhaps, then, it should not be surprising that one consequence of treatment is to increase variability in the treated group (Bergin & Lambert, 1978; Weisz et al., 1987). At times, this phenomenon has been attributed to the misclassification of children or to other child characteristics that moderate treatment effectiveness. Unfortunately, little research has addressed nondiagnostic child characteristics that could influence the impact of child treatments (Kazdin, Bass, et al., 1990). We contend that one important contributor to this phenomenon is the unassessed heterogeneity in pathogenic processes within the same diagnostic group; thus, for some children a prescribed treatment will address an underlying problem; for others it may be irrelevant and essentially inconsequential; and still for others it may be detrimental.

A formulation-based approach to child psychotherapy maintains that it is essential to focus on two levels of children's presenting problems—their focal problems and the pathogenic processes that contribute to them. A basic tenet of this approach is that case formulations provide the framework for the selection of corrective therapeutic processes. In fact, our review of the child psychotherapy literature revealed that change processes typically were developed in concert with formulations of pathogenic processes. Remarkably, this conceptual coupling has been broken in typical studies of child treatment effectiveness and may be lost in the development of prescriptive treatments for children. Instead, child diagnosis has been utilized as the common denominator for comparing the efficacy of treatments—despite the fact that psychiatric diagnoses have been purged of critical dimensions (pathogenic processes) that guide treatment selection. A major thrust of this book has been to restore the role of the case formulation in treatment research and clinical practice. A similar recommendation has been advanced by Evans (1994), who contends that the psychological assessment of children would be strengthened by complementing psychiatric diagnoses with case conceptualizations.

Although early approaches to child treatment suffered from an unfounded optimism that single formulations (e.g., internal conflicts) could account for diverse disorders, we have discovered that the child psychotherapy literature, when viewed collectively, contains multiple basic formulations of pathogenic process. Furthermore, one does not typically find an invariant relation between forms of child psychopathology and types of pathogenic process (Kazdin & Kagan, 1994). Consequently, clinical assessment must involve both the specification of the child's focal problems and the development of a formulation of the underlying pathogenic processes. For the child psychotherapist, this dual approach to assessment is critical; therapeutic interventions are not directed at the focal problems per se, but at the underlying processes that produce or maintain such problems.

Some may be inclined to read this perspective as an indictment of diagnoses or to assume that diagnoses are irrelevant to the practice of child psychotherapy. Certainly others have argued that diagnoses do not entail dimensions that are critical for treatment selection (Beutler, 1989; Persons, 1991). Consistent with such a perspective, we contend that diagnosis, based solely on the covariation of symptoms, is not sufficient for treatment selection in clinical practice or for the selection of homogeneous groups in treatment outcome studies. The degree to which diagnoses are associated with specific pathogenic processes (e.g., dysthymic disorder linked with cognitive biases) will determine whether diagnostic classification provides the clinician with a significant degree of "cognitive economy" in treatment selection. However, it is imperative that we not equate probabilistic relations between diagnoses and pathogenic processes with invariant relations. In brief, research on developmental psychopathology has not revealed patterns of simple one-to-one correspondence between disorders and underlying pathogenic processes (Kazdin & Kagan, 1994). If such a pattern were typical in clinical practice, then diagnosis would provide a more adequate basis for treatment selection.

Nevertheless, diagnoses retain a potentially important place in a formulation-based approach to child psychotherapy. As we have illustrated, case formulations emerge from a consideration of children's focal problems in the context of their developmental and family histories. To the degree that diagnosis captures the salient features of the child's focal problems, then diagnosis provides essential information for the development of case formulations. Conversely, case formulations that are not anchored to specific focal problems are likely to be too generic to be of value clinically. Furthermore, diagnoses may provide valuable prognostic information (Achenbach, 1985); but again, we contend that prognosis will be enhanced with the inclusion of formulations of pathogenic processes in the predictive formula. In summary, although diagnoses retain an elevated place in child therapy research, case formulations should not be treated as the ignored stepchild of clinical assessment or clinical intervention. In contrast, case formulations are essential for the design, selection, and implementation of therapeutic interventions in clinical practice and are likely to enhance the prognostic value of psychiatric diagnoses.

Alternatively, it could be argued that diagnoses represent the logical starting point for treatment selection. This view is based on the assumption that diagnostic judgments, with their focus on observable patterns of behavior, are less inferential than case formulations, which require greater integration of information. To the degree that research reveals probabilistic relations between specific diagnoses and certain pathogenic processes, an accurate diagnosis could orient the clinician to a subset of case formulations. However, given increasing evidence for "subtypes" within child diagnostic groups—some reflecting different developmental pathways and processes (cf. Garland & Weiss, 1995; Loeber, 1990)—the diagnosis is, at best, a starting point for treatment selection (and not the ending point) and must be complemented with a formulation of the pathogenic processes operative in the particular case.

Case Formulations: Directions for Future Research

A major obstacle to the integration of case formulations into outcome research has been the criticism that such formulations are essentially idiographic. Implied in this criticism are a number of concerns: (1) Case formulations cannot be established with any degree of reliability; (2) case formulations are essentially unique and will not generalize from one case to another; and (3) case formulations are specific to particular theoretical models and therefore lack transtheoretical utility. Thus, despite its essential role in clinical practice, the integration of the case formulation into child process and outcome research has been stalled by these criticisms.

However, in recent years there has been a proliferation of case formulation models in the adult psychotherapy literature (Barber & Crits-Christoph, 1993). Models of case formulation have been proposed for dynamic (Perry, 1989), cognitive (Persons, 1989), and behavioral treatment (Turkat, 1985). Within the psychodynamic tradition, for example, there have been systematic efforts to operationalize and validate methods for assessing dynamic formulations (Barber & Crits-Christoph, 1993). In fact, this growing body of research indicates that quantitative methods can be applied to narrative formulations, and that reliability is often as good, if not better, for formulations as it is for psychiatric diagnoses (Luborsky, Barber, & Diguer, 1992). Consequently, it seems premature to dismiss the case formulation on the basis of inherent unreliability.

Nevertheless, research on the reliability of basic level formulations needs to be conducted. As a first pass at this issue, experienced clinicians could be presented with case material—including objective and projective test results, language and pragmatic competence assessments, descriptions or profiles of the child's focal problems, and a detailed developmental history—and be asked to develop for each case a formulation of the key pathogenic process. Independent raters, using the basic prototypes, could then judge the degree to which the formulations correspond with the set described in this work. This preliminary evaluation would provide initial evidence for the degree of inclusiveness and distinctiveness of the proposed basic-level formulations for clinicians who have not been trained in the case formulation approach. Such an analysis could reveal the need for additional basic-level formulations. The study might also be extended (within and/or between subjects) by comparing the same or a different set of experienced clinicians after the completion of training in the use of the basic level case formulation model. Comparisons would not only reveal effects of training, but also variations in the similarities and differences across basic formulations derived by trained and naive clinical judges. For example, trained and untrained clinicians might be rather similar in assessing cases in which emotion regulation problems are key pathogenic processes, but differ considerably in assessing cases with cognitive–language distortions. Furthermore, systematic variation of case histories and focal problems could reveal the featural characteristics of cases that lead to different formulations. Here, hierarchical clustering techniques could be used to define the key content features of each distinctive prototype and to empirically describe the varying relations among them.

With regard to the second concern—that formulations are essentially unique and lack generalizability—we have suggested that case formulations can be made at different levels of analysis. More specifically, we have proposed that meaningful distinctions can be made among child cases at an intermediate level of analysis, what has been referred to as the "basic level" of categorization. One of the virtues of this type of classification is that cases are formulated at a level of abstraction that transcends the unique characteristics of a particular case. Returning to an earlier analogy, bar stools, high chairs, and recliners all possess unique characteristics, but they are also meaningfully classified at an intermediate level—the basic level—as chairs. Similarly, pathogenic processes can be formulated at different levels of analysis, including an analogous intermediate level. Our review has resulted in the identification of six basic-level case formulations. These formulations reflect meaningful differences in the way that under-lying pathogenic processes are conceptualized for particular cases. How-ever, consistent with prototype theory, these clusters of case formulations are not defined by sharp boundaries, but instead represent "fuzzy sets." Although this may prove challenging to reliable classification, we believe that these categories reflect salient differences in pathogenic processes that can easily be identified with appropriate training in the case formulation model, and are commonly, although often implicitly, distinguished in clinical practice. Again, this claim needs to be evaluated empirically, and a starting point would be to elicit commonly used formulations from experienced child psychotherapists. Generalizability might then be as-sessed by asking clinicians who either are or are not trained in the case formulation model to develop case formulations for sets of children with diverse diagnoses. Similar procedures have yielded a high degree of consensus for *categories* of common childhood disorders (Horowitz, Wright, Lowenstein, & Parad, 1981), and it would be useful to see if a comparable pattern emerged for categories of formulations.

Conceptualizing case formulations at the "basic level" of categoriza-tion addresses the problem of uniqueness. Children with diverse focal problems can share similar underlying pathogenic processes. Rather than focusing on the unique features of the case, basic-level formulations reflect core models of pathogenesis (e.g., skills deficits vs. internal conflicts). Clearly such basic-level formulations are more abstract than earlier models of child case formulation (cf. Shapiro, 1989); however, as we have shown, this level of formulation carries important implications for the design and selection of interventions; that is, the child clinician would be directed to different methods and patterns of interaction if a case were formulated in terms of internal conflicts rather than skills deficits.

Again, this claim could be evaluated empirically, perhaps most simply through an analogue study; that is, child clinicians could be given formu-lations for particular cases and then be asked to develop treatment plans with specific aims and procedures. Not only would it be possible to evaluate the degree to which different formulations yield consensus about treatment methods, but one could examine the clinicians' differentiation of treatment strategies, that is, the degree to which clinicians vary their planned interventions as a function of varied formulations. Here one might expect increasing differentiation to be associated with level or breadth of experience.

The degree of abstraction reflected in basic-level formulations also addresses the problem of theoretical breadth. Although some of these formulations are more prominent in specific "brands" of child psychotherapy, our review of this literature indicates that several basic-level formulations appear in more than one therapeutic system. Moreover, because these formulations do not posit processes that are unique to one theoretical model, they appear to be compatible with most approaches to child *psychotherapy.* It is likely that an alternative set of basic-level formulations could be derived for behavior therapy and family therapy; however, within the domain of child psychotherapy these formulations appear to be relevant to a variety of approaches, represent important differences in case conceptualization, and are common in clinical practice. In evaluating these prototypes empirically—for both their relevance and their reliability—it will be essential to include clinician-raters with varied psychotherapeutic preferences.

The development of methods for selecting a formulation for a particular case is an area that deserves considerable attention. It is unlikely that formulations can be derived from a single parent or child interview, or from a structured behavior checklist, although these sources of information will most certainly be relevant. As we have suggested, formulations about pathogenic mechanisms are constructed from a thorough developmental and family history and from opportunities to assess the child's functional capacities and central concerns, including their recurrent interpersonal patterns and points of affect dysregulation. Obviously, such an approach to clinical assessment goes far beyond the structured diagnostic interview and attempts to construct what Kazdin and Kagan (1994) call "a profile of the child's life" that encompasses multiple characteristics of the child, parent, and family context (p. 44). Given the emphasis on developmental and family history in the case formulation approach, a potentially important area for future research involves the construction of a semistructured interview that would systematically assess life events and developmental history. Such information provides the meaningful context for the child's focal problems and is essential for the development of a case formulation. The development of an interview method that is both comprehensive and systematic would enhance the reliability of the formulation process.

Given the assessment of a comprehensive profile of the child's life, including the focal problems, we have suggested several guiding principles for formulating cases. These include the degree of similarity between the particular case and one of the formulation prototypes, the degree of coherence between the focal problems and the underlying pathogenic mechanisms, and the degree to which the postulated pathogenic processes integrate the focal problems with the developmental and family history. In addition, degree of consensus among evaluators would most assuredly increase confidence in the validity of a particular formulation.

Case formulations can also be used to guide process and outcome research. For example, once a case has been formulated, clinician interventions can be assessed for the degree to which they address the underlying pathogenic process. The degree of on-target versus off-target interventions offered by the child therapist could then be related to outcome. The working hypothesis, of course, would be that treatments with more on-target interventions would be more effective than those with a predominant proportion of off-target interventions. With the advent of microanalyses of process data (cf. Russell, 1995), the sequential relations of such on- and off-target interventions to the child's participation in the treatment process can now be assessed as well, revealing characteristic underlying structures of interaction for successful and unsuccessful cases.

Case formulations could also be used prior to therapy to assess the child or the adolescent's awareness of his or her underlying problems and to facilitate their ownership. Using Q-sort methodology, the child or adolescent could be presented with various foil and target case formulations (written in an age-appropriate manner). One might predict that therapy would progress more rapidly for those children who selected formulations that are consistent with the one identified by the treatment team. Such research could also shed light on the developmental parameters of children's awareness of the source of their emotional and behavioral problems. Similarly, the degree to which a case formulation remains accurately descriptive, as assessed by the child, the clinician, and other clinical judges would provide a useful multiperspective assessment of the treatment's progress. In essence, absence of change in the basic formulation would indicate that the case is stuck. Thus, it appears that the case formulation model we have proposed can reinvigorate child process and outcome research, just as it is aimed to revitalize child psychotherapy practice.

FROM TREATMENT BRANDS TO CHANGE PROCESSES

The principal organizing framework for child psychotherapy research and practice has been the clinician's therapeutic orientation. In the practice domain, surveys typically ask child clinicians to report their treatment orientation, despite the fact that many, if not most, child practitioners draw upon methods from a variety of therapeutic systems (Kazdin, Siegel, & Bass, 1990; Tuma & Pratt, 1982). Furthermore, when confronted with critical-choice points in therapy sessions, child clinicians focus on the application of specific techniques or the enactment of specific patterns of interaction. Thus, in practice, the salient construct for the child clinician is not therapeutic orientation per se, but methods of intervention, or what we have called *change processes*. It is noteworthy that studies on the utilization of psychotherapy research by practitioners indicate that clinicians are unlikely to implement a treatment, even a treatment that has been shown to be effective, "if they do not know what the treatment consists of or how it should be delivered" (Cohen, Sargent, & Sechrest, 1986, p. 204). It appears, then, that for treatment research to be relevant to clinical practice, the processes that constitute treatments must be detailed and directly investigated.

In the research domain, the majority of existing studies have focused on the efficacy or comparative efficacy of treatment brands, that is, whole therapies for children. Not only does this type of research stand in sharp contrast to the expressed needs of clinical practitioners, but also it has not yielded consistent results regarding the relative superiority of particular treatment brands for specific childhood disorders. Furthermore, within the domain of child *psychotherapy,* the underrepresentation of certain treatment approaches and modalities, as well as the poor methodological quality of many studies, make it difficult to draw definitive conclusions about the relative effectiveness of various treatments.

Even more striking has been the lack of research on specific therapeutic processes and their relationship with treatment outcome. Our review of research on process–outcome relations yielded only a handful of studies in the child psychotherapy literature that have addressed this question. This is consistent with a review by Kazdin et al. (1990), who found that only about 3% of all child treatment studies utilized a process-oriented strategy. Interestingly, they found that child practitioners viewed research on therapeutic processes and their relation to outcome as a top priority for future research. Consequently, there is a substantial gap between the concerns of clinicians and the type of research that could most directly address their concerns.

It has been our contention that child treatment research must be refocused on the specific interventions delivered by therapists or on patterns of therapist–child interactions within and across sessions. The call for a shift in focus is based on a number of considerations. First, children do not respond to the therapeutic orientation of their therapist, but to the actions, attitudes, and interventions presented by the therapist. As we have contended, the relationship between expressed therapeutic orientation and actual behavior in sessions may only be as strong as the relationship between attitudes and behavior in other domains. In other words, there is not a clear correspondence between treatment brands and treatment processes, in part, because the child exerts an influence over what the therapist is able to do in a particular session or series of sessions. Of equal importance, treatment brands are complex and composed of multiple techniques and patterns of interaction that can be presented in different combinations. Thus, if we are to understand the factors that contribute to therapeutic change, we must redirect our attention to the processes that constitute treatment brands, to their instantiation in actual practice with particular types of children, and to the degree to which these processes are related to outcome. To remain preoccupied with comparisons of treatment brands, that is, with the proverbial "horse-race" question, will only maintain the gap between clinical research and clinical practice.

In an effort to initiate a reorientation of child therapy research and to explicate models of change in child psychotherapy practice, we examined three analytically separable, but interrelated, types of change processes. Our review of interpersonal, emotional, and cognitive processes in child psychotherapy revealed a range of intervention methods that are, at times, poorly elaborated conceptually and rarely investigated empirically.

Some of the conceptual limitations in this literature can be attributed to the failure to recognize continuity between therapeutic processes and similar processes in other developmental or interpersonal contexts. For example, the provision of a supportive relationship has been posited as a critical interpersonal change process in child psychotherapy. However, the role of support in child therapy has not been informed, by and large, by a substantial body of research in developmental and social psychology that could provide new insights into both the dimensions of support and their relations with various outcomes. Instead, models of therapeutic process often appear to develop in isolation from basic research on the psychological processes that constitute them. In contrast, a major thrust of our examination of change processes in child psychotherapy has been to view processes that take place in one social context, the psychotherapy session, as specific instantiations of general psychological processes. It has been our assumption that research on similar processes in other contexts will clarify the operation of change processes in child psychotherapy. To this end, we have reexamined change processes in light of developmental theory and research.

Within the interpersonal, emotional, and cognitive domains we identified a variety of change processes. Thus, unlike early approaches to child treatment, which tended to emphasize one or two methods of intervention, current approaches to child psychotherapy involve multiple techniques and forms of interaction. The major issue, then, for the practicing child clinician is how to select the most useful approach for a particular case. In contrast to matching treatment brands with diagnostic entities, we proposed new elements in the matching equation. As an alternative, change processes, such as interpretation or skills remediation, and case formulations, such as cognitive distortions or self-esteem deficits, have been advanced as the essential ingredients of the matching formula. One virtue of this approach is that both treatments and disorders are conceptualized in terms of component psychological processes; or stated differently, both elements in the matching equation share a common conceptual denominator. Matching, then, is based on the "goodness of fit" between the psychological processes that contribute to maladjustment and the psychological processes aimed at their remediation. Thus, our approach reformulates a number of the elements in Paul's (1967) well-known *matrix* formulation, namely, that effective therapy is a function of who delivers what type of treatment for which individual with what type of problem in which setting, by redefining type of treatment in terms of change processes and type of problem in terms of formulations of pathogenic processes.

THE CONTEXTS OF CHILD PSYCHOTHERAPY

Although our focus has been on the psychological interior of child psychotherapy, the process of child treatment is embedded in, and shaped by, a number of important contexts. Put simply, child psychotherapy does not occur in a vacuum. The formulation, design, and implementation of intervention strategies must take a number of intersecting contexts into consideration; these include the contexts of development, the family, and the child's culture.

The Context of Development

Throughout this volume we have prefaced psychotherapy with a generic developmental modifier, "child." But as both developmentalists and child clinicians remind us, children do not constitute a homogeneous category (Kendall et al., 1984; Shirk, 1988b). In fact, in recent years there has been increasing recognition of the developmental parameters of many interventions for child psychopathology. In many ways this is a rediscovery of some of the insights presented by Anna Freud (1965), who was acutely aware of the role of development in the conduct of child therapy. From her perspective, the child's orientation to the therapist, type of participation in treatment, and degree of interest in focusing on emotional material were all influenced by the child's level of development. In recent years, developmentally oriented clinicians have been concerned primarily with the developmental limits of specific therapeutic techniques (Forehand &

Wierson, 1993; Jessee, Jurkovic, Wilkie, & Chiglinski, 1982; Kendall et al., 1984; Shirk, 1990).

One cluster of techniques that has received some attention from a developmental perspective are the cognitive change processes inherent in many forms of cognitive-behavioral therapy. Based on the assumption that changes in behavior are predicated on changes in cognition, this approach relies heavily on the modification of cognitive patterns and processes. Moreover, most of the therapeutic procedures, such as self-monitoring, problem-solving, and perspective-taking training involve cognitive processes. Not surprisingly, a number of investigators have proposed that children's cognitive developmental status could moderate the effectiveness of cognitive interventions (Kendall, 1985; Meyers & Craighead, 1984).

In an effort to evaluate this hypothesis, Durlak et al. (1991) conducted a meta-analysis of the effectiveness of cognitive-behavioral therapy for maladjusted children. Unique to this meta-analysis was a consideration of child characteristics that could moderate treatment effects. Among the most important was the child's developmental level. Because most studies of cognitive-behavioral therapy, or any child therapy, for that matter, did not directly assess the cognitive developmental level of the treated children, Durlak et al. was forced to rely on age as a proxy for developmental level. Based on Piagetian theory, effect sizes were calculated for children corresponding to three levels of cognitive development—preoperational (ages 5–7), concrete operational (ages 7–11), and formal operational (ages 11–13). Consistent with the hypothesis, Durlak and his colleagues found that the treatment effect for the oldest group—assumed to be formal operational—was over twice as large as the effect for both groups of younger, and presumably, cognitively less advanced children. One implication of this finding is that maladjusted children who enter cognitively oriented therapy with more advanced cognitive abilities are likely to attain greater benefit from treatment than children who are less advanced. In essence, the effectiveness of cognitive change processes varies as a function of developmental level. Younger, cognitively less advanced children may not have the skills or processes to benefit from the cognitive change processes inherent in this form of treatment. Returning to one of our case examples, it is unlikely that the use of "developmental analysis," (i.e., uncovering the origins of dysfunctional cognitions) that was so instrumental in the recovery of a self-critical adolescent would be beneficial for school-age children who are limited in their capacity to evaluate current thoughts and feelings in relation to past events.

Similarly, the effectiveness of interpretation as a change process may be moderated by the child's cognitive developmental level. Shirk (1988a) demonstrated that the causal structure implicit in many therapeutic interpretations is far more complex than the causal reasoning of most "normal" children, let alone disturbed children. Thus, the therapist's use of interpretations that typically connect current behavior or emotion to internal processes or past events that may also be outside the child's awareness is incongruent with the child's tendency to focus on situational and temporally proximal explanations for behavior or emotion. Such discrepancy between the therapist's level of causal understanding and the child's level of causal reasoning may render many interpretations incomprehensible to children. And without comprehension, it is unlikely that interpretations will function as a change process.

As these examples suggest, developmental level can moderate the effectiveness of specific interventions. In designing interventions for children, child therapists must consider the developmental parameters of their interventions. Although a particular type of intervention may be effective for a specific type of problem, this relationship may not be consistent across developmental levels. Thus, the selection of a treatment plan cannot be based on the diagnosis alone, or for that matter, on the formulation of the underlying pathogenic processes alone. Instead, nondiagnostic and nonpathogenic child characteristics must be considered as well. And among the most important is the child's developmental level.

Although "developmental task analyses" of specific therapeutic techniques represent a promising starting point for the design of developmentally sensitive interventions, other aspects of child psychotherapy are affected by the child's developmental level. One of the most important is the *medium* through which the therapist is able to conduct therapy. Many years ago, Anna Freud (1965) observed that the development of child therapy is essentially synonymous with a history of attempts to overcome children's disinclination to *talk* about emotional concerns in treatment. In fact, a variety of conversational substitutes can be found in the practice of child psychotherapy, including puppetry, drawing, games, and most importantly, play. As Kernberg and Chazan (1991) note, "For the troubled, beleaguered child play also provides a safe haven in which reality can be suspended temporarily and new possibilities explored without fear of retaliation" (pp. 23–24). As they point out, therapeutic play provides the child with opportunities for problem solving, practicing, and mastery and can "shed light on hidden meanings with which the child is struggling" (p. 23). We might add that play provides the child with unique opportunities to enact new patterns of relating and to explore the implications of such patterns without concern for real consequences. For example, an inhibited child might "stand up" for herself in the context of a play scenario, but avoid such a behavior in everyday interaction.

Although there are substantial individual differences in children's capacity to play in therapy, and these differences seem largely attributable to the child's comfort with expressing emotion, there are important developmental variations as well. Typically, young children—specifically, preschoolers and early elementary school children—are readily engaged in thematic play. The provision of action or doll figures and relevant props is often enough to stimulate play activity. But with increasing age, thematic play is often supplanted by a growing interest in games and gross motor activities (e.g., playing basketball). Although this shift reflects a common developmental trend, ironically, one cost of maturation is the loss of a unique medium for the communication of emotional concerns. Compounding this loss is the fact that many school-age children remain disinclined to talk about emotional issues. Thus, the developmental shift from play to conversation in child psychotherapy is discontinuous. Interestingly, many children are referred for treatment precisely at a time—during late childhood and preadolescence—when they have lost interest in thematic play but lack the capacity or comfort to talk about their difficulties. These children can be especially challenging for child therapists, who spend what feels like endless sessions involved in repetitive board games. And as Wachtel (1994) has observed, many games are not geared to stimulate meaningful interactions or a deeper understanding of the child's difficulties. Instead, they serve a defensive function and allow the child to avoid dealing with significant issues. Thus, like the techniques of therapy, the medium through which child psychotherapy is conducted is constrained, in part, by the child's developmental level.

A third aspect of child psychotherapy that is affected by developmental level is the child's orientation to the therapist. As Chethik (1989) has noted, the therapist's self-image as a caring and helpful person rarely corresponds to the child's image of the therapist. In part, children who present with psychological problems, particularly behavioral problems, often have faced negative consequences or admonishments from adults in authority roles. Given such experience, children are likely to construe therapists in a similar manner. This may be particularly true for younger children, whose social concepts are less differentiated than their older counterparts.

But of equal importance, children vary in their awareness or recognition of emotional or behavioral problems. As Anna Freud (1965) has observed, owing to their immaturity, children often have "no insight into their abnormalities," and in turn, "they do not develop the same wish to get well" as adults (p. 28). Although Anna Freud contrasts "children" as a group with adults, developmental evidence indicates that the capacity to recognize one's emotional or behavioral problems should be related to the maturation of self-evaluative processes. For example, Selman (1980) has shown that the processes of self-observation and self-awareness follow a predictable developmental sequence. Thus, one would expect older children to have a greater capacity to recognize their difficulties than younger children. Although capacity to recognize problems should not be equated with *problem acknowledgement,* older children's ability to evaluate their own difficulties should increase their willingness to engage in treatment and to perceive the therapist as a potential helper. For the younger child, who fails to recognize the existence of problems, the therapist might be viewed as a benign and attentive adult, but not as a source of help for emotional or behavioral difficulties. Such developmental differences in problem awareness could entail important variations in the type of relationship the child forms with the therapist. For the younger child, the therapist may be primarily a source of gratification (i.e., an attentive playmate), but for the older child, who recognizes his or her problems and wishes to overcome them, the therapist can assume the role of an ally.

As these examples suggest, the techniques, the medium, and the interpersonal framework of child psychotherapy take shape within the context of the child's developmental level. Consequently, the design and implementation of therapeutic interventions must account for developmental variations in the cognitive, emotional, and interpersonal repertoires that children bring to psychotherapy sessions.

The Context of the Family

Child psychotherapy does not occur in an interpersonal vacuum, but instead is embedded in the context of other significant interpersonal relationships, most importantly, relationships within the family. If we return to some of the prototypical cases presented in Chapter 8, we find numerous instances in which family factors appear to be closely connected with the child's focal problems. For example, in the case of Corine, the developmental task of separation and increasing self-reliance was complicated by her mother's overinvolvement and almost exclusive identification as Corine's caregiver. Thus, Corine was caught between the age-appropriate wish to separate from her mother and the fear that such separation would cause excessive pain. In the case of Colin, the proximal cause of his low self-esteem appeared to be the loss of parental availability and support following his parents' divorce. In both cases, the child's relationship with his or her parents was an important component of the case formulation.

The fact that family relationship factors often appear to be involved in children's emotional and behavioral problems has led many child clinicians to redefine the target of intervention as the family, rather than the individual child. However, in general, there is little evidence that family therapy produces larger treatment effects than individual child therapy (Fauber & Long, 1991). In fact, the overall effect sizes for family therapy are very similar to the overall effects of nonbehavioral child psychotherapy (Hazzelrigg, Cooper, & Borduin, 1987). Furthermore, direct comparisons with alternative treatment methods are problematic because of the limited number of studies, and more importantly, because of the broad range of alternative treatments included as such comparisons (e.g., bibliotherapy, group therapy, and problem-solving instruction; Fauber & Long, 1991). In summary, despite compelling conceptualizations of child psychopathology from a family systems perspective, existing research does not support the superiority of treating the whole family over treating the individual child. Of course, the family therapy outcome literature is plagued by many of the same problems that we encountered in the child therapy literature, and there have been relatively fewer controlled studies of family therapy.

It is noteworthy that surveys of child clinicians now indicate that the majority incorporate the family, in some way, into the treatment of individual children (Fauber & Long, 1991). For example, Koocher and Pedulla (1977) find that 94% of all surveyed child psychologists and child psychiatrists routinely see the parents with the child as part of the child's treatment. This finding suggests that some type of collateral intervention with parents is a common part of child psychotherapy as typically practiced. But as Fauber and Long (1991) point out, "The relative efficacy of child treatments as a function of the extent to which they involve family partici-pation, regardless of theoretical orientation, has not been examined" (p. 814). Only Casey and Berman (1985) evaluated the contribution of paren-tal involvement in child treatment, but they failed to uncover a significant difference between treatments that involved collateral parent therapy and those that did not. However, their sample of studies that included parent treatment was quite small, nine to be exact, and typically the type of parental involvement was separate psychotherapy for the parents, which is only one form of parental involvement in treatment (Fauber & Long, 1991).

Returning to our prototypical cases, it is not difficult to image the need for various forms of parental involvement in treatment. In Corine's case, in which her mother's own psychological issues appeared to contribute to her child's conflicts, collateral individual therapy with the parent seems warranted. In Colin's case, in which parental unavailability and lack of support were contributors to his low self-esteem and suicidal thinking, collateral parent–child interaction therapy could prove useful. As these examples suggest, the type of parent or family involvement in child psychotherapy varies as a function of the case formulation.

Fauber and Long (1991) have suggested that a key to deciding what type of family involvement in child treatment is appropriate involves the extent to which "the family is viewed as having a direct role in the etiology and maintenance of the problem" (p. 818). In essence, they propose that family involvement be focused on altering specific interactive processes that contribute to the child's dysfunction, and that it be limited to that endeavor. For the most part, Fauber and Long emphasize interventions into patterns of family interaction or parenting practices as the most valuable forms of family involvement in child treatment. However, it is important to recognize that the immediate impact of family interactions and parenting practices may have their origins in other, less immediate sources. For example, dysfunctional parenting practices may stem from dysregulated parental affect (e.g., low involvement as a function of parental depression) or from beliefs that are rooted in intergenerational patterns (e.g., the belief that disrespect legitimizes punitive practices). As such, direct intervention in family interactions or parenting practices may be insufficient to alter the underlying source of the maladaptive interactional pattern. For example, collateral parent therapy for depression might be more effective than direct interventions to increase parental involvement or alter parenting practices. In summary, the type of parent or family involvement, like the type of individual intervention, must follow from a formulation of the underlying processes that are contributing to the child's focal problem.

It also is important to consider other contributions that parents make to the process of child psychotherapy. First, because children rarely refer themselves for treatment, parents are typically involved in decision making about the need for services. Braswell (1991) suggests that one factor affecting this decision-making process involves parents' expectations about the timing of completion of various developmental tasks; that is, a parent may not view a set of behaviors as problematic until the child has passed the age at which the culture expects a certain task to be resolved. Other factors appear to enter into this process as well. Shirk and Rossman (1989) showed that parents' decisions about the severity of child behavior problems involve judgments about the frequency, the long-term consequences, and causal locus of the problem. There is also emerging data to suggest that the parent's own emotional state and the parent's degree of contribution to the child's problem may influence the extent to which the parent acknowledges a problem and seeks services (Braswell, 1991). Thus, parents play a pivotal role in the definition of the problem and in the decision to seek treatment.

Second, parents are involved in decisions about continuation in treatment. That is, just as parents make decisions about initiating services, they also make decisions about terminating them. Relatively little is known about the factors that influence parents' decisions to continue or terminate therapy, but clinical research indicates that a substantial portion of parents elect not to continue treatment after an initial evaluation (Weisz, Weiss, & Langmeyer, 1987). In fact, this research has revealed a surprising degree of similarity between dropout and continuer groups. For example, even differences in parent perceptions of their child's problems (e.g., "How optimistic or pessimistic do you feel about the concerns that brought your child to the clinic?") or perceptions of the clinic (e.g, "If you were to seek help again for your child, would you go back to the same clinic?") did not discriminate between dropouts and continuers (Weisz et al., 1987).

One possibility is that continuation in child psychotherapy may be predicted from the strength of alliance the therapist forms, not just with the child, but with the parents as well. If this is the case, then collateral parent consultation that keeps the parents informed and involved may be critical for effective child treatment. In fact, in one study we found that children's perception of their parents' alliance with the treatment team was predictive of the quality of their own alliance with their individual therapist (Raney, Shirk, Sarlin, Kaplan, & During, 1991). Therefore, it is possible that the quality of the alliance between therapist and parent affects not just continuation in treatment but also the quality of the treatment process with the individual child. In this respect, child psychotherapy is truly embedded in a broader relational context.

A third and very important area in which parental involvement can affect the process and outcome of treatment is treatment generalization and maintenance. As Braswell (1991) has observed, virtually all forms of child psychotherapy are plagued by problems of generalization and maintenance of treatment gains. Parents play a critical role in both processes. For example, imagine a case in which the clinical focus is on facilitating the expression of feelings. Such work could easily be undermined if parents are not comfortable with the changes initiated in therapy. In fact, such changes could run counter to the family conditions that led the child to treatment in the first place. Such a scenario underscores the importance of parental involvement in both the development and implementation of a treatment plan.

First, agreement on treatment goals is one of the cardinal elements of a positive alliance. Thus, in order to establish a working alliance with parents, the goals of treatment should be made explicit. This means going beyond a discussion of symptom reduction to an explanation of the type of changes that appear to be needed in order to modify the child's presenting problems. Second, as the child begins to demonstrate changes within therapy sessions, for example, to express feelings more freely, parents should be "innoculated" against some of the temporary negative features of such changes (e.g., greater emotionality). As therapy progresses, the involvement of parents in child sessions can be useful for facilitating generalization to other social contexts. Moreover, these sessions can be informative about the degree to which changes will be tolerable within the family context. Viewed from this perspective, the involvement of parents in child psychotherapy can both support the process of individual treatment and reveal countervailing factors that could undermine progress.

The Context of Culture

Tharp (1991) has contended that "individual psychotherapy is a culturally specific form of treatment, just as surely as is a sweat lodge or the herbalism of the curandero . . . " (p. 804). The effectiveness of child psychotherapy, then, can be expected to be moderated by the child's culture; that is, treatments or change processes that have been shown to be effective with children from one culture may not be as useful for children from another. This perspective stands in sharp contrast to the *universalist* position that effective treatments will follow the same course and involve the same processes for children from diverse cultures.

Two major alternatives have been offered to the universalist perspective. The stronger of the two suggests that *culturally specific* forms of therapy that are tailored, or perhaps even unique, to different cultures will produce the most optimal outcomes. An extension of this perspective is that cultural matching of child and therapist is essential because culturally matched therapists are more likely to understand the linguistic and sociocultural codes that will enable them to provide a culturally specific form of intervention (Tharp, 1991). In support of this perspective, Tharp draws on research from child education. Here one finds that cultural conventions of conversation, such as wait time and rhythm of speech, and conventions for participation and listening have a strong impact on the child's reaction to instruction. Analogous patterns might influence children's response to psychotherapy, but research in this area is sorely underdeveloped.

The second alternative to the universalist perspective is captured under the rubric of *culturally sensitive* psychotherapy. This alternative takes two forms. The first involves the selection of treatment modalities that are congruent with the child's cultural context. For example, in recognition of Cubans' strong sense of family, a problem-solving approach to child treatment that involves multiple generations provides greater cultural compatibility than individual treatment with little family involvement (Szapocznik, Rio, Murray, & Cohen, 1989). In fact, Tharp (1991) argues that a more inclusive approach to treatment is indicated when therapists work cross-culturally. As he notes, "Treatment modalities can be arrayed on a continuum of inclusiveness or social contextuality, from individual psychotherapy to group therapy to family therapy to network therapy to community intervention" (p. 809). According to Tharp, because individual therapy depends so heavily on shared values, semiotics, and expectations, it presents a serious challenge for "a therapist facing a client across a cultural chasm" (p. 809). Consequently, it seems advisable to contextualize psychotherapy under these conditions by taking a more inclusive approach, that is, by expanding therapy to include family and community members as resources for commonality.

The second approach to culturally sensitive therapy "takes the client's culture as a point of departure for restructuring therapeutic interventions" (Malgady et al., 1990). In essence, basic change processes are modified to be compatible with the child's (and family's) cultural beliefs and values in order to promote more effective therapeutic gains than would be obtained with standard treatments.

One of the best examples of this approach is illustrated in a program of research on culturally sensitive therapy for Puerto Rican children. In this research (Costantino et al., 1986), storytelling, a common therapeutic method, was adapted by using Puerto Rican *cuentos*, or folktales, to convey a theme or moral to a story. Thus, like other storytelling techniques, narratives were used to illustrate adaptive solutions to problems that children might face. However, the narratives were modified such that the protagonists portrayed beliefs, values, and behaviors that were culturally congruent with the children's own background in order to facilitate identification and imitation. Moreover, the stories themselves were derived from Puerto Rican folktales or were adapted to capture bicultural conflicts of children in the United States. Thus, the treatment method involved the use of a common child therapy process, storytelling, but adapted the process to incorporate the cultural characteristics and dilemmas of the child clients.

Two forms of *cuento* therapy were delivered to high risk kindergarten and early-elementary-school children. The one utilized original Puerto Rican folktales, whereas the other used folktales adapted to bridge Puerto Rican and American cultures. Therapists and mothers read the *cuentos* aloud, then the therapist conducted a group discussion of the main character's feelings and behaviors and the moral of the story. Mother–child dyads then dramatized the stories and resolved the basic conflict. As a comparison treatment, mother–child dyads engaged in play therapy under the supervision of a therapist. In this treatment, mothers and children were also encouraged to dramatize family scenes depicting conflict. A fourth group was randomly assigned to a no-treatment condition.

In brief, results indicated that both forms of *cuento* therapy reduced child anxiety relative to the no-treatment group. The "adapted" *cuento* group showed significantly greater improvement compared to the more traditional play-therapy group as well. In addition, both forms of *cuento* therapy produced gains in social judgment relative to the play therapy and no-treatment groups. These results are especially promising in that they demonstrate that the adaptation of basic therapeutic methods to the cultural characteristics of child clients can promote treatment gains over and above those obtained with standard interventions. The findings also suggest that it is possible, with some creativity, for therapists to import culture into the design and implementation of basic psychotherapeutic interventions for children.

Culture plays an important role, not just in the selection or design of interventions, but also in the development of case formulations. As we have maintained, case formulations typically emerge from a consideration of children's focal problems in the context of their developmental and family history. Consider, first, the impact of culture on the definition of focal problems.

Child clinical problems differ in their power to evoke clinic referral, and one factor that may influence the degree to which problems are regarded as serious enough for referral is the cultural context in which they occur (Weisz & Weiss, 1991). Weisz et al. (1988) examined two models of cultural influence on parental perceptions of child clinical problems. Both models are based on the idea that the threshold for adult distress about child emotional and behavioral problems is set by cultural values and expectations. The first model holds that cultures, and for that matter, subcultures within a single society, set different thresholds of tolerance for clinical problems in general; that is, some cultures may accept wide variations in child behavior, whereas others set more narrow boundaries. The second model, the pattern-specific form, holds that certain types of child problems may be differentially distressing in different cultures; that is, a subset of child problems might arouse distress among parents in one culture, but be tolerated, or in fact, encouraged in another.

To evaluate these models, Weisz and colleagues (1988) compared judgments of problem seriousness in adults from two cultures (Thai and American) in which values and perspectives differ substantially. Parents, teachers, and psychologists rated the seriousness of problems exhibited by two hypothetical children, one with overcontrolled problems (shyness and fear) and one with undercontrolled problems (fighting and disobedience). Overall, the results indicated that Thai adults tolerate wider variation in child behavior than their American counterparts. For both overcontrolled and undercontrolled problems, Thai adults rated them as less serious, unusual, and worrisome than American adults. Interestingly, Thai adults were more likely to believe that the "problems" would improve over time, an idea that is consistent with the Buddhist belief that change is inevitable. Thus, in this study, marked cultural differences emerged in parent and teacher perceptions of common focal problems, and these differences were consistent with the general threshold model of problem perception. Such results suggest that culture may influence the identification and description of focal problems presented by parents to child clinicians.

It is noteworthy that cultural differences also emerged in the causal explanations for child problems given by Thai and American adults. In general, Thai adults were more likely to attribute the cause of the child's problems to faulty parenting or socialization, whereas American adults were more likely to invoke psychodynamic explanations, such as conflicting motives, or in the case of overcontrolled behavior, were more likely to blame the problem on environmental stress. These findings suggest that cultural differences can influence both the identification of focal problems and causal accounts of their origins. The latter effect is especially noteworthy in that cultural factors may influence the salience of specific precipitating events or pathogenic processes for parents, which in turn, affects the presentation of the developmental and family history. Taken together, these findings underscore the fact that clinicians must be aware of the potential impact of culture on parents' (and teachers') descriptions of children's clinical problems.

Of equal importance, child clinicians must also be aware of the impact of their own cultural experience on judgments about problem severity and etiology. One area in which culture is likely to affect clinical judgment is in the evaluation of parent–child relationships. Clearly, many formulations of child psychopathology emphasize the quality of parent–child relationships in the genesis of child maladjustment. Child therapists, through their training and life experience, typically develop a set of "normative" expectations for parent–child relationships. When observed patterns of interaction deviate from these "norms," inferences about their contribution to the child's focal problems frequently follow. However, such inferences could be based on ethnocentric conceptualizations of what constitutes normative interaction. Developmental research has revealed substantial variation in child socialization and parenting practices across cultural contexts (Bornstein, 1991). For example, as Tharp (1991) notes, misunderstanding is potentially very high in two areas in which there is substantial cultural variation: "the degree of responsibility delegated to children and the degree to which children are expected to submit to adult dominance" (p. 801). Thus, in developing a case formulation, child therapists must contextualize their "normative" baselines in order to ensure that culturally prescribed variations in parent–child interaction are not misconstrued as pathogenic processes.

In summary, both the design and implementation of clinical interventions, as well as the development of case formulations, can be affected by cultural factors. Initial research, albeit limited, suggests that adaptation of basic therapeutic techniques to the cultural characteristics of child clients can enhance the effectiveness of intervention. Similarly, culture can influence judgments about the causes and seriousness of specific child clinical problems. Failure to consider culture in the design of interventions or in the formulation of cases involves a variation on the uniformity myth of psychotherapy, in this case, what might be called the "cultural homogeneity myth" of child therapy.

CONCLUSION

Throughout this volume, our focus has been on two basic components of child psychotherapy—change processes and case formulations. However, change processes and case formulations are not disembodied constructs in clinical practice; instead they come to life through the person of the therapist, who constructs the formulations and crafts the interventions. Although a critical part of child psychotherapy involves the skillful formulation of a case and the careful selection of corresponding change processes, child psychotherapy simply cannot be reduced to accurate solutions to this matching problem. Variations in therapist characteristics, including level of skill, exert a significant impact on the efficacy of child psychotherapy. In fact, one of the earliest and most compelling accounts of "therapist effects" comes from the child psychotherapy literature, the often cited "supershrink" study conducted by Ricks (1974).

In this study, the long term outcomes of children treated by two therapists operating within the same therapeutic orientation were examined. Despite comparability in therapists' level of experience, treatment orientation, and caseloads, the outcomes for the two therapists were strikingly different. An analysis of comprehensive process notes revealed notable differences in therapeutic style, delivery, and manner; that is, the two therapists differed, despite shared orientation, not only in what they did, but also in their personal reactions and relationships with their child patients. In essence, long-term outcomes for these children were affected not only by *what* the therapist did, but *who* the therapist was. Moreover, this was by no means an isolated finding. Results from a number of large-scale studies of adult psychotherapy have revealed that the amount of outcome variance attributable to therapist characteristics is substantial, and at times, greater than the amount of variance accounted for by differences in technique (Crits-Christoph & Mintz, 1991; Lambert, 1989).

Relatively little is known about characteristics of effective child therapists. In fact, the only child therapist characteristic that has received more than passing attention has been the level of therapist training. Interestingly, this research has not yielded consistent main effects for therapist experience. Instead, level of therapist training has been shown to interact with child age and problem type, thus suggesting that training may enhance effectiveness with older and overcontrolled children (Weisz et al., 1987). But before one concludes that clinicians with limited training and experience may be as effective as seasoned veterans, it is important to note that treatments delivered by inexperienced clinicians frequently have been conducted in research contexts under the close supervision of experienced professionals.

Almost no attention has been paid to "nontechnical" characteristics of effective child therapists. In one study, Poal and Weisz (1989) found that the number of childhood behavior problems reported by therapists was related to the magnitude of change in their child clients' externalizing problems. This finding suggests that child therapists' personal histories may have an impact on their effectiveness with troubled children. Such an idea is by no means new; in fact, it is a basic tenet of psychoanalytically oriented treatment. Recently, however, there has been growing interest in specifying this relation by considering the impact of therapists' attachment experiences on their interactions with clients. Preliminary findings indicate that therapists attachment status affects both the level of interventions they pursue (Dozier, Cue, & Barnett, 1994) and dropout rates among their clients (Stuart, Pilkonis, Heape, Smith, & Fisher, 1991). These results suggest that therapist characteristics, in the form of personal relationship histories, could have an important impact on both the process and outcome of child psychotherapy. Future child therapy research will need to attend not only to what the therapist does, but also to who the therapist is. In summary, although we have emphasized change processes and case formulations as the essential ingredients of child psychotherapy, to extend the culinary metaphor, the successful outcome of any recipe depends on the experience and expertise of the person who brings the ingredients together.

Finally, it has been our hope that a reformulation of the essential ingredients of child psychotherapy would have an impact on both child psychotherapy research and practice. For the researcher, this reformulation demands a sharper focus on the processes that constitute specific forms of treatment than has been typically found in most child therapy research. Much greater attention must be directed to what actually transpires in and across child therapy sessions. Moreover, variations in the application of specific techniques and patterns of interaction need to be systematically related to treatment outcomes. In addition, researchers must recognize that diagnostically defined groups, even well-defined groups, are often far from homogeneous in terms of underlying pathogenic processes, and that unaccounted variations in these processes are likely to obscure the true effects of specific interventions.

For the practitioner, our approach underscores the fact that there is no substitute for the case formulation in the selection or design of effective interventions. Prescriptive treatments based solely on diagnostic criteria are unlikely to yield consistent results because of substantial variation in the pathogenic processes that produce or maintain children's symptoms. Consequently, diagnosis should not be equated with clinical assessment. The latter process is far more comprehensive and requires the clinician to evaluate children's focal problems in the context of their developmental and family histories. In turn, the development of a case formulation should direct clinicians to corresponding sets of change processes that could correct or compensate for disrupted internal psychological processes. Of course, this implies that child clinicians must be flexible in their approach to child psychotherapy. Allegiance to a single method of treatment or commitment to a "one size fits all" conceptualization of childhood disorders must be replaced by a formulation-guided approach to treatment selection. Given the tendency of most child practitioners to draw upon multiple methods, our recommendations simply amplify what is currently common in clinical practice. However, by no means are we advocating an atheoretical eclecticism. Instead, the choice of interventions must be anchored to formulations of pathogenic process. The theoretical coherence of our approach is based on the coordination of change processes with case formulations. In essence, the practice of child psychotherapy cannot be separated from the insights of developmental psychopathology.

In summary, surveys have revealed troubling gaps between research and practice in child psychotherapy, in part, because clinicians and researchers often find themselves speaking different languages. However, for child psychotherapy to thrive, the dialogic gap between researcher and practitioner must be bridged. It is hoped that our reformulation of the essential ingredients of child psychotherapy in terms of change processes and case formulations will provide these groups with a common dialect.

References

Abbeduto, L., & Rosenberg, S. (1985). Children's knowledge of the presuppositions of *know* and other cognitive verbs. *Journal of Child Language, 12,* 621–641.

Abramowitz, C. V. (1976). The effectiveness of group psychotherapy with children. *Archives of General Psychiatry, 33,* 320–326.

Achenbach, T. (1985). *Assessment and taxonomy of child and adolescent psychopathology.* Beverly Hills, CA: Sage.

Achenbach, T. M. (1990). Developmental psychopathology as a conceptual framework for training in multiple settings. In P. Magreb & P. Wohlford (Eds.), *Improving psychological services for children and adolescents with severe mental disorders: Clinical training in psychology* (pp. 79–84). Washington, DC: American Psychological Association.

Achenbach, T. M., & Edelbrock, C. S. (1981). Behavior problems and competencies reported by parents of normal and disturbed children aged 4 through 16. *Monographs of Society for Research in Child Development, 46* (1, Serial No. 188), 1–120.

Achenbach, T. M., & Edelbrock, C. (1983). *Manual for the Child Behavior Checklist and Revised Child Behavior Profile.* Burlington: University of Vermont.

Ainsworth, M., Blehar, M., Waters, E., & Wall, S. (1978). *Patterns of attachment.* Hillsdale, NJ: Erlbaum.

Alexander, J., & Parsons, B. (1973). Short-term behavioral intervention with delinquent families. *Journal of Abnormal Psychology, 81,* 219–225.

Allen, J. G., Newsom, G. E., Gabbard, G. O., & Coyne, L. (1984). Scales to assess the therapeutic alliance from a psychoanalytic perspective. *Bulletin of the Menninger Clinic, 48,* 383–400.

American Psychiatric Association. (1980). *Diagnostic and statistical manual of mental disorders* (3rd ed.). Washington, DC: Author.

Anderson, J. R. (1980). Concepts, propositions, and schemata: What are the cognitive units? In J. H. Flowers (Ed.), *Nebraska Symposium on Motivation: Cognitive processes* (Vol. 28, pp. 121–162). Lincoln: University of Nebraska Press.

Anthony, E. J. (1986). Contrasting neurotic styles in the analysis of two preschool children. *Journal of the American Academy of Child and Adolescent Psychiatry, 25,* 46–57.

Armsden, G., & Greenberg, M. (1987). Individual differences and their relationship to psychological well-being in adolescence. *Journal of Youth and Adolescence, 16,* 427–453.

Axline, V. (1947). *Play therapy.* Boston: Houghton Mifflin.

Babcock, H., & Levy, L. (1940). *Revision of the Babcock examination for measuring efficiency of mental functioning.* Chicago: Stoelting.

Baker, L., & Cantwell, D. P. (1987). Comparison of well, emotionally disordered and behaviorally disordered children with linguistic problems. *Journal of the American Academy of Child Psychiatry, 26,* 193–196.

Baldwin, J. (1992). Relational schemas and the processing of social information. *Psychological Bulletin, 112,* 461–484.

Banaji, M. R., & Prentice, D. A. (1994). The self in social contexts. *Annual Review of Psychology, 45,* 297–332.

Band, E., & Weisz, J. (1988). How to feel better when it feels bad: Children's perspectives on coping with everyday stress. *Developmental Psychology, 24,* 247–253.

Bandura, A. (1977). Self-efficacy: Toward a unifying theory of behavior change. *Psychological Review, 84,* 191–215.

Barber, J., & Crits-Christoph, P. (1993). Advances in measures of psychodynamic formulations. *Journal of Consulting and Clinical Psychology, 61,* 574–585.

Barden, R., Zelko, F., Duncan, W., & Masters, J. (1980). Children's consensual knowledge about the experiential determinants of emotion. *Journal of Personality and Social Psychology, 39,* 968–976.

Baron-Cohen, S. (1991). The theory of mind deficit in autism: How specific is it? *British Journal of Developmental Psychology, 9,* 301–314.

Baron-Cohen, S., Leslie, A. M., & Frith, U. (1986). Mechanical, behavioural, and intentional understanding of picture stories in autistic children. *British Journal of Developmental Psychology, 4,* 113–125.

Barrett, C., Hampe, I., & Miller, L. (1978). Research on child psychotherapy. In S. L. Garfield & A. E. Bergin (Eds.), *Handbook of psychotherapy and behavior change: An empirical analysis* (2nd ed., pp. 411–435). New York: Wiley.

Barrnett, R. J., Docherty, J. P., & Frommelt, G. M. (1991). A review of child clinical psychotherapy research since 1963. *Journal of the American Academy of Child and Adolescent Psychiatry, 30*(1), 1–14.

Bateson, M. C. (1979). "The epigenesis of conversational interaction": A personal account of research development. In M. Bullowa (Ed.), *Before speech: The beginning of interpersonal communication* (pp. 63–78). Cambridge, England: Cambridge University Press.

Baurer, P. J., & Wewerka, S. S. (1995). One- to two-year olds' recall of events: The more expressed, the more impressed. *Journal of Experimental Child Psychology, 59,* 475–496.

Baymur, F. B., & Patterson, C. H. (1960). A comparison of three methods of assisting underachieving high school students. *Journal of Counseling Psychology, 7,* 83–90.

Beck, A. (1967). *Depression: Clinical experimental and theoretical aspects.* New York: Hoeber.

Beck, A. (1976). *Cognitive therapy and the emotional disorders.* New York: Meridian.

Beck, A., Rush, H., Shaw, B., & Emery, A. (1979). *Cognitive therapy of depression.* New York: Guilford Press.

Bellack, L. (1986). *The TAT, CAT, and SAT in clinical use* (4th ed., rev.). Orlando, FL: Grune & Stratton.

Bennet-Kastor, T. (1983). Noun phrases and coherence in child narratives. *Journal of Child Language, 10,* 135–149.

Berger, M., & Kennedy, H. (1975). Pseudobackwardness in children. *Psychoanalytic Study of the Child, 30,* 279–306.

Bergin, A. E., & Garfield, S. L. (1971). *Handbook of psychotherapy and behavior change.* New York: Wiley.

Bergin, A. E., & Lambert, M. J. (1978). The evaluation of therapeutic outcomes. In S. L. Garfield & A. E. Bergin (Eds.), *Handbook of psychotherapy and behavior change: An empirical analysis* (2nd ed., pp. 139–189). New York: Wiley.

Berman, J. S., Miller, C. R., & Massman, J. (1985). Cognitive therapy versus systematic desensitization: Is one treatment superior? *Psychological Bulletin, 97,* 451–461.

Beutler, L. (1989). Differential treatment selection: The role of diagnosis in psychotherapy. *Psychotherapy: Theory, Research, Practice, and Training, 26,* 271–281.

Beutler, L. (1991). Have all won and must all have prizes? Revisiting Luborsky et al.'s verdict. *Journal of Consulting and Clinical Psychology, 59,* 226–232.

Bixler, R. (1949). Limits are therapy. *Journal of Consulting Psychology, 13,* 1–11.

Blatt, S. (1974). Levels of object representation in anaclitic and introjective depression. *Psychoanalytic Study of the Child, 24,* 107–157.

Boll, T. J. (1971). Systematic observation of behavior change with older children in group therapy. *Psychological Reports, 28,* 26.

Bonner, B., & Everett, F. (1982). Influence of client preparation and therapist prognostic expectations on children's attitudes and expectations of psychotherapy. *Journal of Clinical Child Psychology, 11,* 202–208.

Bordin, E. S. (1979). The generalizability of the psychoanalytic concept of working alliance. *Psychotherapy: Theory, Research, and Practice, 16,* 252–260.

Bornstein, M. (Ed.). (1991). *Cultural approaches to parenting.* Hillsdale, NJ: Erlbaum.

Boutte, M. A. (1971). Play therapy practices in approved counseling agencies. *Journal of Clinical Psychology, 27,* 150–152.

Bowlby, J. (1958). The nature of the child's tie to his mother. *International Journal of Psycho-Analysis, 39,* 350–373.

Bowlby, J. (1973). *Attachment and loss: Vol. 2. Separation anxiety and anger.* New York: Basic Books.

Bowlby, J. (1980). *Attachment and loss: Vol. 3. Loss, sadness, and depression.* New York: Basic Books.

Bowlby, J. (1988). *A secure base: Parent–child attachment and healthy human development.* New York: Basic Books.

Braswell, L. (1991). Involving parents in cognitive-behavioral therapy with children and adolescents. In P. Kendall (Ed.), *Child and adolescent therapy: Cognitive-behavioral procedures* (pp. 316–351). New York: Guilford Press.

Bretherton, I. (1991). Intentional communication and the development of an understanding of mind. In D. Frye and C. Moore (Eds.), *Children's theories of mind: Mental states and social understanding* (pp. 49–75). Hillsdale, NJ: Erlbaum.

Bretherton, I., & Beeghly, M. (1982). Talking about internal states: The acquisition of an explicit theory of mind. *Developmental Psychology, 18,* 906–921.

Bretherton, I., Fritz, J., Zahn-Waxler, C., & Ridgeway, D. (1986). Learning to talk about emotions: A functionalist perspective. *Child Development, 57,* 529–548.

Brody, L., & Carter, A. (1982). Children's emotional attributions to self versus other: An exploration of an assumption underlying projective techniques. *Journal of Consulting and Clinical Psychology, 50,* 665–671.

Brody, L., Rozek, M., & Muten, E. (1985). Age, sex, and individual differences in children's defense styles. *Journal of Clinical Child Psychology, 14,* 132–138.

Brown, A. L., & Ferrara, R. A. (1985). Diagnosing zones of proximal development. In J. V. Wertsch (Ed.), *Culture, communication, and cognition: Vygotskian perspectives* (pp. 273–305). Cambridge, MA: Cambridge University Press.

Brown, J. R., & Dunn, J. (1991). "You can cry, mum": The social and developmental implications of talk about internal states. *British Journal of Developmental Psychology, 9,* 237–256.

Brown, R. (1977). Introduction. In C. E. Snow & C. A. Ferguson (Eds.), *Talking to children: Language input and acquisition* (pp. 1–27). Cambridge, England: Cambridge University Press.

Bruner, J. (1983). *Child's talk: Learning to use language.* New York: Norton.

Bruner, J. (1986). *Actual minds, possible worlds.* Cambridge, MA: Harvard University Press.

Buchsbaum, H., Toth, S., Clyman, R., Cicchetti, D., & Emde, R. (1992). The use of narrative story stem technique with maltreated children: Implications for theory and practice. *Development and Psychopathology, 4,* 603–625.

Burke, A. E., Crenshaw, D. A., Green, J., Schlosser, M. A., & Strocchia-Rivera, L. (1989). Influence of verbal ability on the expression of aggression in physically abused children. *Journal of the American Academy of Child and Adolescent Psychiatry, 28,* 215–218.

Burns, D., & Nolen-Hoeksema, S. (1992). Therapeutic empathy and recovery from depression in cognitive-behavioral therapy: A structural equation model. *Journal of Consulting and Clinical Psychology, 60,* 441–449.

Campagna, A. F., & Harter, S. (1975). Moral judgment in sociopathic and normal children. *Journal of Personality and Social Psychology, 31,* 199–205.

Campos, J. (1983). The importance of affective communication in social referencing: A commentary of Feinman. *Merrill–Palmer Quarterly, 29,* 83–87.

Camras, L., Grow, G., & Ribordy, S. (1983). Recognition of emotional expression by abused children. *Journal of Clinical Child Psychology, 12,* 325–328.

Cantor, N., Smith, E., French, R., & Mezzich, J. (1980). Psychiatric diagnosis as prototype categorization. *Journal of Abnormal Psychology, 89,* 181–193.

Cantwell, D. P., & Baker, L. (1987). *Developmental speech and language disorders.* New York: Guilford Press.

Carkhuff, R., & Berenson, B. (1967). *Beyond counseling and therapy.* New York: Holt, Rinehart & Winston.

Carroll, J., & Steward, M. (1984). The role of cognitive development in children's understanding of their own feelings. *Child Development, 55,* 1486–1492.

Casey, R. J., & Berman, J. (1985). The outcome of psychotherapy with children. *Psychological Bulletin, 98,* 388–400.

Cassidy, J., & Kobak, R. (1988). Avoidance and its relation to other defensive processes. In J. Belsky & T. Neworski (Eds.), *Clinical implications of attachment* (pp. 300–323). Hillsdale, NJ: Erlbaum.

Cattell, R. B., & Luborsky, L. B. (1950). P-technique demonstrated as a new clinical method for determining personality and symptom structure. *Journal of General Psychology, 42,* 3–24.

Chandler, M. (1973). Egocentrism and anti-social behavior: The assessment and training of social perspective taking skills. *Developmental Psychology, 9,* 326–332.

Chandler, M., Greenspan, S., & Barenboim, C. (1974). Assessment and training of role-taking and referential communication skills in institutionalized emotionally-disturbed children. *Developmental Psychology, 10,* 546–553.

Chandler, M., Paget, K., & Koch, D. (1978). The child's demystification of psychological defense mechanisms: A structural and developmental analysis. *Developmental Psychology, 14,* 197–205.

Chethik, M. (1989). *Techniques of child therapy: Psychodynamic strategies.* New York: Guilford Press.

Cicchetti, D., Ganiban, J., & Barnett, D. (1991). Contributions from the study of high risk populations to understanding the development of emotion regulation. In J. Garber & K. Dodge (Eds.), *The development of emotion regulation and dysregulation* (pp. 15–48). New York: Cambridge University Press.

Cohen, L., Sargent, M., & Sechrest, L. (1986). Use of psychotherapy research by professional psychologists. *American Psychologist, 41,* 188–197.

Cohen, S., & Wills, T. (1985). Stress, social support, and the buffering hypothesis. *Psychological Bulletin, 98,* 310–357.

Cohler, B. J. (1982). Personal narrative and life discourse. In P. B. Baltes & O. G. Brim, Jr. (Eds.), *Life span development and behavior* (Vol. 4, pp. 205–241). New York: Academic Press.

Cole, P., Michel, M., & O'Donnell, L. (1994). The development of emotion regulation and dysregulation: A clinical perspective. In N. Fox (Ed.), *Monographs of the Society for Research on Child Development, 59,* 73–100.

Cole, P., & Zahn-Waxler, C. (1992). Emotional dysregulation in disruptive behavior disorders. In D. Cicchetti & S. Toth (Eds.), *Rochester symposium on developmental psychopathology* (Vol. 4, pp. 173–209). Rochester, NY: University of Rochester Press.

Coleman, D., & Kaplan, M. (1990). Effects of pretherapy videotape preparation on child therapy outcomes. *Professional Psychology: Research and Practice, 21,* 199–203.

Collins, N., & Read, S. (1990). Adult attachment, working models, and relationship quality in dating couples. *Journal of Personality and Social Psychology, 58,* 644–663.

Collins, J. T., Day, J. R., & Russell, R. L. (1993). *Sincerity, appropriateness, and truth in the Gloria Tapes: Tracking the pulse of therapeutic interaction.* Paper presented at the Ninth Annual Conference of the Society for the Exploration of Psychotherapy Integration, New York.

Compas, B. (1987). Coping with stress during childhood and adolescence. *Psychological Bulletin, 101,* 393–403.

Condon, W. (1979). Neonatal entrainment and enculturation. In M. Bullowa (Ed.), *Before speech: The beginning of interpersonal communication* (pp. 131–148). Cambridge, England: Cambridge University Press.

Conti, D. J., & Camras, L. A. (1984). Children's understanding of conversational principles. *Journal of Experimental Child Psychology, 38,* 456–463.

Cooley, C. H. (1902). *Human nature and the social order.* New York: Charles Scribner's Sons.

Costantino, G., Malgady, R., & Rogler, L. (1986). Cuento therapy: A culturally sensitive modality for Puerto Rican children. *Journal of Consulting and Clinical Psychology, 5,* 639–645.

Cowan, P. (1988). Developmental psychopathology: A nine-cell map of the territory. In E. Nannis & P. Cowan (Eds.), *Developmental psychopathology and its treatment* (pp. 5–30). San Francisco: Jossey-Bass.

Cramer, P. (1979). Defense mechanisms in adolescence. *Developmental Psychology, 15,* 476–477.

Cramer, P. (1983). Children's use of defense mechanisms in reaction to displeasure caused by others. *Journal of Personality, 51,* 78–94.

Cramer, P. (1987). The development of defense mechanisms. *Journal of Personality, 55,* 597–614.

Cramer, P., & Carter, T. (1978). The relationship between sexual identification and the use of defense mechanisms. *Journal of Personality Assessment, 42,* 63–73.

Crick, N., & Dodge, K. (1994). A review and reformulation of social information-processing mechanisms in children's social adjustment. *Psychological Bulletin, 115,* 74–101.

Crits-Christoph, P., Cooper, A., & Luborsky, L. (1988). The accuracy of therapists' interpretations and the outcome of dynamic psychotherapy. *Journal of Consulting and Clinical Psychology, 56,* 490–495.

Crits-Christoph, P., & Mintz, J. (1991). Implications of therapist effects for the design and analysis of comparative studies of psychotherapies. *Journal of Consulting and Clinical Psychology, 59,* 20–26.

Czogalik, D., & Russell, R. L. (1994a). Key processes of client participation in psychotherapy: Chronography and narration. *Psychotherapy: Theory, Research, Practice, and Training, 31,* 170–182.

Czogalik, D., & Russell, R. L. (1994b). Structures of therapist participation in psychotherapy. *Psychotherapy Research, 4,* 75–94.

Czogalik, D., & Russell, R. L. (1995). Interactional structures of therapist and client participation in adult psychotherapy: P-technique and chronography. *Journal of Consulting and Clinical Psychology, 63,* 28–36.

Dana, R. H., & Dana, J. M. (1969). Systematic observation of children's behavior in group therapy. *Psychological Reports, 24,* 134.

Danish, S. J., & Kagan, N. (1971). Measurement of affective sensitivity: Toward a valid measure of interpersonal perception. *Journal of Counseling Psychology, 18,* 51–54.

Davis, A., Singer, D., & Morris-Friehe, M. (1991). Language skills of delinquent and nondelinquent adolescent males. *Journal of Communicative Disorders, 24,* 251–266.

Day, L., & Reznikoff, M. (1980). Preparation of children and parents for treatment at a children's psychiatric clinic through videotaped modeling. *Journal of Consulting and Clinical Psychology, 48,* 303–304.

Demos, V. (1986). Crying in early infancy: An illustration of the motivational function of affect. In T. Brazelton & M. Yogman (Eds.), *Affective development in infancy* (pp. 39–74). Norwood, NJ: Ablex.

Dennis, M., Jacennik, B., & Barnes, M. A. (1994). The content of narrative discourse in children and adolescents after early-onset hydrocephalus and in normally developing age peers. *Brain and Language, 46,* 129–165.

Densmore, A., & McCabe, A. (1994). *Up in the air: Contrastive narrative form in inpatient children with and without post-traumatic stress disorder.* Paper presented at Eastern Psychological Association, Boston, MA.

DiGiuseppe, R. (1981). Cognitive therapy with children. In G. Emery, S. Hollon, & R. Bedrosian (Eds.), *New directions in cognitive therapy* (pp. 50–67). New York: Guilford Press.

Dodge, K. A. (1980). Social cognition and children's aggressive behavior. *Child Development, 51,* 162–170.

Dodge, K. A. (1985). Attributional bias in aggressive children. In P. Kendall (Ed.), *Advances in cognitive-behavioral research and therapy* (Vol. 4, pp. 73–110). New York: Academic Press.

Dodge, K. A. (1991). Emotion and social information processing. In J. Garber & K. A. Dodge (Eds.), *The development of emotion regulation and dysregulation* (pp. 159–181). New York: Cambridge University Press.

Dodge, K. A., & Frame, C. (1982). Social cognitive biases and deficits in aggressive boys. *Child Development, 53,* 620–635.

Dodge, K. A., & Garber, J. (1991). Domains of emotion regulation. In J. Garber & K. A. Dodge (Eds.), *The development of emotion regulation and dysregulation.* New York: Cambridge University Press.

Dodge, K. A., Price, J., Bachorowski, J., & Newman, J. (1990). Hostile attribution biases in severely aggressive adolescents. *Journal of Abnormal Psychology, 99,* 385–392.

Donaldson, S., & Westerman, M. (1986). Development of children's understanding of ambivalence and causal theories of emotion. *Developmental Psychology, 26,* 655–662.

Dorfman, E. (1951). Play therapy. In C. Rogers (Ed.), *Client-centered therapy* (pp. 237–277). Boston: Houghton Mifflin.

Dozier, M., Cue, K., & Barnett, L. (1994). Clinicians as caregivers: Role of attachment organization in treatment. *Journal of Consulting and Clinical Psychology, 62,* 793–800.

Durlak, J., Fuhrman, T., & Lampman, C. (1991). Effectiveness of cognitive-behavioral therapy for maladapting children: A meta-analysis. *Psychological Bulletin, 110,* 204–214.

Eisemajer, R., & Prior, M. (1991). Cognitive linguistic correlates of "theory of mind" ability in autistic children. *British Journal of Developmental Psychology, 9,* 351–354.

Ellis, P. L. (1982). Empathy: A factor in antisocial behavior. *Journal of Abnormal Child Psychiatry, 12,* 385–395.

Eltz, M., Shirk, S., & Sarlin, N. (1995). Alliance formation and treatment outcome among maltreated adolescents. *Child Abuse and Neglect, 19,* 419–431.

Erikson, E. (1963). Play and cure. In *Childhood and society* (pp. 222–234). New York: Norton.

Erikson, E. (1964). Clinical observations of play disruption in young children. In M. Haworth (Ed.), *Child psychotherapy* (pp. 264–276). New York: Basic Books.

Essig, T., & Russell, R. L. (1990). Analyzing subjectivity in therapeutic discourse: Rogers, Pearls, Ellis, and Gloria revisited. *Psychotherapy: Theory, Research, Practice and Training, 27,* 271–281.

Estrada, A. U., Russell, R. L., Durlak, J., Elling, K., Piette, J., & Jones, M. E. (1994a, July). *Interactional structures of therapist and client participation in child psychotherapy.* Paper presented at the Society for Psychotherapy Research, York, England.

Estrada, A. U., Russell, R. L., Durlak, J., Elling, K., Piette, J., & Jones, M. E. (1994b, November). *Structures of child participation in psychotherapy.* Paper presented at the North American Society for Psychotherapy Research, Santa Fe, NM.

Estrada, A. U., Russell, R. L., Durlak, J., Elling, K., Piette, J., & Jones, M. E. (1994c, November). *Structures of therapist participation in child psychotherapy.* Paper presented at the North American Society for Psychotherapy Research, Santa Fe, NM.

Estrada, A. U., Russell, R. L., McGlinchey, K., & Hoffman, L. (1994, October). *The development of the Loyola child and child therapist psychotherapy process scales.* Paper presented at the First Kansas Conference on Clinical Child Psychology, Lawrence, KS.

Evans, I. (1994). *Principles and criteria for science-based education: Psychological assessment and diagnosis.* Paper presented at meetings of Council of University Directors of Clinical Psychology (CUDCP). San Antonio, TX.

Evans, M. A. (1987). Discourse characteristics of reticent children. *Applied Psycholinguistics, 8,* 171–184.

Eysenck, H. J. (1952). The effects of psychotherapy: An evaluation. *Journal of Consulting Clinical Psychology, 16,* 319–324.

Eysenck, H. J. (1961). The effects of psychotherapy. In H. J. Eysenck (Ed.), *Handbook of abnormal psychology.* New York: Basic Books.

Eysenck, H. J. (1966). *The effects of psychotherapy (with commentary).* New York: International Universities Press.

Eysenck, H. J. (1978). An exercise in mega-silliness. *American Psychologist, 33,* 517.

Eysenck, H. J. (1995). Meta-analysis squared: Does it make sense? *American Psychologist, 50,* 110–111.

Fauber, R., & Long, N. (1991). Children in context: The role of the family in child psychotherapy. *Journal of Consulting and Clinical Psychology, 59,* 813–820.

Feldman, C. F. (1988). Early forms of thought about thoughts: Some simple linguistic expressions of mental state. In J. Astington, P. Harris, & D. Olson (Eds.), *Developing theories of mind* (pp. 126–137). Cambridge, England: Cambridge University Press.

Ferguson, C. A. (1977). Baby talk as a simplified register. In C. E. Snow & C. A. Ferguson (Eds.), *Talking to children: Language input and acquisition* (pp. 219–236). Cambridge, England: Cambridge University Press.

Filmer-Bennett, G., & Hillson, J. S. (1959). Some child therapy practices. *Journal of Clinical Psychology, 15,* 105–106.

Fischer, K. (1980). A theory of cognitive development: The control and construction of hierarchies of skills. *Psychological Review, 87,* 477–531.

Fisher, E. P. (1992). The impact of play on development: A meta-analysis. *Play and Culture, 5,* 159–181.

Fisher, W. R. (1984). Narration as a human communication paradigm: The case of public moral argument. *Communication Monographs, 52,* 347–367.

Fivush, R. (1991). The social construction of personal narratives. *Merrill–Palmer Quarterly, 37,* 59–81.

Fivush, R., & Fromhoff, F. A. (1988). Style and structure in mother–child conversations about the past. *Discourse Processes, 11,* 337–355.

Fivush, R., & Slackman, E. A. (1986). The acquisition and development of scripts. In K. Nelson (Ed.), *Event memory* (pp. 71–96). Hillsdale, NJ: Erlbaum.

Flavell, J. (1977). *Cognitive development.* Englewood Cliffs, NJ: Prentice-Hall.

Fonagy, P., & Target, M. (1994). The efficacy of psychoanalysis for children with disruptive disorders. *Journal of the American Academy of Child and Adolescent Psychiatry, 33,* 45–55.

Forehand, R., & Wierson, M. (1993). The role of developmental factors in planning behavioral interventions for children: Disruptive behavior as an example. *Behavior Therapy, 24,* 117–141.

Frank, J. (1974). Therapeutic components of psychotherapy. *Journal of Nervous and Mental Disease, 159,* 325–342.

Franzke, E. (1989). *Fairy tales in psychotherapy: The creative use of old and new tales.* Lewiston, NY: Hogrefe & Huber.

Freud, A. (1946). *The psychoanalytical treatment of children.* New York: International Universities Press.

Freud, A. (1965). *Normality and pathology in childhood: Assessments of development.* New York: International Universities Press.

Freud, A. (1966). *The ego and the mechanisms of defense.* New York: International Universities Press.

Freud, A. (1968). Indications and contraindications for child analysis. *Psychoanalytic Study of the Child, 23,* 37–46.

Freud, A. (1971). The infantile neurosis—Genetic and dynamic considerations. *Psychoanalytic Study of the Child, 26,* 79–90.

Freud, S. (1909). Phobia in a five year old boy. In *Collected papers* (Vol. 3, pp. 149–295). London: Basic Books.

Freud, S. (1940). *An outline of psychoanalysis.* New York: Norton.

Freud, S. (1946). *New introductory lectures.* London: Hogarth Press.

Freud, S. (1949). *An outline of psychoanalysis.* New York: Norton.

Friedman, R. J. (1975). The young child who does not talk. *Clinical Pediatrics, 14,* 403–406.

Frieswyk, S., Allen, J., Colson, D., Coyne, L., Gabbard, G., Horowitz, L., & Newsome, G. (1986). Therapeutic alliance: Its place as a process and outcome variable in psychotherapy research. *Journal of Consulting and Clinical Psychology, 54,* 32–38.

Garber, J., Braafladt, N., & Zeman, J. (1991). The regulation of sad affect: An information processing perspective. In J. Garber & K. Dodge (Eds.), *The development of emotion regulation and dysregulation* (pp. 208–242). New York: Cambridge University Press.

Gardner, R. A. (1971). *Therapeutic communication with children: The mutual storytelling technique.* New York: Science House.

Garfield, S. L., & Bergin, A. E. (Eds.). (1978). *Handbook of psychotherapy and behavior change* (2nd ed.). New York: Wiley.

Garland, E., & Weiss, M. (1995). Subgroups of adolescent depression. *Journal of the American Academy of Child and Adolescent Psychiatry, 34,* 831.

Garmezy, N. (1985). Stress-resilient children: The search for protective factors. In J. E. Stevenson (Ed.), *Recent research in development psychopathology* (pp. 213–233). Oxford: Pergamon Press.

Garvey, C. (1977). *Play.* Cambridge, MA: Harvard University Press.

Gerlsma, C., Emmelkamp, P., & Arrindell, W. (1990). Anxiety, depression, and perception of early parenting: A meta-analysis. *Clinical Psychology Review, 10,* 251–277.

Gendlin, E. (1974). Client-centered and experiential psychotherapy. In D. Wexler & L. Rice (Eds.), *Innovations in client-centered therapy* (pp. 211–246). New York: Wiley.

Genlette, G. (1980). *Narrative discourse.* Ithaca, NY: Cornell University Press.

Gibbons, J., & Foreman, S. (1989, June). *Advances in child psychotherapy research using the Mt. Zion Psychotherapy Research Model.* Panel presented at meetings of the Society for Psychotherapy Research, Wintergreen, VA.

Ginott, H. (1964). The theory and practice of 'therapeutic intervention' in child treatment. *Journal of Consulting Psychology, 23,* 160–166.

Glasberg, R., & Aboud, F. (1982). Keeping one's distance from sadness: Children's reports of emotional experience. *Developmental Psychology, 18,* 287–293.

Gomes-Schwartz, B. (1978). Effective ingredients in psychotherapy: Prediction of outcome from process variables. *Journal of Consulting and Clinical Psychology, 46,* 1023–1035.

Gottman, J. (1986). Merging social cognition and behavior. *Monographs of the Society for Research in Child Development, 51*(2, Serial No. 213).

Greenberg, L., & Safran, J. (1987). *Emotion in psychotherapy.* New York: Guilford Press.

Greenberg, L., & Safran, J. (1989). Emotion in psychotherapy. *American Psychologist, 44,* 19–29.

Greenwald, S., & Russell, R. L. (1991). *Psychotherapy Research, 1,* 17–24.

Grice, H. P. (1975). Logic and conversation. In P. Cole & J. L. Morgan (Eds.), *Syntax and semantics* (Vol. 3, pp. 41–58). New York: Academic Press.

Guerney, B., Jr., Burton, J., Silverberg, D., & Shapiro, E. (1965). Use of adult responses to codify children's behavior in a play situation. *Perceptual and Motor Skills, 20,* 614–616.

Guidano, V. F., & Liotti, G. (1983). *Cognitive processes and emotional disorders.* New York: Guilford Press.

Guidano, V. F., & Liotti, G. (1985). A constructivistic foundation for cognitive therapy. In M. Mahoney & A. Freeman (Eds.), *Cognition and psychotherapy* (pp. 101–142). New York: Plenum Press.

Gumaer, J. (1984). *Counseling and therapy for children.* New York: Free Press.

Guntrip, H. (1971). *Psychoanalytic theory, therapy, and the self.* New York: Basic Books.

Gurman, A. S., & Kniskern, D. P. (1978). Research on marital and family therapy: Progress, perspective, and prospect. In S. L. Garfield & A. E. Bergin (Eds.), *Handbook of behavior therapy and behavior change: An empirical analysis* (2nd ed., pp. 817–901). New York: Wiley.

Halberstadt, A. G. (1986). Family socialization of emotional expression and nonverbal communication skills. *Journal of Personality and Social Psychology, 51,* 827–836.

Hambleton, G., Wandrei, M., & Russell, R. L. (in press). Narrative performance as a predictor of psychopathology. *Journal of Narrative and Life History.*

Harris, P. (1983). Children's understanding of the link between situation and emotion. *Journal of Experimental Child Psychology, 36,* 490–509.

Harris, P., & Lipian, M. (1989). Understanding emotion and experiencing emotion. In C. Saarni & P. Harris (Eds.), *Children's understanding of emotion* (pp. 241–258). New York: Cambridge University Press.

Harris, P., Olthot, T., & Meerum Terwogt, M. (1981). Children's knowledge of emotion. *Journal of Child Psychology and Psychiatry, 45,* 247–261.

Harter, S. (1977). A cognitive-developmental approach to children's expression of conflicting feelings and a technique to facilitate such expression in play therapy. *Journal of Consulting and Clinical Psychology, 45,* 417–432.

Harter, S. (1985). *The Self-Perception Profile for Children.* University of Denver, Denver, CO.

Harter, S. (1986). Processes underlying the construction, maintenance, and enhancement of the self-concept in children. In J. Suls & A. Greenwald (Eds.), *Psychological perspectives on the self* (Vol. 3). Hillsdale, NJ: Erlbaum.

Harter, S. (1988). Developmental and dynamic changes in the nature of the self-concept: Implications for child psychotherapy. In S. Shirk (Ed.), *Cognitive development and child psychotherapy* (pp. 119–160). New York: Plenum Press.

Harter, S., & Buddin, B. (1987). Children's understanding of the simultaneity of two emotions: A five stage developmental acquisition sequence. *Developmental Psychology, 23,* 388–399.

Harter, S., & Whitesell, N. (1989). Developmental changes in children's understanding of single, multiple, and blended emotion concepts. In C. Saarni & P. Harris (Eds.), *Children's understanding of emotion* (pp. 81–116). New York: Cambridge University Press.

Hartmann, H. (1939). *Ego psychology and the problem of adaptation.* New York: International Universities Press.

Hay, D. F. (1994). Prosocial development. *Journal of Child Psychology and Psychiatry, 35*(1), 29–77.

Hazzelrigg, M., Cooper, H., & Borduin, C. (1987). Evaluating the effectiveness of family therapies: An integrative review and analysis. *Psychological Bulletin, 101,* 428–442.

Heinicke, C. M., & Goldman, A. (1960). Research on psychotherapy with children: A review and suggestions for further study. *American Journal of Orthopsychiatry, 30,* 483–494.

Heinicke, C. M., & Strassman, L. H. (1975). Toward more effective research on child psychotherapy. *Journal of the American Academy of Child Psychiatry, 14,* 561–588.

Henry, W. E. (1973). *The analysis of fantasy.* Huntington, NY: Krieger.

Hinshaw, S. P. (1992). Externalizing behavior problems and academic under-achievement in childhood and adolescence: Causal relationships and under-lying mechanisms. *Psychological Bulletin, 111,* 127–155.

Hood-Williams, J. (1960). The results of psychotherapy with children: A re-evaluation. *Journal of Consulting Psychology, 24,* 84–88.

Horowitz, L., Post, D., French, R., Wallis, K., & Siegelman, E. (1981). The prototype as a construct in abnormal psychology: Clarifying disagreements in psychiatric judgments. *Journal of Abnormal Psychology, 90,* 575–585.

Horowitz, L., Wright, J., Lowenstein, E., & Parad, H. (1981). The prototype as a construct in abnormal psychology: A method for deriving prototypes. *Journal of Abnormal Psychology, 90,* 568–574.

Horvath, A., & Luborsky, L. (1993). The role of the therapeutic alliance in psychotherapy. *Journal of Consulting and Clinical Psychology, 61,* 561–573.

Howe, P. A., & Silvern, L. E. (1981). Behavioral observation of children during play therapy: Preliminary development of a research instrument. *Journal of Personality Assessment, 45*(2), 168–182.

Hudson, J. A. (1991). Learning to reminisce: A case study. *Journal of Narrative and Life History, 1,* 295–324.

Jessee, E., Jurkovic, G., Wilkie, J., & Chiglinski, M. (1982). Positive reframing with children: Conceptual and clinical issues. *American Journal of Orthopsychiatry, 52,* 314–322.

Johnson, C. J., & Wellman, H. M. (1982). Children's developing conceptions of the mind and brain. *Child Development, 53,* 222–234.

Jones, M. C. (1924). A laboratory study of fear: The case of Peter. *Pedagogical Seminary, 31,* 308–315.

Jurkovic, C. J., & Prentice, N. M. (1977). Relation of moral and cognitive development to dimensions of juvenile delinquency. *Journal of Abnormal Psychology, 86,* 414–420.

Kahn, E. (1985). Heinz Kohut and Carl Rogers: A timely comparison. *American Psychologist, 40,* 893–904.

Kane, M., & Kendall, P. (1989). Anxiety disorders in children: A multiple-baseline evaluation of a cognitive-behavioral treatment. *Behavior Therapy, 20,* 499–508.

Kaplan, A. (1983). Empathic communication in the psychotherapy relationship. In J. Jordan, J. Surrey, & A. Kaplan (Eds.), *Women and empathy* (pp. 12–16). Wellesley, MA: Stone Center for Developmental Services and Studies.

Kaslow, N., Rehm, L., & Siegel, A. (1984). Social-cognitive and cognitive correlates of depression in children. *Journal of Abnormal Child Psychology, 12,* 605–620.

Kaslow, N., Stark, K., Printz, B., Livingston, R., & Tsai, S. (1992). Cognitive triad inventory for children: Development and relation to depression and anxiety. *Journal of Clinical Child Psychology, 21,* 339–347.

Kazdin, A. (1988). *Child psychotherapy: Developing and identifying effective treatments.* New York: Pergamon Press.

Kazdin, A. E. (1990a). Premature termination from treatment among children referred for anti-social behavior. *Journal of Child Psychology, 31,* 415–425.

Kazdin, A. E. (1990b). Psychotherapy for children and adolescents. *Annual Review of Psychology, 41,* 21–54.

Kazdin, A. E. (1991). Effectiveness of psychotherapy with children and adolescents. *Journal of Consulting and Clinical Psychology, 59,* 785–789.

Kazdin, A. E. (1993a). Adolescent mental health prevention treatment programs. *American Psychologist, 48*(2), 127–141.

Kazdin, A. E. (1993b). Psychotherapy for children and adolescents' current progress and future directions. *American Psychologist, 48*(6), 644–657.

Kazdin, A. E., Bass, D., Ayers, W. A., & Rodgers, A. (1990). Empirical and clinical focus of child and adolescent psychotherapy research. *Journal of Consulting and Clinical Psychology, 58*(6), 729–740.

Kazdin, A., French, N., & Sherick, R. (1981). Acceptability of alternative treatments for children: Evaluations by inpatient children, parents, and staff. *Journal of Consulting and Clinical Psychology, 49,* 900–907.

Kazdin, A., French, N., Unis, A., & Esveldt-Dawson, K. (1983). Child, mother, father evaluations of depression in psychiatric inpatient children. *Journal of Abnormal Child Psychology, 11,* 167–180.

Kazdin, A., & Kagan, J. (1994). Models of dysfunction in developmental psychopathology. *Clinical Psychology: Science and Practice, 1,* 35–52.

Kazdin, A., Siegel, T., & Bass, D. (1990). Drawing upon clinical practice to inform research on child and adolescent psychotherapy. *Professional Psychology: Research and Practice, 21,* 189–198.

Kemple, K., Speranza, H., & Hazen, N. (1992). Cohesive discourse and peer acceptance: Longitudinal relations in the preschool years. *Merrill–Palmer Quarterly, 38*(3), 364–381.

Kendall, P. (1981). Cognitive-behavioral interventions with children. In B. Lahey & A. Kazdin (Eds.), *Advances in clinical child psychology* (Vol. 4, pp. 53–90). New York: Plenum Press.

Kendall, P. C. (1984). Social cognition and problem solving: A developmental and child-clinical interface. In B. Gholson & T. Rosenthal (Eds.), *Applications of cognitive-developmental theory* (pp. 115–148). New York: Academic Press.

Kendall, P. (1985). Toward a cognitive-behavioral model of child psychopathology and a critique of related interventions. *Journal of Abnormal Child Psychology, 31,* 357–372.

Kendall, P. (Ed.). (1991a). *Child and adolescent therapy: Cognitive-behavioral procedures.* New York: Guilford Press.

Kendall, P. C. (1993). Cognitive-behavioral therapies with youth: Guiding theory, current status, and emerging developments. *Journal of Consulting and Clinical Psychology, 61,* 235–247.

Kendall, P., Chansky, T., Freidman, M., Kim, R., Kortlander, E., Sessa, F., &

Siqueland, L. (1991). Treating anxiety disorders in children and adolescents. In P. Kendall (Ed.), *Child and adolescent therapy: Cognitive-behavioral procedures* (pp. 131–164). New York: Guilford Press.

Kendall, P., Kane, M., Howard, B., & Siqueland, L. (1989). *Cognitive-behavioral therapy for anxious children: Treatment manual.* Unpublished treatment manual. Temple University, Philadelphia: PA.

Kendall, P., Lerner, R., & Craighead, W. (1984). Human development and intervention in child psychopathology. *Child Development, 55,* 71–82, 777–784.

Kendall, P., & Panichelli-Mendel, S. (1995). Cognitive-behavioral treatments. *Journal of Abnormal Child Psychology, 23,* 107–124.

Kendall, P. C., Stark, K. D., & Adam, T. (1990). Cognitive deficit or cognitive distortion in childhood depression. *Journal of Abnormal Child Psychology, 18,* 255–270.

Kennedy, H. (1971). Problems in reconstruction in child analysis. *The Psychoanalytic Study of the Child, 26,* 386–402.

Kennedy, H. (1979). The role of insight in child analysis: A developmental viewpoint. *Journal of the American Psychoanalytic Society, 27,* 9–29.

Kernberg, P. F. (1992). Discussion of "A re-evaluation of estimates of child therapy effectiveness." *Journal of the American Academy of Child and Adolescent Psychiatry, 31*(4), 710.

Kernberg, P. F., & Chazan, S. (1991). *Children with conduct disorders: A psychotherapy manual.* New York: Basic Books.

Kiesler, D. (1966). Some myths of psychotherapy research and a search for a paradigm. *Psychological Bulletin, 65,* 110–136.

Kiesler, D. J. (1988). Therapeutic metacommunication: Therapist impact disclosure as feedback in psychotherapy. Palo Alto, CA: Consulting Psychologists Press.

Klein, G. (1954). Need and regulation. In M. R. Jones (Ed.), *Nebraska Symposium on Motivation* (Vol. 2, pp. 224–274). Lincoln: University of Nebraska Press.

Klein, M. H. (1975). *The psychoanalysis of children.* London: Hogarth Press.

Klein, M. H., Mathieu, P. L., Gendlin, E. T., & Kiesler, D. J. (1969). *The Experiencing Scale: A research and training manual* (2 vols.). Madison: Bureau of Audio Visual Instruction, University of Wisconsin.

Kobak, R., Cole, H., Ferenz-Gillies, R., Fleming, W., & Gamble, W. (1993). Attachment and emotion regulation during mother–teen problem-solving: A control theory analysis. *Child Development, 64,* 231–245.

Kobak, R., & Sceery, A. (1988). Attachment in late adolescence: Working models, affect regulation, and representations of self and other. *Child Development, 59,* 135–146.

Kobak, R., Sudler, N., & Gamble, W. (1991). Attachment and depressive symptoms in adolescence: A developmental pathways analysis. *Development and Psychopathology, 3,* 461–474.

Kobak, R., & Waters, D. (1984). Family therapy as a rite of passage: The play's the thing. *Family Process, 23,* 89–100.

Kohut, H. (1977). *The restoration of the self.* New York: International Universities Press.

Kolvin, L., Garside, R. F., Nicol, A. R., MacMillan, A., Wolstenholme, F., & Leitch, I. M. (1981). *Help starts here: The maladjusted child in the ordinary school.* London: Tavistock.

Koocher, G., & Pedulla, B. (1977). Current practices in child psychotherapy. *Professional Psychology, 8,* 275–287.

Kopp, C. (1989). Regulation of distress and negative emotions: A developmental view. *Developmental Psychology, 25,* 343–354.

Kreutzer, M., & Charlesworth, W. (1973). *Infants' reactions to different expressions of emotions.* Paper presented at the annual meeting of the Society for Research in Child Development, Philadelphia.

Kurdek, L., & Rodgon, M. (1975). Perceptual, cognitive, and affective perspective taking in kindergarten through sixth grade children. *Developmental Psychology, 11,* 643–650.

Labov, W., & Fanshel, D. (1977). *Therapeutic discourse.* New York: Academic Press.

Lamb, S. (1991). Internal state words: Their relation to moral development and to maternal communications about moral development in the second year of life. *First Language, 11, 391–406.*

Lambert, M. (1989). The individual therapist's contribution to psychotherapy process and outcome. *Clinical Psychology Review, 9,* 217–224.

Landisberg, S., & Snyder, W. U. (1946). Nondirective play therapy. *Journal of Clinical Psychology, 2*(3), 203–214.

Leahy, R. (1985). The costs of development: Clinical implications. In R. Leahy (Ed.), *The development of the self* (pp. 267–294). New York: Academic Press.

Leahy, R. (1988). Cognitive therapy of childhood depression: Developmental considerations. In S. Shirk (Ed.), *Cognitive development and child psychotherapy* (pp. 187–206). New York: Plenum Press.

Lebo, D. (1952). The relationship of response categories in play therapy to chronological age. *Journal of Child Psychiatry, 2,* 330–336.

Lebo, D. (1953). The present status of research on nondirective play therapy. *Journal of Consulting Psychology, 17*(3), 177–183.

Lebo, D. (1955). Quantification of the nondirective play therapy process. *Journal of Genetic Psychology, 86,* 375–378.

Lebo, D. (1956). Age and suitability for nondirective play therapy. *Journal of Genetic Psychology, 89,* 231–238.

Lebo, D., & Lebo, E. (1957). Aggression and age in relation to verbal expression in nondirective play therapy. *Psychological Monographs: General and Applied, 71*(20), 1–12.

Lehrman, L. J., Sirluck, H., Black, B. J., & Glick, S. J. (1949). Success and failure of treatment of children in the child guidance clinics of the Jewish Board of Guardians, New York City. *Jewish Board of Guardians Research Monographs, 1,* 1–87.

Leitenberg, H., Yost, L., & Carroll-Wilson, M. (1986). Negative cognitive errors in children: Questionnaire development, normative data, and comparisons between children with and without symptoms of depression, low self-esteem, and evaluation anxiety. *Journal of Consulting and Clinical Psychology, 54,* 528–536.

Levitt, E. E. (1957). The results of psychotherapy with children: An evaluation. *Journal of Consulting Psychology, 21*(3), 189–196.

Levitt, E. E. (1963). Psychotherapy with children: A further evaluation. *Behaviour Research Theory, 1,* 45–51.

Levitt, E. E. (1971). Research on psychotherapy with children. In S. L. Garfield & A. E. Bergin (Eds.), *Handbook of psychotherapy and behavior change: An empirical analysis* (1st ed., pp. 475–494). New York: Wiley.

Levitt, E. E., Beiser, H. R., & Robertson, R. E. (1959). A follow-up evaluation of cases treated at a community child guidance clinic. *American Journal of Orthopsychiatry, 29,* 347–377.

Levy, D. (1963). *Psychological interpretation.* New York: Holt, Rinehart & Winston.

Lewis, M. (1992). The role of the self in social behavior. In F. S. Kessel, D. M. Cole, & D. L. Johnson (Eds.), *Self and consciousness: Multiple perspectives* (pp. 19–44). Hillsdale, NJ: Erlbaum.

Lewis, M., Feiring, C., McGoffog, C., & Jaskir, J. (1984). Predicting psychopathology in six-year-olds from early social relations. *Child Development, 55,* 123–136.

Lochman, J., & Curry, J. (1986). Effects of social problem-solving training and self-instructional training with aggressive boys. *Journal of Clinical Child Psychology, 15,* 159–164.

Lochman, J., & Dodge, K. (1994). Social-cognitive processes of severely violent, moderately aggressive, and nonaggressive boys. *Journal of Consulting and Clinical Psychology, 62,* 366–374.

Lochman, J., White, K., & Wayland, K. (1991). Cognitive-behavioral assessment and treatment with aggressive children. In P. Kendall (Ed.), *Child and adolescent therapy: Cognitive-behavioral procedures* (pp. 25–65). New York: Guilford Press.

Loeber, R. (1990). Development and risk factors of juvenile antisocial behavior and delinquency. *Clinical Psychology Review, 10,* 1–42.

Lord, J. J., Castelino, C. T., & Russell, R. L. (1991, June). *Linguistic aspects of client discourse: Affect, subjectivity, and client experiencing levels.* Paper presented at the meeting of the Society for Psychotherapy Research, Wintergreen, VA.

Luborsky, L., Barber, J., & Diguer, L. (1992). The meanings of narratives told during psychotherapy: The fruits of a new observational unit. *Psychotherapy Research, 2,* 277–290.

Luborsky, L., Chandler, M., Auerbach, A., Cohen, J., & Bachrach, H. (1971). Factors influencing the outcome of psychotherapy: A review of quantitative research. *Psychological Bulletin, 75,* 145–185.

Luborsky, L., Crits-Christoph, J., Mintz, J., & Huerbach, A. (1988). *Who will benefit from psychotherapy: Predicting therapeutic outcomes.* New York: Basic Books.

Luborsky, L., & Crits-Christoph, P. (1990). *Understanding transference: The Core Conflictual Relationship Theme method.* New York: Basic Books.

Luborsky, L., Singer, B., & Luborsky, L. (1975). Comparative studies of psychotherapies. *Archives of General Psychiatry, 42,* 995–1008.

Luria, A. R. (1961). *The role of speech in the direction of normal and abnormal behavior.* New York: Pergamon Press.

Lynch, M., & Cicchetti, D. (1991). Patterns of relatedness in maltreated and nonmaltreated children: Connections among multiple representational models. *Development and Psychopathology, 3,* 207–226.

Lyons-Ruth, K., Alpern, L., & Rapaholi, B. (1993). Disorganized infant attachment classification and maternal psychosocial problems as predictors of hostile–

aggressive behavior in the preschool classroom. *Child Development, 64,* 572–585.

Maccoby, E., & Martin, J. H. (1983). Socialization in the context of the family: Parent–child interaction. In P. Mussen (Ed.), *Handbook of child psychology: Vol. 4. Socialization, personality, and social development.* New York: Wiley.

MacIntyre, A. (1980). Epistemological crises, dramatic narrative, and the philosophy of science. In G. Gutting (Ed.), *Paradigms and revolutions* (pp. 54–73). Notre Dame, IN: University of Notre Dame Press.

Mahoney, M. (1985). Psychotherapy and human change processes. In M. Mahoney & A. Freeman (Eds.), *Cognition and psychotherapy* (pp. 3–48). New York: Plenum Press.

Main, M., Kaplan, N., & Cassidy, J. (1985). Security in infancy, childhood, and adulthood: A move to the level of representation. In I. Bretherton & E. Waters (Eds.), Growing points of attachment theory and research. *Monographs of the Society for Research in Child Development, 50*(1–2, Serial No. 209).

Malatesta, C., & Wilson, A. (1988). Emotion cognition interaction in personality development: A discrete emotions functional analysis. *British Journal of Social Psychology, 27,* 91–112.

Malgady, R., Rogler, L., & Costantino, G. (1990). Culturally sensitive psychotherapy for Puerto Rican children and adolescents: A program of treatment outcome research. *Journal of Consulting and Clinical Psychology, 58,* 704–712.

Mann, B. J., & Borduin, C. M. (1991). A critical review of psychotherapy outcome studies with adolescents, 1978–1988. *Adolescence, 26,* 506–535.

Marks, S., & Tolsma, R. (1986). Empathy research: Some methodological considerations. *Psychotherapy, 23,* 4–20.

McCloskey, M., & Glucksberg, S. (1978). Natural categories: Well-defined or fuzzy sets? *Memory and Cognition, 6,* 462–472.

Mead, G. (1934). *Mind, self, and society.* Chicago: University of Chicago Press.

Meichenbaum, D. (1977). *Cognitive-behavioral modification: An integrative approach.* New York: Plenum Press.

Meichenbaum, D. (1979). Teaching children self-control. In B. Lahey & A. Kazdin (Eds.), *Advances in clinical child psychology* (Vol. 2, pp. 1–35). New York: Plenum Press.

Meltzoff, A. N., & Moore, M. K. (1983). Newborn infants imitate adult facial gestures. *Child Development, 54,* 702–709.

Mervis, C., & Crisati, M. (1982). Order of acquisition of subordinate-, basic-, and superordinate-level categories. *Child Development, 53,* 258–266.

Meyers, A., & Craighead, W. (Eds.). (1984). *Cognitive behavior therapy with children.* New York: Plenum Press.

Miller, P. H., & Aloise, P. A. (1989). Young children's understanding of the psychological causes of behavior: A review. *Child Development, 60,* 255–285.

Miller, P. J., Mintz, J., Hoogstra, L., Fung, H., & Potts, R. (1992). The narrated self: Young children's construction of self in relation to others in conversational stories of personal experience. *Merrill–Palmer Quarterly, 38,* 45–67.

Mischel, W. (1973). Toward a cognitive social learning reformulation of personality. *Psychological Review, 80,* 252–283.

Mishne, J. (1983). *Clinical work with children.* New York: Free Press.

Mitchell, K. M., Bozarth, J. D., & Krauft, C. C. (1977). A reappraisal of the therapeutic effectiveness of accurate empathy, nonpossessive warmth and genuineness. In A. S. Gurman & A. M. Razins (Eds.), *Effective psychotherapy: A handbook of research* (pp. 482–502). New York: Pergamon.

Mook, B. (1982a). Analyses of therapist variables in a series of psychotherapy sessions with two child clients. *Journal of Clinical Psychology, 38,* 63–76.

Mook, B. (1982b). Analyses of client variables in a series of psychotherapy sessions with two child clients. *Journal of Clinical Psychology, 38,* 263–274.

Morisset, C. E., Barnard, K. E., Greenberg, M. T., Booth, C. L., & Spieker, S. J. (1990). Environmental influences on early language development: The context of social risk. *Development and Psychopathology, 2*(2), 127–149.

Moustakas, C. E. (1955). The frequency and intensity of negative attitudes expressed in play therapy: A comparison of well-adjusted and disturbed young children. *Journal of Genetic Psychology, 86,* 309–325.

Moustakas, C. (1959). *Children in play therapy.* New York: McGraw-Hill.

Moustakas, C. E., & Schalock, H. D. (1955). An analysis of therapist–child interaction in play therapy. *Child Development 26*(2), 143–157.

Moustakas, C. E., Sigel, I. E., & Schalock, H. D. (1956). An objective method for the measurement and analysis of child–adult interaction. *Child Development, 27,* 109–134.

Nachman, P., & Stern, D. N. (1983). *Recall memory of emotional experience in pre-linguistic infants.* Paper presented at the National Clinical Infancy Fellows Conference, Yale University, New Haven, CT.

Nannis, E. (1988). A cognitive-developmental view of emotional understanding and its implications for child psychotherapy. In S. Shirk (Ed.), *Cognitive development and child psychotherapy* (pp. 91–118). New York: Plenum Press.

Neisser, U. (1992). The development of consciousness and the acquisition of skill. In F. S. Kessel, P. M. Cole, & D. L. Johnson (Eds.), *Self and consciousness: Multiple perspectives* (pp. 1–18). Hillsdale, NJ: Erlbaum.

Neitzel, M. T., Russell, R. L., Hemmings, K. A., & Gretter, M. L. (1987). Clinical significance of psychotherapy for unipolar depression: A meta-analytic approach to social comparison. *Journal of Consulting and Clinical Psychology, 55,* 156–381.

Newman, D. (1986). The role of mutual knowledge in the development of perspective taking. *Developmental Review, 6,* 122–145.

Noam, G., & Recklitis, C. (1990). The relationship between defenses and symptoms in adolescent psychopathology. *Journal of Personality Assessment, 54,* 311–327.

Nuffield, E. (1988). Psychotherapy. In J. Matson (Ed.), *Handbook of treatment approaches in child psychopathology* (pp. 135–160). New York: Plenum Press.

Olson, D. R. (1993). The development of representations: The origins of mental life. *Canadian Psychology, 43,* 293–306.

Olson, S. L., Bates, J. E., & Kaskie, B. (1992). Caregiver–infant interaction antecedents of children's school-aged cognitive ability. *Merrill–Palmer Quarterly, 38,* 309–330.

Orlinsky, D. E., & Howard, K. (1978). The relation of process to outcome in psychotherapy. In S. L. Garfield & A. E. Bergin (Eds.), *Handbook of psychotherapy and behavior change* (2nd ed., pp. 283–329). New York: Wiley.

Orlinsky, D. E., & Howard, K. I. (1986). Process and outcome in psychotherapy. In S. L. Garfield & A. E. Bergin (Eds.), *Handbook of psychotherapy and behavior change* (3rd ed., pp. 311–381). New York: Wiley.

Orlinsky, D. E., & Russell, R. L. (1994). Tradition and change in psychotherapy research: Notes on the fourth generation. In R. L. Russell (Ed.), *Reassessing psychotherapy research* (pp. 185–214). New York: Guilford Press.

Parloff, M. B. (1984). Psychotherapy research and its incredible credibility crisis. *Clinical Psychology Review, 4,* 95–109.

Parten, M. (1932). Social participation among preschool children. *Journal of Abnormal and Social Psychology, 27,* 243–269.

Paul, G. (1967). Strategy of outcome research in psychotherapy. *Journal of Consulting Psychology, 31,* 109–118.

Perry, J. C. (1989). Scientific progress in psychodynamic formulation. *Psychiatry, 52,* 245–249.

Perry, J. C., Augusto, F., & Cooper, S. (1989). Assessing psychodynamic conflicts: Reliability of the Idiographic Conflict Formulation Method. *Psychiatry, 52,* 289–301.

Persons, J. (1986). The advantages of studying psychological phenomena rather than psychiatric diagnoses. *American Psychologist, 41,* 1252–1260.

Persons, J. (1989). *Cognitive therapy in practice: A case formulation approach.* New York: Norton.

Persons, J. (1991). Psychotherapy outcome studies do not accurately represent current models of psychotherapy. *American Psychologist, 46,* 99–106.

Persons, J. (1993). The process of change in cognitive therapy: Schema change or acquisition of compensatory skills? *Cognitive Therapy and Research, 17,* 123–137.

Pfeiffer, S. I., & Strzelecki, S. C. (1990). Inpatient psychiatric treatment of children and adolescents: A review of outcome studies. *Journal of the American Academy of Child and Adolescent Psychiatry, 29*(6), 847–853.

Phillips, R. D. (1985). Whistling in the dark?: A review of play therapy research. *Psychotherapy, 22,* 752–760.

Piaget, J. (1932/1965). *The moral judgment of the child.* New York: Free Press.

Piel, J. A. (1990). Unmasking sex and social class differences in childhood aggression: The case for language maturity. *Journal of Educational Research, 84*(2), 100–106.

Pine, F. (1976). Therapeutic change: A parent–child model. *Psychoanalysis and Contemporary Science, 5,* 127–147.

Piper, W., Joyce, A., McCallum, M., & Azim, H. (1993). Concentration and correspondence of transference interpretations in short-term psychotherapy. *Journal of Consulting and Clinical Psychology, 61,* 586–595.

Platt, J. J., & Spivak, G. (1975). *Manual for the Means–Ends Problem-Solving Procedures (MEPS): A measure of interpersonal cognitive problem solving skills.* Camden, NJ: University of Medicine and Dentistry of New Jersey.

Poal, P., & Weisz, J. (1989). Therapists' own childhood problems as predictors of their effectiveness in child psychotherapy. *Journal of Clinical Child Psychology, 18,* 202–205.

Pope, A., McHale, S., & Craighead, W. E. (1988). *Self-esteem enhancement with children and adolescents.* Boston: Allyn & Bacon.

Premack, D. (1991). The infant's theory of self-propelled objects. In D. Frye & C. Moore (Eds.), *Children's theories of mind: Mental states and social understanding* (pp. 39–48). Hillsdale, NJ: Erlbaum.

Quay, H. C., & Peterson, D. R. (1967). *Manual for the Behavior Problem Checklist.* Champaign: University of Illinois Children's Research Center.

Rabian, B., Petersen, R., Richters, J., & Jensen, P. (1993). Anxiety sensitivity among anxious children. *Journal of Clinical Child Psychology, 22,* 441–446.

Rachman, S. (1971). *The effects of psychotherapy.* Oxford: Pergamon Press.

Raney, D., Shirk, S., Sarlin, N., Kaplan, D., & During, L. (1991, March). *Parent collaboration as a predictor of adolescent inpatient treatment process and progress.* Paper presented at meetings of the Society for Adolescent Medicine, Denver, CO.

Ratner, N. B. (1984). Phonological rule usage in mother–child speech. *Journal of Phonetics, 12*(3), 245–254.

Reisman, J. (1973). *Principles of psychotherapy with children.* New York: Appleton-Century-Crofts.

Renouf, A., & Harter, S. (1990). Low self-worth and anger as components of the depressive experience in young adolescents. *Development and Psychopathology, 2,* 293–310.

Rice, L., & Greenberg, L. (1984). The new research paradigm. In L. Rice & L. Greenberg (Eds.), *Patterns of change: Intensive analysis of psychotherapy process* (pp. 1–25). New York: Guilford Press.

Ricks, D. (1974). Supershrink: Methods of a therapist judged successful on the basis of adult outcomes of adolescent patients. In D. Ricks, M. Rott, & A. Thomas (Eds.), *Life history research in psychopathology,* (Vol. 3, pp. 275–297). Minneapolis: University of Minnesota Press.

Robinson, N. (1989, April). *The impact of different types of parent and peer support on global self-worth.* Poster presented at meetings of the Society for Research on Child Development, Kansas City, MO.

Rogers, C. (1939). *The clinical treatment of the problem child.* Boston: Houghton Mifflin.

Rogers, C. (1942). *Counseling and psychotherapy.* Boston: Houghton Mifflin.

Rogers, C. (1951). *Client-centered therapy.* Boston: Houghton Mifflin.

Rogers, C. (1957). The necessary and sufficient conditions for personality change. *Journal of Consulting and Clinical Psychology, 21,* 95–103.

Rogers, C. (1961). *On becoming a person.* Boston: Houghton Mifflin.

Rogers, C. (1977). *Carl Rogers on personal power.* New York: Delta.

Rogoff, B. (1990). *Apprenticeship in thinking.* New York: Oxford University Press.

Rosch, E. (1973). On the internal structure of perceptual and semantic categories. In T. E. Moore (Ed.), *Cognitive development and the acquisition of language* (pp. 111–144). New York: Academic Press.

Rosch, E. (1978). Principles of categorization. In E. Rosch & B. Lloyd (Eds.), *Cognition and categorization* (pp. 27–48). Hillsdale, NJ: Erlbaum.

Rosch, E., Mervis, C., Gray, W., Johnson, D., & Boyes-Braem, P. (1976). Basic objects in natural categories. *Cognitive Psychology, 8,* 382–439.

Rosenberg, M. (1979). *Conceiving the self.* New York: Basic Books.

Rossman, R. (1992). School-age children's perceptions of coping and distress:

Strategies for emotion regulation and the moderation of adjustment. *Journal of Child Psychology and Psychiatry, 33,* 1373–1397.

Roth, D., & Leslie, A. M. (1991). The recognition of attitude conveyed by utterance: A study of preschool and autistic children. *British Journal of Developmental Psychology, 9,* 315–330.

Ruddy, M. G., & Bornstein, M. H. (1982). Cognitive correlates of infant attention and maternal stimulation over the first year of life. *Child Development, 53,* 183–188.

Russ, S. W. (1995). Play psychotherapy research: State of the science. In T. Ollendick & R. Prinzer (Eds.), *Advances in clinical child psychology, 17* (pp. 365–391). New York: Plenum Press.

Russell, J., & Ridgeway, D. (1983). Dimensions underlying children's emotion concepts. *Developmental Psychology, 19,* 795–804.

Russell, R. L. (1984). *Empirical investigations of psychotherapeutic techniques: A critique of and prospects for language analysis.* Ann Arbor, MI: University Microfilms International.

Russell, R. L. (1991). Narrative in views of humanity, science, and action: Lessons for cognitive therapy. *Journal of Cognitive Psychotherapy, 5,* 241–256.

Russell, R. L. (1995). Introduction to the special section on multivariate psychotherapy process research: Structure and change in the talking cure. *Journal of Consulting and Clinical Psychology, 63,* 3–5.

Russell, R. L., Bryant, F., & Estrada, A. U. (in press). Confirmatory P-technique analyses of therapist discourse in child psychotherapy: High versus low quality sessions. *Journal of Consulting and Clinical Psychology.*

Russell, R. L., Castelino, C. C., Wandrei, M., & Jones, M. (1995). *Building theories of mind through narrative exchange.* Manuscript submitted for publication.

Russell, R. L., Greenwald, S., & Shirk, S. R. (1991). Language in child psychotherapy: A meta-analytic review. *Journal of Consulting and Clinical Psychology, 6,* 916–919.

Russell, R. L., Stokes, J., Czogalik, D., Jones, M. E., & Rohleder, L. (1993). The role of nonverbal sensitivity in childhood psychopathology. *Journal of Nonverbal Behavior, 17*(1), 69–83.

Russell, R. L., & van den Broek, P. (1988). A cognitive-developmental account of storytelling in child psychotherapy. In S. R. Shirk (Ed.), *Cognitive development and child psychotherapy* (pp. 19–52). New York: Plenum Press.

Russell, R. L., & van den Broek, P. (1992). Changing narrative schemas in psychotherapy. *Psychotherapy Research: Theory, Research, Practice, and Training, 29,* 344–354.

Russell, R. L., van den Broek, P., Adams, S., Rosenberger, K., & Essig, C. (1993). Analyzing narratives in psychotherapy: A formal framework and empirical analysis. *Journal of Narrative and Life History, 3,* 337–360.

Safran, J. (1990a). Towards a refinement of cognitive therapy in light of interpersonal theory: Theory. *Clinical Psychology Review, 10,* 87–105.

Safran, J. (1990b). Towards a refinement of cognitive therapy in light of interpersonal theory: Practice. *Clinical Psychology Review, 10,* 107–121.

Sandler, J., Kennedy, H., & Tyson, R. L. (1980). *The techniques of child psychoanalysis–discussions with Anna Freud.* Cambridge, MA: Harvard University Press.

Santostephano, S. (1985). *Cognitive control therapy with children and adolescents.* New York: Pergamon.

Santostephano, S. (1989). Cognitive control therapy with children: Rationale and technique. *Psychotherapy, Theory, Research, and Practice, 21,* 76–91.

Schafer, R. (1981). Narration in psychoanalytic dialogue. In W. J. T. Mitchell (Ed.), *On narrative* (pp. 25–49). Chicago: University of Chicago Press.

Scherer, N. J., & Olswang, L. B. (1984). Role of mothers' expansions in stimulating children's language production. *Journal of Speech and Hearing Research, 27,* 387–396.

Seligman, M., Peterson, C., Kaslow, N., Tanenbaum, R., Alloy, L., & Abramson, L. (1984). Explanatory style and depressive symptoms among school children. *Journal of Abnormal Psychology, 93,* 235–238.

Selman, R. (1980). *The growth of interpersonal understanding: Developmental and clinical analyses.* New York: Academic Press.

Selman, R., & Demorest, A. (1984). Observing troubled children's interpersonal negotiation strategies: Implications of and for a developmental model. *Child Development, 55,* 288–304.

Selman, R., Schorin, M., Stone, C., & Phelps, E. (1983). A naturalistic study of children's social reasoning. *Developmental Psychology, 19,* 82–102.

Selman, R., & Schultz, L. (1988). Interpersonal thought and action in the case of a troubled early adolescent. In S. Shirk (Ed.), *Cognitive development and child psychotherapy* (pp. 207–246). New York: Plenum Press.

Shadish, W. R., & Sweeney, R. B. (1991). Mediators and moderators in meta-analysis: There's a reason we don't let dodo birds tell us which psychotherapies should have prizes. *Journal of Consulting and Clinical Psychology, 59,* 883–893.

Shapiro, D. A. (1985). Recent applications of meta-analysis in clinical research. *Clinical Psychology Review, 5,* 13–34.

Shapiro, D. A., Harper, H., Startup, M., Reynolds, S., Bird, D., & Suokas, A. (1994). The high-water mark of the drug metaphor: A meta-analytic critique of process–outcome research. In R. L. Russell (Ed.), *Reassessing psychotherapy research* (pp. 1–35). New York: Guilford Press.

Shapiro, D. A., & Shapiro, D. (1982). Meta-analysis of comparative therapy outcome studies: A replication and refinement. *Psychological Bulletin, 92,* 581–604.

Shapiro, D. A., & Shapiro, D. (1983). Comparative therapy outcome research: Methodological implications of meta-analysis. *Psychological Bulletin, 92,* 581–604.

Shapiro, T. (1989). The psychodynamic formulation in child and adolescent psychiatry. *Journal of the American Academy of Child and Adolescent Psychiatry, 28,* 675–680.

Shirk, S. R. (1988a). Causal reasoning and children's comprehension of therapeutic interpretations. In S. Shirk (Ed.), *Cognitive development and child psychotherapy* (pp. 53–90). New York: Plenum Press.

Shirk, S. (1988b). The interpersonal legacy of physical abuse of children. In M. Straus (Ed.), *Abuse and victimization across the life span* (pp. 57–81). Baltimore: Johns Hopkins University Press.

Shirk, S. (Ed.). (1988c). *Cognitive development and child psychotherapy.* New York: Plenum Press.

Shirk, S. (1990). Cognitive processes in child psychotherapy: Where are the developmental limits? In J. Dewit, W. Slot, H. van Leeuwen, & M. Terwogt (Eds.), *Developmental psychopathology and clinical practice* (pp. 19–31). Amsterdam, The Netherlands: Acco.

Shirk, S., & Eltz, M. (in press). Multiple victimization and the process and outcome of child psychotherapy. In B. B. Rossman & M. Rosenberg (Eds.), *Multiple victimization of children: Conceptual, research, and treatment issues.* New York: Haworth Press.

Shirk, S., & Harter, S. (1996). Treatment of low self-esteem. In M. A. Reinecke, F. M. Dattilio, & A. Freeman (Eds.), *Cognitive therapy with children and adolescents: A casebook for clinical practice* (pp. 175–198). New York: Guilford Press.

Shirk, S., & Rossman, B. B. (1989, April). *Discrepancies between parents' and children's appraisals of problem behaviors.* Paper presented to the Society for Research on Child Development, Kansas City, MO.

Shirk, S., & Russell, R. (1992). A re-evaluation of estimates of child therapy effectiveness. *Journal of the American Academy of Child and Adolescent Psychiatry, 31,* 703–709.

Shirk, S. R., Saiz, C., & Sarlin, N. (1993, June). *The therapeutic alliance in child and adolescent treatment: Initial studies with inpatients.* Paper presented at meetings of the Society for Psychotherapy Research, Pittsburgh, PA.

Shirk, S. R., & Eason, A. P. (1993, April). *Emotional and caregiving characteristics associated with self/other representations in young adolescents.* Poster presented at meetings of the Society for Research in Child Development, New Orleans, LA.

Shirk, S. R., & Russell, R. L. (1995). Reply to Weiss and Weisz: Effectiveness of psychotherapy. *Journal of the American Academy of Child and Adolescent Psychiatry, 34,* 972.

Shirk, S. R., & Saiz, C. C. (1992). Clinical, empirical, and developmental perspectives on the therapeutic relationship in child psychotherapy. *Development and Psychopathology, 4,* 713–728.

Shure, M., & Spivack, G. (1978). *Problem-solving techniques in childrearing.* San Francisco: Jossey-Bass.

Siegel, C. L. F. (1972). Changes in play therapy behaviors over time as a function of differing levels of therapist-offered conditions. *Journal of Clinical Psychology, 28,* 235–236.

Silberschatz, G., Fretter, P., & Curtis, J. (1986). How do interpretations influence the process of psychotherapy? *Journal of Consulting and Clinical Psychology, 54,* 646–652.

Silver, L. B., & Silver, B. J. (1983). Clinical practice of child psychiatry: A survey. *Journal of the American Academy of Child and Adolescent Psychiatry, 22,* 573–579.

Silverstein, A. (1988). An Aristotelian resolution of the idiographic versus nomothetic tension. *American Psychologist, 43,* 425–430.

Smith, M. L., & Glass, G. V. (1977). Meta-analysis of psychotherapy outcome studies. *American Psychologist, 37,* 752–760.

Smith, M. L., Glass, G. V., & Miller, T. I. (1980). *The benefits of psychotherapy.* Baltimore: Johns Hopkins University Press.

Smith, W., & Rossman, R. (1986). Developmental changes in trait and situational denial under stress during childhood. *Journal of Child Psychology and Psychiatry, 27,* 227–235.

Smith-Acuna, S., Durlak, J. A., & Kaspar, C. J. (1991). Development of child psychotherapy process measures. *Journal of Clinical Child Psychology, 20,* 126–131.

Snow, J., & Paternite, C. (1986). Individual and family therapy in the treatment of children. *Professional Psychology: Research and Practice, 17,* 242–250.

Spitz, R. A. (1945). Hospitalism: An inquiry into the genesis of psychiatric conditions in early childhood. *Psychoanalytic Study of the Child, 1,* 53–74.

Spivack, G., Platt, J., & Shure, M. (1976). *The problem-solving approach to adjustment.* San Francisco: Jossey-Bass.

Spivack, G., & Shure, M. (1974). *Social adjustment of young children.* San Francisco: Jossey-Bass.

Sroufe, A., & Waters, E. (1977). Attachment as an organizational construct. *Child Development, 48,* 1184–1199.

Stark, K., Humphrey, L., Laurent, J., Livingston, R., & Christopher, J. (1993). Cognitive, behavioral, and family factors in the differentiation of depressive and anxiety disorders during childhood. *Journal of Consulting and Clinical Psychology, 61,* 878–886.

Stark, K., Rouse, L., & Livingston, R. (1991). Treatment of depression during childhood and adolescence: Cognitive-behavioral procedures for the individual and the family. In P. Kendall (Ed.), *Child and adolescent therapy: Cognitive-behavioral procedures* (pp. 165–208). New York: Guilford Press.

Stein, N. L., & Glenn, C. G. (1979). An analysis of story comprehension in elementary school children. In R. O. Freedle (Ed.), *New directions in discourse processing* (Vol. 2, pp. 53–120). (In the series *Advances in discourse processes*). Norwood, NJ: Ablex.

Stern, D. (1985). *The interpersonal world of the infant: A view from psychoanalysis and developmental psychology.* New York: Basic Books.

Stevenson, J., Richman, N., & Graham, P. (1985). Behaviour problems and language abilities at three years and behavioural deviance at eight years. *Journal of Child Psychology and Psychiatry, 26,* 215–230.

Stiles, W. B. (1988). Psychotherapy process–outcome correlations may be misleading. *Psychotherapy, 25,* 27–35.

Stiles, W., Shapiro, D., & Elliott, R. (1986). Are all psychotherapies equivalent? *American Psychologist, 41,* 165–180.

Stolorow, R., & Lachman, F. (1978). The developmental prestages of defenses: Diagnostic and therapeutic implications. *Psychoanalytic Quarterly, 47,* 73–102.

Stone, C. A., & Wertsch, J. V. (1990). A social interactional analysis of learning disabilities remediation. *Journal of Learning Disabilities, 17,* 194–199.

Strauss, M. (Ed.). (1988). *Abuse and victimization across the life-span.* Baltimore: Johns Hopkins University Press.

Strayhorn, J. (1988). *The competent child: An approach to psychotherapy and preventive mental health.* New York: Guilford Press.

Strube, M. J., Gardner, W., & Hartmann, D. P. (1985). Limitations, liabilities, and obstacles in reviews of the literature: The current status of meta-analysis. *Clinical Psychology Review, 5,* 63–78.

Strupp, H. (1973). On the basic ingredients of psychotherapy. *Journal of Consulting and Clinical Psychology, 41,* 1–8.

Strupp, H. (1989). Psychotherapy: Can the practitioner learn from the researcher. *American Psychologist, 44,* 717–724.

Strupp, H. J. (1986). The nonspecific hypothesis of therapeutic effectiveness: A current assessment. *American Journal of Orthopsychiatry, 56,* 513–520.

Strupp, H. J., Hartley, D., & Blackwood, G. L., Jr. (1974). *Vanderbilt Psychotherapy Process Scale.* Unpublished manuscript, Vanderbilt University, Nashville, TN.

Stuart, S., Pilkonis, P., Heape, C., Smith, K., & Fisher, B. (1991). *The patient–therapist match in psychotherapy: Effects of security of attachment and personality style.* Paper presented at meetings of the North American Chapter of the Society for Psychotherapy Research, Lyons, France.

Szapocznik, J., Rio, A., Murray, E., & Cohen, R. (1989). Structural family versus psychodynamic child therapy for problematic Hispanic boys. *Journal of Consulting and Clinical Psychology, 57,* 571–578.

Tant, J., & Douglas, V. (1982). Problem-solving in hyperactive, normal, and reading disabled boys. *Journal of Abnormal Child Psychology, 10,* 285–306.

Target, M., & Fonagy, P. (1994). Efficacy of psychoanalysis for children with emotional disorders. *Journal of the American Academy of Child and Adolescent Psychiatry, 33,* 361–371.

Taylor, D., & Harris, P. (1983). Knowledge of the link between emotion and memory among normal and maladjusted boys. *Developmental Psychology, 19,* 832–838.

Tharp, R. (1991). Cultural diversity and treatment of children. *Journal of Consulting and Clinical Psychology, 59,* 799–812.

Thompson, R. (1989). Causal attributions and children's emotional understanding. In C. Saarni & P. Harris (Eds.), *Children's understanding of emotion* (pp. 117–150). New York: Cambridge University Press.

Tolpin, M. (1978). Self objects and Oedipal objects. *Psychoanalytic Study of the Child, 33,* 167–184.

Tramontana, M. G. (1980). Critical review of research on psychotherapy outcome with adolescents: 1967–1977. *Psychological Bulletin, 88*(2), 429–450.

Traux, C., Wargo, D., & Silber, L. (1966). Effects of group psychotherapy with accurate empathy and nonpossessive warmth upon female institutionalized delinquents. *Journal of Abnormal Psychology, 71,* 267–274.

Truax, C. B., Altman, H., Wright, L., & Mitchell, K. M. (1973). Effects of therapeutic conditions in child therapy. *Journal of Community Psychology, 1*(3), 313–318.

Truax, C. B., & Wittmer, J. (1973). The degree of the therapist's focus in defense mechanisms and the effect on therapeutic outcome with institutionalized juvenile delinquents. *Journal of Community Psychology, 1,* 201–203.

Tuma, J. (1989). Mental health services to children: State of the art. *American Psychologist, 44,* 188–199.

Tuma, J., & Pratt, J. (1982). Clinical child psychology practice and training: A survey. *Journal of Clinical Child Psychology, 11,* 27–34.

Turkat, I. (Ed.). (1985). *Behavioral case formulation.* New York: Plenum Press.

Urbain, E., & Kendall, P. (1980). Review of social-cognitive problem-solving interventions with children. *Psychological Bulletin, 88,* 109–143.

Vaillant, G. (1971). Theoretical hierarchy of adaptive ego mechanisms. *Archives of General Psychiatry, 24,* 107–118.

Vaillant, G. (1977). *Adaptation to life.* Boston: Little, Brown.

Vaillant, G. (1986). A brief history of empirical assessment of defense mechanisms. In G. Vaillant (Ed.), *Empirical studies of ego mechanisms of defense* (pp. viii–xx). Washington, DC: American Psychiatric Press.

van den Broek, P., & Thurlow, R. (1991). The role and structure of personal narratives. *Journal of Cognitive Psychotherapy, 5,* 257–274.

Vaux, A. (1988). *Social support: Theory, research, and intervention.* New York: Praeger.

Vygotsky, L. (1962). *Thought and language.* New York: Wiley.

Vygotsky, L. (1978). *Mind in society.* Cambridge, MA: Harvard University Press.

Vygotsky, L. (1936/1986). *Thought and language.* Cambridge, MA: MIT Press.

Wachtel, E. F. (1994). *Treating troubled children and their families.* New York: Guilford Press.

Watt, N., Anthony, E., Wynne, L., Rolf, J. (Eds.). (1984). *Children at risk: A longitudinal perspective.* New York: Cambridge University Press.

Wechsler, D. (1945). A standardized memory scale for clinical use. *Journal of Psychology, 19,* 87–95.

Weinstein, M. (1988). Preparation of children for psychotherapy through videotaped modeling. *Journal of Clinical Child Psychology, 17,* 131–136.

Weiss, B., & Weisz, J. R. (1990). The impact of methodological factors on child psychotherapy outcome research: A meta-analysis for researchers. *Journal of Abnormal Child Psychology, 18*(6), 639–670.

Weiss, B., & Weisz, J. R. (1995). Relative effectiveness of behavioral versus nonbehavioral child psychotherapy. *Journal of Consulting and Clinical Psychology, 63,* 317–320.

Weiss, J., Sampson, H., & the Mt. Zion Psychotherapy Research Group (1986). *The psychoanalytic process: Theory, clinical observations, and empirical research.* New York: Guilford Press.

Weisz, J., Suwanlert, S., Chaiyasit, W., Weiss, B., Walter, B., & Anderson, W. (1988). Thai and American perspectives on over- and undercontrolled child behavior problems: Exploring the threshold model among parents, teachers, and psychologists. *Journal of Consulting and Clinical Psychology, 56,* 601–609.

Weisz, J., & Weiss, B. (1991). Studying the "referability" of child clinical problems. *Journal of Consulting and Clinical Psychology, 59,* 266–273.

Weisz, J., Weiss, B., Alicke, M., & Klotz, M. (1987). Effectiveness of psychotherapy with children and adolescents: A meta-analysis for clinicians. *Journal of Consulting and Clinical Psychology, 55,* 542–549.

Weisz, J. R., Weiss, B., & Donnenberg, G. R. (1992). The lab versus the clinic effects of child and adolescent psychotherapy. *American Psychologist, 47*(12), 1578–1585.

Weisz, J., Weiss, B., & Langmeyer, D. (1987). Giving up on child psychotherapy: Who drops out? *Journal of Consulting and Clinical Psychology, 55,* 916–918.

Werner, H. (1957). The concept of development from a comparative and organismic point of view. In D. Harris (Ed.), *The concept of development* (pp. 125–148). Minneapolis: University of Minnesota Press.

Werry, J. S., Elkind, G. S., & Reeves, J. C. (1987). Attention deficit, conduct, oppositional, and anxiety disorders in children: III Laboratory differences. *Journal of Abnormal Child Psychotherapy, 15,* 409–428.

Wertsch, J. (1985). *Vygotsky and the social formation of mind.* Cambridge, MA: Harvard University Press.

Westen, D. (1988). Transference and information processing. *Clinical Psychology Review, 8,* 161–179.

White, H. (1980). The value of narrativity in the representation of reality. *Critical Inquiry, 7,* 5–27.

Wilkinson, L. C., & Milosky, L. M. (1987). School-age children's metapragmatic knowledge of requests and responses in the classroom. *Topics in Language Disorders, 7,* 61–70.

Winfrey, N. (1993). *Self-perceptions and defensive styles in children with signs of psychopathology.* Unpublished doctoral dissertation, University of Denver, CO.

Winnicott, D. (1964). *The child, the family, and the outside world.* London: Penguin Books.

Winnicott, D. (1965). *The maturational process and the facilitating environment.* New York: International Universities Press.

Witmer, H. L., & Keller, J. (1942). Outgrowing childhood problems: A study in the value of child guidance treatment. *Smith College Study Social Work, 13,* 74–90.

Wolfe, V., Finch, A., Saylor, C., Blount, R., Pallmeyer, T., & Carek, D. (1987). Negative affectivity in children: A multitrait–multimethod investigation. *Journal of Consulting and Clinical Psychology, 55,* 245–250.

Worman, P. N. (1983). Meta-analysis: A validity perspective. *Annual Review of Psychology, 34,* 223–260.

Wright, L., Everett, F., & Roisman, L. (1986). *Experiential therapy with children.* Baltimore: Johns Hopkins University Press.

Wright, L., Truax, C. B., & Mitchell, K. M. (1972). Reliability of process ratings of psychotherapy with children. *Journal of Clinical Psychology, 28,* 232–234.

Yeaton, W. H., & Sechrest, L. (1981). Critical dimension in the choice and maintenance of successful treatments. *Journal of Consulting and Clinical Psychology, 49,* 156–160.

Zabel, R. (1979). Recognition of emotions in facial expressions by emotionally disturbed and nondisturbed children. *Psychology in the Schools, 16,* 119–126.

Zahn-Waxler, C., Cummings, E. M., & Cooperman, G. (1984). Emotional development in childhood. In G. Whitehurst (Ed.), *Annals of child development* (Vol. 1, pp. 45–106). London: JAI Press.

Zahn-Waxler, C., & Radke-Yarrow, M. (1990). The origins of empathic concern. *Motivation and Emotion, 14*(2), 107–130.

Index